S0-ESG-311

Herb-Drug Interaction Handbook

2nd edition

Sharon M. Herr, RD, CDN

Editors:

Edzard Ernst, MD, PhD, FRCP
Veronica S. L. Young, PharmD

Published and distributed by:

Church Street Books   (518) 766-4200
7 Church St.   csbooks@NYCAP.rr.com
P. O. Box 527   http://home.NYCAP.rr.com/csbooks
Nassau, NY 12123-0527

Cataloging-in-publication data available from the Library of Congress
ISBN: 0-9678773-1-8

Second Edition

Editors:
Prof. Edzard Ernst, MD, PhD, FRCP (Edin.) Veronica Young, Pharm.D.
Department of Complementary Medicine   Assistant Director, Drug Information Service
School of Sport and Health Sciences   The University of Texas Health Science Center
University of Exeter   San Antonio, TX
England   Clinical Assistant Professor, College of Pharmacy
                                         The University of Texas at Austin, San Antonio, TX

This book is not intended to take the place of a physician. Always consult your physician before combining herbs/dietary supplements and drugs. The publisher, editors and author do not accept responsibility for injury or damages incurred from the use of the information in this book; its accuracy and completeness, and conclusions based thereon are not guaranteed. As every effort has been made to provide accurate information in this publication, we would appreciate it if readers would call our attention to any errors that may occur by communicating with Sharon M. Herr, RD, CDN (sharon@onlineRD.com).

Table of Contents

Preface

This handbook was compiled to meet the needs of health care professionals. It was designed as an aid in the safe integration of herbal supplements with pharmaceuticals in patient care. The author's goal was to provide this aid in a format which could be readily consulted in the clinical setting, thus a book which readily fits in a lab coat pocket.

Use, part used, contraindications, safety and adverse reactions are provided for screening purposes only. The material contained in these sections should not be relied upon for making clinical decisions, which is beyond the scope of a book this size. Recommendations for the use of herbs should only be made after carefully studying each herb. Herbs are complex mixtures of chemicals and use should be based on a thorough knowledge of all aspects of a particular herb. The author suggests compiling relevant references and filing by either herb or use. No one reference is sufficient to completely understand the complexity of herbal medicine. The **potential interactions** listed in this book were compiled from numerous sources and do not represent every possible interaction between herbal supplements and drugs. References are located on pages 303 through 371, and are indicated throughout the handbook in parentheses. Some references may be mutually contradictory. One source may find no interaction while another source reports that an interaction exists. It is important to review the References section to determine which sources you feel most comfortable with.

To obtain maximum value from this book, patients must be questioned on their supplement use. Patients are often reluctant to discuss their use of supplements and may not report an adverse reaction unless open discussion is promoted. Even when the patient makes full disclosure, drawing conclusions from patient histories is made difficult by the current lack of regulation of dietary supplements in the U.S. Numerous adulterations of dietary supplements have occurred, and there are instances where a substance on the label is totally absent from the product.

Although the practitioner must always be looking for the possibility of adverse herb-drug interactions, these interactions may also be positive in their effects. For example, herbs that have a hypoglycemic effect may be used to enhance blood glucose control. However, such a use should be monitored by a qualified health care professional to ensure that safe and optimal blood glucose levels are achieved. Prescribed herb doses commonly exceed those used in cooking, and the risk of interaction increases with larger quantities of both herbs and drugs. Any heretofore unreported interactions should be reported to FDA Medwatch (800-FDA-1088).

Comments or suggestions regarding this publication may be directed to the author at sharon@onlineRD.com. We look forward to providing the most current information available via the Internet to the purchasers of our publication. Updates, with references, will be periodically posted at the author's web page, http://www.herbdrug.org.

Acknowledgments

The author would like to express thanks to the librarians of Schaffer Library at Albany Medical College, Albany, New York, for their assistance in locating books and journal articles. Invaluable comments were made by Dr. Aaron Burstein, formerly of NIH, and Forest Batz, PharmD. Special thanks to the editors, Veronica Young, PharmD and Dr. Edzard Ernst, for doing their editing under tight deadlines. Their suggestions have been incorporated in the final version. The encouragement of Zaneta Pronsky, MS, RD, FADA, throughout the writing of this book was invaluable. I must also express my sincere gratitude to Carol Sokolik, MS, RD, Maria Stanish, MS, RD and Shahla Wunderlich, PhD, RD, FACN, of Montclair State University, without whom this book would not have been possible.

Drugs that may form insoluble complexes with herbs and decrease absorption of herbs (separate by at least 4 hours)

Carafate (sucralfate)   Colestid (colestipol)
Cholestyramine (Questran)   Tetracycline

Drugs that may decrease stomach acid and decrease absorption of some herbs

H2 blockers

Cimetidine (Tagamet)   Famotidine (Pepcid)
Nizatidine (Axid)   Ranitidine (Zantac)

Proton pump inhibitors

Omeprazole (Prilosec)   Lansoprazole (Prevacid)
Rabeprazole (Aciphex)

Drugs that increase intestinal motility and may decrease absorption of herbs

Alosetron (Lotronex)   Bethanechol (Urecholine)
Erythromycin (Erythrocin, Ilotycin)   Metoclopramide (Reglan)

Drugs that decrease intestinal motility and may decrease absorption of herbs

Anticholinergic drugs (see Appendix 5)

Drugs that decrease intestinal motility and may increase absorption of herbs

Haloperidol (Haldol)

<u>Drugs that may alter metabolism of herbs</u>

Inducers of the following P450 enzymes

1A2: ß-myrcene, caffeine, insulin, modafinil (Provigil), omeprazole (Prilosec), tobacco

2C9: Rifampin (Rifadin), secobarbital (Seconal)

3A4,5,7: Barbiturates (see Appendix 12), ß-myrcene, carbamazepine (Tegretol), glucocorticoids, modafinil (Provigil), phenobarbital (Nembutal), phenytoin (Dilantin), pioglitazone (Actos), rifampin (Rifadin)

Inhibitors of the following P450 enzymes

1A2: Cimetidine (Tagamet), felbamate (Felbatol), fluoxetine (Prozac), fluvoxamine (Luvox), indomethacin (Indocin), ketoconazole (Nizoral), lansoprazole (Prevacid), modafinil (Provigil), omeprazole (Prilosec), paroxetine (Paxil), ticlopidine (Ticlid), topiramate (Topamax)

2C9: Amiodarone (Cordarone), fluconazole (Diflucan), fluvastatin (Lescol), fluvoxamine (Luvox), isoniazid (Nydrazid), lovastatin (Mevacor), paroxetine (Paxil), phenylbutazone, sertraline (Zoloft), teniposide (Vumon), zafirlukast (Accolate)

2D6: Amiodarone (Cordarone), celecoxib (Celebrex), chlorpheniramine, cocaine, fluoxetine (Prozac), halofantrine (Halfan), haloperidol (Haldol), methadone, paroxetine (Paxil), quinidine (Quinaglute), ranitidine (Zantac), ritonavir (Norvir), terbinafine (Lamisil)

3A4: Antivirals (see Appendix 22), amiodarone (Cordarone), cimetidine (Tagamet), ciprofloxacin (Cipro), clarithromycin (Biaxin), diltiazem (Cardizem), erythromycin (Erythrocin, Ilotycin), fluconazole (Diflucan), fluvoxamine (Luvox), grapefruit juice, itraconazole (Sporanox), ketoconazole (Nizoral), mifepristone (Mifeprex), nefazodone (Serzone), norfloxacin (Noroxin), troleandomycin (TAO)

1994 Dietary Supplement Health and Education Act

~ Gives FDA authority to establish GMPs.
~ Defines dietary supplements and ingredients.
~ Makes manufacturer responsible for ensuring safety.
~ Allows third-party literature at point of sale.
~ Regulates support statements.
~ Establishes label requirements.
~ Requires that new ingredients be submitted to the FDA 75 days prior to marketing product.
~ Establishes the Office of Dietary Supplements and the Commission on Dietary Supplements.

Dietary Supplement Label Requirements

~ Identity.
~ Contents.
~ Structure-function claim.
~ Directions.
~ Facts panel.
~ Ingredients in descending order.
~ Correspondence address.

Safety Issues
~ Lack of quality control.
~ Misidentification of plants.
~ Contents not verified.
~ Potential allergic reactions.
~ Adulteration with prescription drugs.
~ Lack of regulation.
~ Contamination with heavy metals and pesticides.
~ Raw animal parts. Obscure labeling. No restriction on source of animal tissues.
~ Variation in chemical composition of plants.
~ Over-harvesting of endangered species.
~ Substitution of herbs.
~ Standardized to only one component.
~ Lack of research supporting use.
~ Effective dosage not established.
~ Misleading labels and advertising.

High Risk Patients
~ Elderly and children.
~ Taking prescription or OTC medicines, especially if more than 3 drugs or high-risk
  drugs are involved.
~ Pregnant or breastfeeding.
~ Chronically ill.
~ Kidney disease. Diazability of herbs is unknown.

4

High Risk Drugs
~ Digoxin.
~ Transplantation drugs.
~ Rifamycin agents.
~ Theophylline.
~ Antifungals.

~ NNRTIs & PIs.
~Chemotherapy agents.
~Macrolides.
~Warfarin.
~Antiepileptics.

Pharmacokinetic Interactions
~ Altered absorption or distribution.
~ Inhibition or induction of metabolism.

~Alteration in protein-binding sites.
~Altered renal elimination.

Pharmacodynamic Interactions
~ Additive activity.

~Synergistic activity.

Herbs Which May Have Adverse Health Effects
~ Chaparral.
~ Ephedra.
~ Lobelia.
~ Slimming/Dieter's tea.
~ Wormwood.
~ *Bragantia wallichii.*[1]
~ Asarum spp.[1]
~ *Cocculus* spp.[1]
~ *Menispernum dauricum.*[1]

~Comfrey.
~Germander.
~Magnolia-Stephania preparations.
~Willow Bark.
~*Aristolochia* spp.[1]
~*Akebia* spp.[1]
~*Clematis* spp.[1]
~*Diploclisia spp.*[1]
~*Saussurea lappa.*[1]

Herbs Which May Have Adverse Health Effects (cont'd.)

~ *Sinomenium acutum.*[1]   ~*Stephania* spp.[1]

~ *Vladimiria souliei.*[1]   ~Triatricol.

[1] - May contain or be adulterated with aristolochic acid

Herb Safety

~ Encourage patients to discuss supplements with their physician.

~ Don't combine herbs and drugs having similar actions.

~ Urge caution with patients taking drugs with a narrow margin of safety, on multiple drugs or scheduled for elective surgery.

~ Don't exceed dosages on supplement label.

~ Use nationally known brands or brands tested by independent labs, such as Consumer Labs.

~ Collect data on supplement use. Compare supplement use against verifiable changes in health status.

~ Report any suspected interactions to MedWatch at the FDA.

~ Keep up-to-date information on dietary supplements.

Communicating with Patients

~ Ask patient about supplement use. Patient may consider herbs natural and safe.

~ Patient might not acknowledge the need to report use to health care providers. Review ingredients in vitamin/mineral supplements. Ask about herbal teas and their ingredients. Examine how you feel about complementary and alternative medicine.

~ Don't be judgmental. Body language is as important as words.

Communicating with Patients (cont'd.)

~ Assess patient's knowledge about supplements used. Who recommended supplement? Is scientific research available to support that use?

~ Provide reliable resources for patients.

<u>Section 3</u> Internet resources

Dr. Duke's Phytochemical and Ethnobotanical Databases
http://www.ars-grin.gov/duke/
FDA Special Nutritionals Adverse Event Monitoring System Web Report
http://vm.cfsan.fda.gov/~dms/aems.html#search
Longwood Herbal Taskforce
http://www.mcp.edu/herbal/
Consumer Labs
http://www.consumerlabs.com/
HerbMed
http://www.herbmed.org/index.html
University of Texas Center for Alternative Medicine Research in Cancer
http://www.sph.uth.tmc.edu/utcam/therapy.htm
Self-Instructional Curriculum in Holistic Pediatrics – Children's Hospital of Boston
http://www.childrenshospital.org/holistic/educat.html
NIH Office of Dietary Supplements - IBIDS database
http://dietary-supplements.info.nih.gov/databases/ibids.html
A Healthcare Professional's Guide to Evaluating Dietary Supplements - ADA/APhA
http://www.eatright.com/members/career/supplguide.html
American Botanical Council
http://www.herbalgram.org/
HIV ReSources, Inc. —Dietary Supplement Information
http://www.hivresources.com/Supps.html#Information%20
National Cancer Institute Office of Cancer Complementary and Alternative   8

Medicine

http://occam.nci.nih.gov/

National Center for Complementary and Alternative Medicine (NCCAM)
http://nccam.nih.gov/

Nutrition in Complementary Care
http://www.complementarynutrition.org/index.cfm

Natural Medicine News® by Forrest Batz, PharmD (free newsletter)
Send email with name, academic degree, institutional affiliation, location and title to
fbatz@sonic.net

Herb Research Foundation
http://www.herbs.org/

<u>Section 4</u>   Herbs containing vitamin K, potassium and phosphorus

406,716,719,916,923,930

Herbs containing variable amounts of vitamin K (clinical significance not established)

Alfalfa

Black tea leaf (not brewed)

Cruciferous vegetables

Juniper

Parsley

Purslane

Soybeans

Stinging Nettles

Watercress

Amaranth leaf

Coriander

Green tea leaf (not brewed)

Mint

Passion flower (extract)

Seaweed (Nori)

Spring onions

Verbena

Herbs containing potassium

Alfalfa (20,300 ppm)

Bai Zhi (root 26,600 ppm)

Black Mustard (leaf 28,215 ppm)

Catnip (23,500 ppm)

Celery (plant 57,800 ppm; root 56,360 ppm)

Chicory (leaf 37,128 ppm)

Coriander (leaf 48,177 ppm)

Dandelion (root 75,000 ppm; leaf 27,569 ppm)

American Ginseng (33,800 ppm)

Bitter melon (fruit 45,000, leaf 33,117 ppm)

Blessed Thistle (26,000 ppm)

Cayenne (fruit 34,272 ppm)

Chervil (leaf 51,200 ppm)

Chinese Boxthorn (leaf 49,808 ppm)

Cumin (20,916 ppm)

Dill (76,450 ppm)

Dulse (22,700 ppm)

Evening Primrose (35,100 ppm)

Fennel (39.700 ppm)

Feverfew (22,500 ppm)

Garlic (leaf 23,971 ppm)

Genipap (fruit 22,900 ppm)

Ginger (rhizome 25,079 ppm)

Goto Kola (38,693 ppm)

Guava (fruit 21,658 ppm)

Hops (fruit 20,350 ppm)

Horseradish (root 31,150 ppm)

Japanese Honeysuckle (flower 20,100 ppm)

Kelp (21,100 ppm)

Kudzu (shoot 36,050 ppm)

Lemongrass (23,000 ppm)

Mint (35,100 ppm)

Mugwort (22,000 ppm - 41,000ppm)

Noni

Oats (78,900 ppm)

Onions (bulb 22,164 ppm)

Papaya (leaf 28,978 ppm; fruit 25,469 ppm)

Parsley (53,833 ppm)

Peppermint (leaf 22,600 ppm)

Purslane (81,200 ppm)

Red Clover (20,000-25,700 ppm)

Rhubarb (plant 66,400 ppm)

Safflower (flower 22,400 ppm)

Sage (leaf 24,700 ppm)

Sassafras (leaf 21,760 ppm)

Scullcap (21,800 ppm)

Shepherd's Purse (33,390 ppm)

Soybeans (seed 27,600 ppm)

Stinging Nettle (leaf 37,220 ppm)

Sweet basil (leaf 42,900 ppm)

Tarragon (32,719 ppm)

Turmeric (rhizome 42,371 ppm)

Watercress (66,000 ppm)

Water Lotus (34,925 ppm)

Wild carrot (root 46,360 ppm)

Herbs containing phosphorus

American Ginseng (5,200 ppm)

Borage (leaf 7,579 ppm)

Celery (plant 6,849 ppm; root 7,900 ppm; seed 6,843 ppm)

Cocoa (seed 5,571 ppm)

Cumin (fruit 5,673 ppm)

Evening Primrose (seed 7,257 ppm)

Feverfew (5,010 ppm)

Garlic (bulb 5,220 ppm)

Horseradish (root 5,000 ppm)

Milk Thistle (7,060 ppm)

Onion (leaf 5,513 ppm)

Parsley (6,425 ppm)

Pokeweed (shoot 5,238 ppm)

Shepherd's Purse (7,288 ppm)

Soybean (5,410-8,040 ppm)

Sunflower (seed 7,449 ppm)

Turmeric (rhizome 6,307 ppm)

Wild Carrot (root 5,090 ppm)

Bitter Melon (8,333ppm - 33,467 ppm)

Buchu (leaf 6,780 ppm)

Coriander (leaf 6,452 ppm)

Dill (7,625 ppm)

Fennel (fruit 5,960 ppm; plant 5,100 ppm)

Flaxseed (seed 20,335 ppm)

Ginger (rhizome 5,323 ppm)

Indian Sorrel (seed 6,000 ppm)

Oats (plant 8,800 ppm; seed 10,200 ppm)

Papaya (leaf 6,311 ppm)

Peppermint (leaf 7,720 ppm)

Purslane (7,740 ppm)

Silk Cotton Tree (seed 9,700-12,690 ppm)

Stinging Nettle (leaf 6,800 ppm)

Sweet Basil (leaf 5,168 ppm)

Water Lotus (seed 7,130 ppm)

Yellow Dock (7,568-7,570 ppm)

Data listed under Uses, Contraindications, Safety and Adverse Reactions are for screening purposes only. Clinical decisions and patient instruction should be based on comprehensive data obtained from various current well documented sources. Where there is no entry for a particular supplement, there was insufficient data to evaluate it.

USES: (H) = based on human research or case studies. (A) = based on animal research.

CONTRAINDICATIONS: Little data exists for safety in pregnancy, lactation, children and various chronic illnesses.

SAFETY: Key to data listed as AHPA Class (from American Herbal Products Association):[66]

Class 1 Safe when consumed appropriately.

Class 2 Use restricted, unless directed by qualified prescriber

2a External use only.

2b Not during pregnancy.

2c Not while nursing.

2d Other specified.

Class 3 Recommends the following labeling, with dosage, contraindications, adverse effects and drug interactions: "To be used only under the supervision of an expert qualified in the appropriate use of this substance."

Class 4 Insufficient data to classify.

ADVERSE REACTIONS: Adverse reactions reported.

INTERACTIONS: These include efficacy enhancement via synergistic or additive mechanisms as well as antagonistic effects with concurrent use of herbs and drugs.

Section 6 Herb-drug interactions

5-HTP (5-hydroxytryptophan)
  USES: Anxiety (H), cerebellar ataxia (H), depression (H), fibromyalgia (H), insomnia (H), obesity (H), tension headache (H).
  CONTRAINDICATIONS: Angina, carcinoid tumors, cardiovascular disease, Down's syndrome, heart disease, hypertension. Safety in pregnancy and lactation not established.
  SAFETY: Some 5-hydroxytryptophan supplements have been found to contain peak X, a contaminant. The effect of peak X in humans has not been studied.
  ADVERSE REACTIONS: Anorexia, arrhythmias, breathing difficulty, diarrhea, eosinophilia myalgia syndrome, GI distress, muscle incoordination, N&V, neurological changes, pupil dilation, hyporeflexes and blurring of vision.
  INTERACTIONS:
   Serotonin antagonist (see Appendix 34)[2] Drug is a competitive antagonist of peripheral serotonin and may also affect CNS serotonin. Theoretically, 5-HTP drug may decrease effectiveness of drug.

   Antidepressants (see Appendix 9)[2] Theoretical risk of serotonin excess or serotonin syndrome.

   Carbidopa (lodosyn, larodopa)[2] Case report of scleroderma-like illness after concurrent use of L-5-HTP and carbidopa for intention myoclonus, most likely due to abnormality of enzymes that catabolize kynurenine. Carbidopa inhibits the peripheral, but not CNS, conversion of 5-HTP to serotonin.

5-HTP (cont'd.)

L-Tryptophan[2] Theoretical serotonin excess or serotonin syndrome with concurrent use.

Sibutramine (Meridia)[2] Theoretical serotonin excess or serotonin syndrome with concurrent use.

Tramadol (Ultram)[2] Theoretical serotonin excess or serotonin syndrome with concurrent use.

Triptans (see Appendix 37)[2] Theoretical serotonin excess or serotonin syndrome with concurrent use.

Acacia *Acacia senegal*

USES: Chronic renal failure (H), fecal incontinence (H), hypercholesterolemia (H-equivocal).

PART USED: Gum.

CONTRAINDICATIONS: Intestinal obstruction. Safety in pregnancy and lactation not established. May form salts with minerals, thereby decreasing absorption.

SAFETY: GRAS (flavoring and emulsifier).

ADVERSE REACTIONS: Allergic reaction.

INTERACTIONS:

Herb may reduce intestinal absorption of other drugs.[4]

Alcohol[4] When acacia is exposed to alcohol, it becomes insoluble and will form a precipitate.

Aceitilla *Bidens pilosa*
  USES: HTN (A).
  PART USED: Leaf.
  INTERACTIONS:
    Insulin/Oral hypoglycemic agents (see Appendix 24)[6,88] Ethanolic extract decreased blood glucose in mice. Anorexic effect of herb may, at least in part, be responsible for hypoglycemia in treated animals.

Ackee Apple Seed *Blighia sapida*
  USES: Ripe fruit in Jamaican cooking.
  PART USED: Cooked ripe fruit.
  CONTRAINDICATIONS: Children, pregnancy, lactation (especially unripe fruit).
  SAFETY: Unripe fruit contains hypoglycin, which can cause severe hypoglycemia by inhibiting gluconeogenesis. Other symptoms of poisoning include vomiting, coma and seizures and death. Children and the malnourished are most susceptible.
  ADVERSE REACTIONS: Unripe fruit and seed may cause hypoglycemia, seizures, vomiting, coma and possibly death.
  INTERACTIONS:
    Insulin/Oral hypoglycemic agents (see Appendix 24)[5,173] Consumption of unripe fruit and seeds (hypoglycin A and hypoglycin B) may lead to severe hypoglycemia. May be additive with diabetes medications.

Aconite *Aconitum napellus, Aconitum spp.*
ADVERSE REACTIONS: Aconitine, contained in aconite, is a cardiotoxin, which may cause tachyarrhythmias. Fatal outcome from ingestion has occurred.
SAFETY: Toxic internally and externally. AHPA Class: 3.[66]
INTERACTIONS:
Antiarrhythmics, Antihypertensives, Digoxin/Cardiac glycosides[7] (see Appendix 6,[11,14]) Aconitine, a component of aconite, is a cardiotoxin that can cause tachyarrhythmias.

Agar *Gelidium spp., Gracilaria spp.*
USES: Constipation.
PART USED: Thallus.
CONTRAINDICATIONS: GI obstruction, swallowing difficulty. Safety of therapeutic dosage in pregnancy, lactation and children not established.
ADVERSE REACTIONS: Possible GI tract obstruction with inadequate concurrent fluid. May form salts with minerals, thereby decreasing absorption.
SAFETY: Take with at least 8 oz. fluid. AHPA Class: 2d.[66]
INTERACTIONS:
Herb may reduce intestinal absorption of other drugs.[4]
Alcohol[4] Agar contains a large amount of pectin, which may precipitate when exposed to alcohol.

Agrimony *Agrimonia eupatoria, Agrimonia procera*
  USES: Diabetes (A), diarrhea (H).
  PART USED: Herb.
  CONTRAINDICATIONS: Pregnancy, lactation, allergy to rose family.
  SAFETY: Tannin content (50,000 - 80,000 ppm). Avoid high dose for extended period. Furanocoumarin content increases photosensitivity. AHPA class: 1.[66]
  ADVERSE REACTIONS: Photodermatitis, photosensitivity.
  INTERACTIONS:
  Alkaloids (see Appendix 4)[4] High tannin content of plant may cause alkaloids to become insoluble and precipitate.
  Anticoagulants and drugs that increase the risk of bleeding[8,923] (see Appendix 8) Herb contains coumarins, which may increase the risk of bleeding.
  Insulin/Oral hypoglycemic agents[82,107,173] (see Appendix 24) Possible hypoglycemia or loss of blood glucose control.

Alfalfa *Medicago sativa*
  USES: Diabetes (A), hypercholesterolemia (A), menopause (H), type II hyperlipoproteinemia (H).
  PARTS USED: Herb.
  CONTRAINDICATIONS: Children, endometriosis, estrogen-sensitive cancers, lupus, lactation, pregnancy.
  SAFETY: Contains the protein canavanine, which may cause flare-up in lupus patients. Heating will denature the protein canavanine. Some vitamin B supplements contain alfalfa. There have been cases of bacterial contamination of alfalfa tablets. GRAS

(as flavoring and spice). AHPA Class: 1.[66]

ADVERSE REACTIONS: Large amounts of seed may cause pancytopenia and increase photosensitivity.

INTERACTIONS:

Drugs that induce photosensitivity[9] (see Appendix 29) Large amounts of herb, if allowed to become moldy, may increase photosensitivity, as seen in animals. It is unknown if effect may be additive when consumed concurrently with drugs that also increase photosensitivity.

Insulin/Oral hypoglycemic agents[12] (see Appendix 24) Aqueous extract lowered blood glucose in diabetes-induced mice. The hypoglycemic action is believed to be induced by a potentiation of insulin secretion and a decrease in insulin resistance.

Lipid-lowering drugs[13] (see Appendix 25) Herb has lipid-lowering effect. It is not known if lipid-lowering effect of drug is enhanced by alfalfa.

Oral contraceptives/Estrogen replacement therapy[15] Alfalfa contains estrogenic substances, such as coumestrol.

Warfarin (Coumadin)[10] (see Appendix 8) Herb contains vitamin K, which may antagonize warfarin.

Algin/Alginate *Macrocystis pyrifera*

USES: Hypercholesterolemia (A), HTN (A).

PART USED: Carbohydrate from brown seaweed.

INTERACTIONS:

Herb may reduce intestinal absorption of other drugs.[4]

Algin/Alginate (cont'd.)

Antihypertensives[17] (see Appendix 11) Herb may decrease blood pressure, which may enhance hypotensive effect of drug.

Antacids such as Gavison[18] Effectiveness of antacids is improved when combined with alginic acid.

Alkali Seepweed *Suaeda fruticosa*

USES: Hypercholesterolemia (A).

PART USED: Aqueous extract.

SAFETY: Safety in humans not established.

INTERACTIONS:

Insulin/Oral hypoglycemic agents[301] (see Appendix 24) Aqueous extract of alkali seepweed reduced blood glucose in normal and STZ-induced rats. No significant change in serum insulin was noted. Use of herb with insulin should only be made under the supervision of a knowledgeable health care professional.

Aloe (gel) *Aloe spp., Aloe vera*

TOPICAL USES: Burns (H), genital herpes (H), psoriasis (H), prevention of radiation-induced skin injury (H), wound healing (H).

PART USED: Gel (topical).

CONTRAINDICATIONS: Allergy to *Liliaceae* family. Safety in pregnancy, lactation and children not established.

SAFETY: GRAS (*A. barbadensis* as flavoring). AHPA Class: 1 (internal), 2d (external).

ADVERSE REACTIONS: Allergic response, contact dermatitis, urticaria.

Aloe (gel) (cont'd.)

INTERACTIONS:

Hydrocortisone (Cortef, Hydrocortone)[20]   Combination may decrease inflammation and enhance wound healing.

Aloe (dried juice of leaf) *Aloe spp., Aloe vera*

USES: Constipation (H).

PART USED: Leaf juice.

CONTRAINDICATIONS: Safety in lactation and children not established. Abdominal pain of unknown origin, appendicitis, Crohn's disease, diverticulitis, GI obstruction or stenosis, hemorrhoids, hypokalemia, IBS, ileus, kidney disease, pregnancy, severe dehydration, ulcerative colitis.

SAFETY: Short-term use only. Chronic use may increase the risk of hepatitis. Anthraquinone, a component of aloe, is a cathartic laxative. GRAS *(Aloe barbadensis* as flavoring). AHPA Class: 2b, 2c, 2d.

ADVERSE REACTIONS: Abdominal pain and spasm, cramps, excretion of calcium in stools. Long-term use is associated with more serious reactions: albuminuria, electrolyte imbalance, hematuria, hypokalemia, laxative dependence, malabsorption, melanosis coli, metabolic acidosis, orthostatic hypotension, osteomalacia, protein-losing gastroenteropathy, renal tubular damage, steatorrhea, weakness, weight loss.

INTERACTIONS:

Aloe may reduce intestinal absorption of drug by reducing transit time.[116]

Antiarrhythmics[1] (see Appendix 6)   Aloe may increase potassium loss in GI, which may be additive with potassium loss due to antiarrhythmics, thereby increasing the

Aloe (dried juice of leaf) (cont'd.)

risk of hypokalemia.

Corticosteroids[1] (see Appendix 18) Possible additive loss of potassium with concurrent use of aloe and corticosteroids, which may increase the risk of hypokalemia. (dried latex from leaf)

Digoxin/Cardiac glycosides[1] Aloe increases potassium loss in GI, which may increase the risk of hypokalemia with long-term use. Dosage of drug may need to be adjusted for patients with hypokalemia.

Diuretics[1] (see Appendix 11) Loss of potassium from use of aloe and drug may increase risk of hypokalemia.

Insulin/Oral hypoglycemic agents[105,162,173,287] (see Appendix 24) In human research, glibenclamide (glyburide) combined with aloe had greater hypoglycemic effect than glibenclamide (glyburide) alone. In research using streptozotocin-induced diabetic rats (type 1 diabetes model) administered aloe leaf pulp extract, blood glucose was significantly decreased at 2 and 6 hours after glucose administration. Therapeutic use of aloe should only be made under professional supervision. The effect when combined with diabetes medications is unknown and may require an alteration of insulin drug dosage.

Licorice[116] Both licorice and aloe may increase the loss of potassium, which may lead to hypokalemia with concurrent use over an extended period of time.

Alpha-lipoic acid

USES: Diabetic neuropathy (H), type 2 diabetes (H).

CONTRAINDICATIONS: Safety in pregnancy and lactation not established. Take on empty stomach.

INTERACTIONS:

Alcohol[21] Lipoic acid was protective against ethanol-induced gastric ulcers.

Chemotherapy[24] (see Appendix 16) In mice, supplement at low doses antagonized doxorubicin and had an additive effect at high doses. Urge caution in use by cancer patients until more research is completed on humans.

Oral hypoglycemic agents[29,30] (see Appendix 24) Alpha-lipoic acid may decrease insulin resistance. It is not known if hypoglycemia may result from concurrent administration. Monitor blood glucose. In one human study, no pharmacokinetic interaction was found with glibenclamide (glyburide) or acarbose. IV Administration showed the most reduction in insulin resistance.

Andrographis *Andrographis paniculata*

USES: Cold (H), HIV (H-andrographolide), upper respiratory tract infection (H).

PART USED: Herb.

CONTRAINDICATIONS: Bleeding disorders, hypotension, male infertility. Safety in pregnancy and lactation not established.

SAFETY: Infertility in laboratory animals. AHPA Class: 2b.[66]

ADVERSE REACTIONS: Anaphylaxis, GI distress, infertility.

INTERACTIONS:

Acetaminophen/Paracetamol[31] Andrographolide, isolated from herb, decreased

Andrographis (cont'd.)
hepatotoxicity of drug.

Anticoagulants and drugs that increase the risk of bleeding[32] (see Appendix 8) Andrographolide, a component of andrographis, inhibits platelet aggregation.

Antihypertensives[35] (see Appendix 11) Research using laboratory animals showed a lowering of blood pressure, which may be additive with antihypertensive medications.

Immunosuppressants[33] (see Appendix 23) Herb has immunostimulant activity, which theoretically may decrease effectiveness of immunosuppressants.

Insulin/Oral hypoglycemic agents[36] (see Appendix 24) Ethanolic extract of herb decreased blood glucose in laboratory animals. Effect of concurrent use not known. Monitor blood glucose closely.

Angelica *Angelica archangelica, Angelica spp.*

USES: Gastric ulcers (A), premature ejaculation (H-root as part of cream composed of multiple herbs).

PART USED: Root, herb, fruit/seed.

CONTRAINDICATIONS: Bleeding disorders, GERD (essential oil), peptic ulcers, pregnancy.

SAFETY: Root contains furanocoumarins (angelicin, bergapten, imperatorin, and xanthotoxin), which increase photosensitivity. Avoid prolonged exposure to sunlight and UV radiation. GRAS (spice, seasoning, flavoring). AHPA Class: 2b, 2d—increased photosensitivity.[66]

ADVERSE REACTIONS: Photosensitivity.

INTERACTIONS:

Anticoagulants and drugs that increase the risk of bleeding[37] (see Appendix 8) Herb contains osthole (coumarin-like substance), which may have an additive effect with anticoagulants.

Photosensitizing drugs[39] (see Appendix 29) Furanocoumarin content of herb may increase photosensitizing effect of drug.

Anise *Pimpinella anisum*

USES: Expectorant (H-pinene).

PART USED: Fruit/seed, oil.

CONTRAINDICATIONS: Therapeutic amounts during pregnancy, bleeding disorders, catecholamine-sensitive and estrogen-sensitive cancers.

SAFETY: Undiluted oil may be unsafe. Excessive amount may cause neurological abnormalities. GRAS (spice, seasoning, flavoring, oil, extract, oleoresin). AHPA Class: 2b.[66]

ADVERSE REACTIONS: Allergic reaction, large amounts of oil may cause N&V, neurological abnormalities, photosensitivity (topical), pulmonary edema, seizures.

INTERACTIONS:

Anticoagulants and drugs that increase the risk of bleeding[40] (see Appendix 8) Scopoletin, one of the coumarins present in herb, had antiplatelet activity in rabbits. Concurrent use with drugs that also increase bleeding may be additive.

Anticonvulsants[42] (see Appendix 10) Fruit essential oil had an anticonvulsant effect in mice. It is not known if concurrent use with anticonvulsants is additive.

Anise (cont'd.)

Estrogen replacement therapy/Oral contraceptives[41] Herb contains anethole, which has estrogenic activity. Effect of concurrent use with hormone therapy is not known.

Iron[43] Beverage extract of anise enhanced absorption of iron in rats.

MAOIs[117] (see Appendix 9) MAOIs increase catecholamines at the synapse. Anise contains catecholamines, and action with concurrent use is not known.

Annatto *Bixa orellana*
PART USED: Seed.

SAFETY: AHPA Class: 1.[66]

ADVERSE REACTIONS: Anaphylaxis due to annatto dye allergy.

INTERACTIONS:

Insulin/Oral hypoglycemic agents[44,162] (see Appendix 24) Bixin, a component of annatto, has a hyperglycemic effect. High intakes of annatto may disturb blood glucose control.

Arnica *Arnica montana*
PART USED: Flower, plant, rhizome.

CONTRAINDICATIONS: Pregnancy. Allergy to *Asteraceae/Compositae* family.

SAFETY: May be toxic when administered orally (gastroenteritis, nervousness, tachycardia, muscular weakness, and possibly death) or on broken skin. AHPA Class: External 2d—use only on intact skin.[66]

ADVERSE REACTIONS: Allergic response, cardiac arrest, coma, death, dermatitis, diarrhea, drowsiness, dyspnea, eczema, gastroenteritis, gastric distress, mucous membrane irritation, N&V.

INTERACTIONS:

Anticoagulants and drugs that increase the risk of bleeding[45] (see Appendix 8) Helenalin and 11 alpha,13-dihydrohelenalin, contained in arnica, may alter platelet function. Amounts in homeopathic preparations are too small to cause increased bleeding.

Surgery[286] In a double blind study of 130 patients undergoing surgery for varicose veins, homeopathic arnica CH5 was administered prior to surgery. No significant reduction in postoperative hematomas was found in group taking homeopathic remedy.

Artichoke *Cynara scolymus*

USES: Hypercholesterolemia (H), IBS (H-preliminary post marketing).

PARTS USED: Leaf, root stem.

CONTRAINDICATIONS: Allergy to *Compositae* family, gallbladder disease, gallstones and obstruction of common bile duct. Safety in pregnancy and lactation not established.

SAFETY: GRAS (flavoring in alcoholic beverage).

ADVERSE REACTIONS: Allergic reaction, contact dermatitis, urticaria.

INTERACTIONS:

Lipid-lowering drugs[46] (see Appendix 25) In research using humans with hyperlipoproteinemia, use of dry extract of artichoke resulted in a decrease in total

Artichoke (cont'd.)

cholesterol and LDL cholesterol. It is not known whether effect is additive if combined with lipid-lowering drugs.

Asafoetida *Ferula assafoetida, Ferula spp.*
PART USED: Root, rhizome, resin.
CONTRAINDICATIONS: Bleeding disorders, children, pregnancy, infectious or inflammatory GI diseases.
SAFETY: GRAS (oil, extract, oleoresins). AHPA Class: 2b, 2d—not for infant colic.[66]
ADVERSE REACTIONS: Possible methemoglobinemia. Convulsions, headache, swelling of lips.

Ashwagandha *Withania somnifera*
PARTS USED: Berry, root.
CONTRAINDICATIONS: Pregnancy.
SAFETY: AHPA Class: 2b, 2d—potentiates barbiturates.[66]
ADVERSE REACTIONS: Sedation.
INTERACTIONS:

Azathioprine (Imuran)[47] Herb prevented myelosuppression of drug in mice. An increase in hemoglobin concentration, RBC, WBC, platelet count and weight occurred in mice treated with ashwagandha.

Barbiturates[48,52] (see Appendix 12) Theoretically, herb may potentiate drug.

Benzodiazepines[48,52] (see Appendix 13) Theoretically, herb may increase effect of drug.

Ashwagandha (cont'd.)

CNS depressants[48,52] (see Appendix 15) Herb may be sedating, which theoretically may be additive with drug.

Cyclophosphamide (Cytoxan, Neosar)[47,245,276] Herb may decrease urotoxicity of drug. Research using rats found herb to have immunopotentiating and myeloprotective effects as well as increasing hemoglobin concentration, RBC, WBC, platelet count and weight.

Immunosuppresants, also see **Azathioprine** and **Paclitaxel**[245,276] (see Appendix 16 and 23) Theoretical antagonism based on immune stimulating effect of herb.

Insulin/Oral hypoglycemic agents[50] (see Appendix 24) In research using humans with mild diabetes, root was found to decrease blood glucose.

Paclitaxel (Taxol)[59] In mice, aqueous extract of herb decreased the neutropenic effect of drug. Herb may prevent bone marrow suppression associated with paclitaxel. More research is need in humans before using as adjunct to chemotherapy.

Prednisolone[47] Herb prevented myelosuppression of drug in mice. An increase in hemoglobin concentration, RBC, WBC, platelet count and weight occurred in mice treated with ashwagandha.

Thyroid replacement therapy[194] Herb may increase serum T_4.

Astragalus *Astragalus membranaceus*

PART USED: Root.

CONTRAINDICATIONS: Safety in pregnancy and lactation not established. Theoretically, in autoimmune diseases and transplant patients. AHPA Class: 1.[66]

Astragalus (cont'd.)
INTERACTIONS:
Acyclovir (Zovirax)[60] In research using mice, herb was found to be synergistic with drug against herpes simplex virus type 1.

Anticoagulants and drugs that increase the risk of bleeding[61] (see Appendix 8) In in vitro research, astragaloside IV increased the fibrinolytic potential. Theoretically, herb may potentiate drug.

Cyclophosphamide (Cytoxan, Neosar)[64] Concurrent use of herb with cyclophosphamide, an immunosuppressant, decreased effectiveness of drug.

Immunosuppressants[64] (see Appendix 23) Concurrent use of herb with cyclophosphamide decreased effectiveness of drug.

Recombinant interferon alpha 1[65] Herb was found to be synergistic with drug in treatment of papillomavirus, herpes simplex virus type 2 and cytomegalovirus.

Recombinant interleukin-2[67] In in vitro research, herb was found to potentiate effect of drug.

Autumn Crocus *Colchicum autumnale*
SAFETY: Most likely unsafe for consumption. Contains colchicine, which may be toxic.

ADVERSE REACTIONS: Abdominal pain, diarrhea, organ failure and N&V. Prolonged use may cause agranulocytosis, aplastic anemia and peripheral nerve inflammation.

Ayahuasca Harmala alkaloids from *Banisteriopsis caapi*, Malpighiaceous liana, *Psychotria viridis* and *Psychotria carthagenensis or Diplopterys cabrerana*

SAFETY: Contains beta-carboline, harmine and n,n-dimethyltryptamine (DMT).

INTERACTIONS:

Fluoxetine (Prozac)[305] (see Appendix 9 for list of other SSRIs) Case report of 36 year old male taking fluoxetine 20 mg/d and ayahuasca 100ml/d reported tremors, shivering, sweating, severe N&V. Symptoms consistent with serotonin syndrome, which improved after 4 hours with no long-lasting effects. Herb preparation is believed to block the breakdown of neurotransmitters, which may increase the risk of interaction with other antidepressants.

MAOIs[68] (see Appendix 9) Herb has been shown to inhibit MAO in vitro. Beta-carbolines and tryptamine are believed to be the components responsible for inhibition.

Bai Zhi *Angelica dahurica*

PART USED: Root.

SAFETY: AHPA Class: 1.[66]

INTERACTIONS:

Drugs metabolized by the P450 CYP2C, CYP3A, and CYP2D1[74,237] (see Appendix 38) Research suggests that herb extract may inhibit the above, P450 isozymes. Serum levels of drugs metabolized by these isozymes may be elevated.

Bufuralol[237] Herb extract inhibits the metabolism of drug.

Diazepam (Valium)[237] Herb extract delays the elimination of oral dose of drug.

Nifedipine (Adalat, Procardia)[237] Herb extract inhibits the metabolism of drug.

Tolbutamide (Orinase)[237] Herb extract delays elimination of drug.

Bai Zhu *Atractylodes ovata, Atractylodes macrocephala*
   PART USED: Rhizome.
   SAFETY: AHPA Class: 1.[66]
   ADVERSE REACTIONS: Allergic reaction, GI distress, increased BP.
   INTERACTIONS:
      Insulin/Oral hypoglycemic agents[105] (see Appendix 24) Herb has had
      hypoglycemic activity in animals. Monitor patients with diabetes.

Baikal Skullcap *Scutelleria baicalensis*
Part of formula called PC-SPES and Sho-saiko-To
   USES: See PC-SPES and Sho-saiko-To.
   PART USED: Root.
   SAFETY: AHPA Class: 1.[66]
   INTERACTIONS:
      Drugs metabolized by P450 CYP1A1/2[85] (see Appendix 38) Extract of root had an
      inhibitory effect on CYP1A1/2 in research using rat liver microsomes.

      5-Fluorouracil[90] In research using rats, herb decreased myelotoxicity and
      decreased life span of tumor.
      Anticoagulants[94] (see Appendix 8) Baicalein and oroxylin contained in herb may
      inhibit vitamin K reductase, which may increase risk of bleeding.
      Benzodiazepines[97] (see Appendix 13) Wogonin, baicalein, scutellarein and
      baicalin, components of herb, can interact with benzodiazepine site on the GABA-A
      receptor and theoretically may produce additive effect.
      CNS depressants[97] (see Appendix 15) Wogonin, baicalein, scutellarein and

baicalin, components of herb, can interact with benzodiazepine site on the GABA-A receptor and theoretically may produce additive effect.

Cyclophosphamide (Cytoxan, Neosar)[90] In research using rats, herb decreased myelotoxicity and decreased life span of tumor.

Insulin/Oral hypoglycemic agents[89] (see Appendix 24) Baicalein, a component of herb, has alpha-glucosidase inhibitor activity. The oral hypoglycemic, acarbose, is an alpha-glucosidase inhibitor. It is not known if concurrent use is additive, and it should be monitored by a qualified health care provider.

Balloon Cotton *Asclepias fruticosa*
SAFETY: Contains cardiac glycosides.
INTERACTIONS:
Digoxin/Cardiac glycosides[34,100] Herb contains cardiac glycosides. Do not use concurrently with other cardiac glycosides.

Balloon Flower *Platycodon grandiflorum*
USES: Hyperinsulinemia (A).
PART USED: Root. AHPA Class: 2d—not with TB. Caution with peptic ulcers.[66]
INTERACTIONS:
Acetaminophen/Paracetamol[102] Aqueous extract protected against drug-induced hepatotoxicity in mice, most likely due to herb's ability to block P450 bioactivation.
Alcohol[116] Increased sedation.
CNS depressants[116] (see Appendix 15) Increased sedation.

Banana *Musa sapientum*

    USES: Diarrhea in enterally fed (H-flakes), hypercholesterolemia induced by diet (A).

    PART USED: Flowers, pulp, root.

    INTERACTIONS:

    Aspirin[288] In research using male Wistar rats, administration of green unripe dried powder of plantain bananas was protective against aspirin-induced ulcerations. Benefit of plantain bananas is lost if cooked. Flavonoid leucocyanidin is believed to be responsible for protective action.

    Indomethacin (Indocin)[106] In research using animals, herb protected against drug-induced ulcer formation.

    Insulin/Oral hypoglycemic agents[108] (see Appendix 24) Banana flowers and roots have hypoglycemic action. Theoretical increase in hypoglycemic action of diabetes medications. Monitor blood glucose.

    Phenylbutazone[106] In research using animals, herb protected against drug-induced ulcer formation.

    Prednisolone[106] In research using animals, herb protected against drug-induced ulcer formation.

    Cysteamine (Cystagon)[106] In research using animals, herb protected against drug-induced ulcer formation.

    Enteral nutrition support[115] Enterally fed, critically ill patients had decreased diarrhea when administered banana flakes.

    Insulin/Oral hypoglycemic agents[55,105,108] (see Appendix 24) In research using rats, chloroform extract of flowers decreased blood glucose.

Banyan Stem *Ficus bengalensis*

USES: Diarrhea (A).

PART USED: Bark.

INTERACTIONS:

Insulin/Oral hypoglycemic agents[105,119,120,173] (see Appendix 24) Leucodelphinidin and bengalenoside derived from *Ficus bengalensis* decreased blood glucose in research animals. It is not known if hypoglycemia will occur if herb is taken concurrently with diabetes medications.

Barberry *Berberis vulgaris*

PART USED: Berries, root, root bark.

CONTRAINDICATIONS: Safety in pregnancy and lactation not established. Gallbladder disease, kidney disease, liver disease.

SAFETY: Contains berberine, which has a hypotensive effect. AHPA Class: 2b.[66]

ADVERSE REACTIONS: Consumption of large amount may cause lethargy, skin and eye irritation, cardiac damage, decreased blood pressure, dyspnea, GI distress, nose bleed, nephritis, N&V, breathing difficulties and stupor. Caution is urged with use of other herbs containing berberine (Amur cork tree, celandine, goldthread, goldenseal, Oregon grape). Berberine may increase the risk of photosensitivity.

INTERACTIONS:

Drugs metabolized by P450 enzymes[121] (see Appendix 38) Berberine, a component of barberry, may inhibit P450 enzymes.

Acetaminophen/Paracetamol[121] Berberine, a component of herb, decreased the hepatotoxicity of acetaminophen.

Barberry (cont'd.)

Alpha-adrenergic agonist[122,123] (see Appendix 36) Berberine, a component of herb, blocked contraction by phenylephrine, norepinephrine and caffeine.

Antiarrhythmics[130] (see Appendix 6) Berberine, a component of herb, has antiarrhythmic activity, which theoretically may be additive with antiarrhythmic drugs.

Antibiotics See **Tetracycline** and **Pyrimethamine**, below. Herb increased effectiveness of antibiotics.

Anticoagulants and drugs that increase the risk of bleeding[133,923] (see Appendix 8) Berberine, a component of herb, may inhibit platelet aggregation, which may increase bleeding.

Antihypertensives[130] (see Appendix 11) Berberine, a component of herb, has hypotensive effect, which theoretically may be additive with antihypertensive drugs. Berberine blocks calcium channels.

CNS depressants[129] (see Appendix 15) Components of barberry (berberine, caffeic acid, hydrastine) have a sedative effect, which theoretically may be additive with drugs causing sedation.

Cyclophosphamide (Cytoxan, Neosar)[124,128] Berberine, a component of herb, decreased urotoxicity of drug in rats. In another study, berberine decreased retention of chemotherapeutic agents. Concurrent use is not suggested.

Digoxin/Cardiac glycosides[130] Berberine, a component of herb, may have an additive effect with cardiac glycosides.

General anesthetics[130] (see Appendix 20) Berberine, a component of herb, may potentiate hypotensive action of anesthetics.

Barberry (cont'd.)

MAOIs[134] (see Appendix 9) Berberine, a component of herb, competitively inhibited MAO-A in rat brain mitochondria. Avoid concurrent use.

Pentobarbital[121] Berberine, a component of herb, increased pentobarbital-induced sleep time.

Photosensitivity, drugs causing[127] (see Appendix 29) Preliminary research revealed a potential increase in photosensitivity with use of berberine (a component of herb), which theoretically may be additive with drugs that also increase photosensitivity. Avoid concurrent use.

Pyrimethamine (Daraprim, Fansidar)[126] Berberine, a component of herb, when combined with drug was more effective than combinations with other antibiotics in treating chloroquine-resistant malaria.

Tetracyclines[125] (see Appendix 7) Simultaneous administration of tetracycline and herb (berberine) decreased efficacy of drug.

Barleria Plant Hygrophila auriculata

INTERACTIONS:

Acetaminophen/Paracetamol[136] Methanolic extract of seed decreased hepatotoxicity of drug.

Thioacetamine[136] Methanolic extract of seed decreased hepatotoxicity of drug.

Barley Sprouts *Hordeum vulgare*
 USES: Hypercholesterolemia (A).
 PART USED: Sprouted seed, seed.
 CONTRAINDICATIONS: Safety of medicinal amounts in pregnancy, lactation and children not established. Celiac disease (seed contains gliadin, a component of gluten).
 SAFETY: GRAS (oil, extract, oleoresin). AHPA CLASS: 2b.[66]
 ADVERSE REACTIONS: Anaphylaxis, contact dermatitis.
 INTERACTIONS:

   May decrease/delay absorption of drugs.[4] Based on fiber content.

   Insulin/Oral hypoglycemic agents[105,137] (see Appendix 24) Postprandial response to barley is lower than that to white flour. Research suggests that replacement of white flour with barley may assist in blood glucose control for those with type 2 diabetes.

   Sympathomimetics[138] (see Appendix 36) Hordenine in barley may liberate norepinephrine from stores.

Bay *Laurus nobilis*
 PART USED: Leaf.
 SAFETY: Bay leaf may perforate GI tract. GRAS (oil—extract, spice, flavoring, oleoresin). AHPA Class: 1.[66]
 ADVERSE REACTIONS: Allergic reaction, dermatitis (oil).
 INTERACTIONS:

Bay (cont'd.)

Alcohol[139] In research using animals, herb provided gastroprotection against ethanol.

Drugs metabolized by P450 CYP2B[262] (see Appendix 38) ß-Myrcene (acyclic monoterpene in essential oil of bay) may induce CYP2B isozymes, which may decrease serum level of drugs metabolized by these enzymes. This research was conducted on rat hepatic microsomes. Monitor concurrent use with substrates of this isozyme.

Bayberry *Myrica cerifera*

PART USED: Bark, berries, root.

CONTRAINDICATIONS: Pregnancy, lactation, HTN.

SAFETY: Contains tannins; avoid high dose for extended period. Safety of internal use not established. Large doses may have a mineralocorticoid effect. AHPA Class: 1, 66

ADVERSE REACTIONS: Allergic response, GI irritation, vomiting.

INTERACTIONS:

Corticosteroids[117] (see Appendix 18) High doses of herb may have a mineralocorticoid effect, which may increase side effects of drug.

Belladonna *Atropa belladonna*

PART USED: Leaf, root.

CONTRAINDICATIONS: Safety in pregnancy, lactation and in children 6 years old and under has not been established. GI stenosis, megacolon, narrow-angle glaucoma, GI

Belladonna (cont'd.)

obstruction, prostate adenoma, respiratory edema, tachyarrhythmias, urinary retention.

SAFETY: Use only under supervision of qualified health care professional. AHPA Class: 3.[66]

ADVERSE REACTIONS: A case report of an overdose of belladonna, which was resolved with administration of 2 mg physostigmine. Blurred vision, decreased perspiration, difficulty urinating, dry skin, hallucinations, hyperthermia, spasms, tachycardia, xerostomia.

INTERACTIONS:

Anticholinergic drugs[140] (see Appendix 5) Potential additive anticholinergic effect .

Betel Nut *Areca catechu*

PART USED: Nut.

CONTRAINDICATIONS: Safety in pregnancy and lactation not established. Asthma, thyroid disease.

SAFETY: Not for long-term use or for extended period of time. Long-term use may be linked to an increased risk of cardiovascular disease, diabetes and asthma. High tannin content.

ADVERSE REACTIONS: Altered heart rate, CNS stimulation, diarrhea, convulsions (large amounts), increased GI motility, leukoplakia, nausea, oral submucous fibrosis, red stain, vomiting.

INTERACTIONS:

Alkaloids (see Appendix 4)[4] High tannin content of nut may cause alkaloids to become insoluble and precipitate.

Betel Nut (cont'd.)

Anticholinergic drugs[141] (see Appendix 5) Arecoline, a component of betel nut, has been found to have anticholinergic action, which may be additive with anticholinergic drugs.

Cholinergic drugs[141] (see Appendix 17) Theoretically, based on anticholinergic effect of betel nut, herb may antagonize effect of drug.

Procyclidine (Kemadrin)[141] Arecoline, a component of betel nut, may antagonize the anticholinergic effect of drug.

Thyroid medications[142] In mice, betel leaf extract was found to decrease T_4 and increase T_3 at low doses. The opposite was found at higher doses. Monitor patients who use betel leaf extract and are on thyroid medications.

Bilberry *Vaccinium myrtillus*

USES: Atherosclerosis (H), diabetes (A) diabetic retinopathy (H–preliminary evidence), cataracts (H), easy bruising (H), hemorrhoids (H), hypertriglyceridemia (A), macular degeneration (H–anthocyanoside), poor night vision (H–equivocal), varicose veins (H).

PART USED: Fruit.

CONTRAINDICATIONS: Safety in children, pregnancy and lactation not established. Contraindicated for those with bleeding disorders.

SAFETY: Large amounts may cause GI distress or increase risk of bleeding (extract). Monitor patients with hypoglycemia. AHPA Class: 4.[66]

INTERACTIONS:

Alkaloids[4] (see Appendix 4) High tannin content of herb may cause alkaloids to become insoluble and precipitate.

Bilberry (cont'd.)

Anticoagulants and drugs that increase the risk of bleeding[143] (see Appendix 8) Anthocyanidins, components of bilberry, inhibit platelet aggregation and thrombus formation, which increases the risk of bleeding.

Insulin/Oral hypoglycemic agents[92,107,144,173] (see Appendix 24) Blood glucose lowered in study using rats. Monitor concurrent use of bilberry leaf with diabetes medications.

Bishop's Weed *Ammi visnaga*

PART USED: Ripe fruit (dried).

CONTRAINDICATIONS: Safety in pregnancy not established. Gallbladder disease, jaundice, liver disease, long periods of time in the sun.

SAFETY: Herb has caused elevated liver enzymes. Herb contains khellin, which increases photosensitivity.

ADVERSE REACTIONS: Elevated liver enzymes (SGOT and SGPT), N&V, photosensitivity.

INTERACTIONS:

Drugs that are substrates of P450 isozymes[591] (see Appendix 38) Khellin, and other components of herb, inhibited P450 enzymes, which may increase serum level of drugs that are substrates of these enzymes.

Antihypertensives[584,590] (see Appendix 11) Visnadine, a component of herb, has a vasodilator effect on vascular smooth muscles, which may be additive when combined with antihypertensive drugs.

Calcium channel blockers[589] (see Appendix 11) Visnadin, a component of

Bishop's Weed (cont'd.)

herb, may have calcium-blocking activity. Theoretical, possible additive effect.

Digoxin/Cardiac glycosides[584,586] Visnagin, a component of herb, when used concurrently with cardiac glycoside may cause an additive decrease in heart rate.

Hepatotoxic drugs[588] (see Appendix 21) In one study, 2 out of 14 subjects had an elevation of SGOT and SGPT. Monitor patients using both herb and hepatotoxic drugs.

Photosensitivity, drugs causing[587] (see Appendix 29) Furanocoumarin content of herb may increase photosensitivity, which theoretically may be additive.

Bitter Melon / Bitter Gourd *Momordica charantia*

USES: Type 2 diabetes (under medical supervision only). May be useful for those at high risk of developing type 2 diabetes, such as those with syndrome X and polycystic ovary disease.

PART USED: Fruit, seeds.

CONTRAINDICATIONS: Safety in pregnancy not established. Red arils should not be consumed by children.

SAFETY: Consumed as a food in Asia.

ADVERSE REACTIONS: Excessive amounts can cause diarrhea and GI distress.

INTERACTIONS:

Insulin/Oral hypoglycemic agents[53,76,83,95,105,107,145, 62,173,257,304,324] (see Appendix 24) In one study, the herb was observed to have hypoglycemic effects in 86% of participants. Use of herb with oral hypoglycemic agents should only be made under the supervision of a knowledgeable health care professional, as herb may increase

Bitter Melon (cont'd.)

secretion of insulin by beta cells and may increase the risk of hypoglycemia in laboratory animals.

Bitter Orange *Citrus aurantium*

USES: Antifungal (H-topical oil).
PART USED: Peel.
CONTRAINDICATIONS: Not large amounts in children. Safety in pregnancy and lactation not established. HTN, narrow-angle glaucoma, tachyarrhythmias.
SAFETY: Not excessive doses. GRAS (oil, extract, oleoresin).   AHPA Class: 1.[66]
ADVERSE REACTIONS: Cardiovascular toxicity, HTN, photosensitivity.
INTERACTIONS:

Decongestants containing ephedrine[146] Bitter orange contains m-synephrine, which is a stimulant. Effects may be additive with ephedrine.

Drugs metabolized by P450 CYP3A4[147] (see Appendix 38) In research using felodipine (CYP3A4 substrate), AUC was decreased 76%, which suggests induction of intestinal CYP3A4. Use caution in concurrent use of drugs which are substrates of CYP3A4, as serum levels may be increased.

MAOIs[146] (see Appendix 9) Bitter orange contains m-synephrine, which is a stimulant. Concurrent use with MAOIs may theoretically lead to hypertensive crisis.

Photosensitivity, drugs causing[147] (see Appendix 29) Herb increases risk of phototoxicity, which may be additive with drugs that increase photosensitivity.

Black Cohosh *Cimicifuga racemosa, Actaea racemosa*
USES: Menopausal symptoms (H).
PART USED: Rhizome.
CONTRAINDICATIONS: Estrogen-sensitive cancers, pregnancy (has been used during labor, but safety of this use has not been established), lactation.
SAFETY: Commission E suggests limiting use to 6 months. AHPA Class: 2b, 2c.[66]
ADVERSE REACTIONS: Headache, hypotension, mild GI distress. Large amounts may cause dizziness, N&V, vertigo.

Black Currant *Ribes nigrum*
USES: Rheumatoid arthritis (H).
PART USED: Fruit/seed oil.
CONTRAINDICATIONS: Bleeding disorders.
SAFETY: GRAS (buds and leaves as flavoring). AHPA Class: 1.[66]
INTERACTIONS:
Anticoagulants and drugs that increase the risk of bleeding[148] (see Appendix 8)
Linolenic acid may inhibit platelet aggregation, which may increase the risk of bleeding.
Diuretics[226] (see Appendix 11) No interactions reported. Black currant has diuretic action, which may be additive with drugs.

Black Hellebore *Helleborus niger*
PART USED: Flower, rhizome, seed.
CONTRAINDICATIONS: Pregnancy, lactation, children.

Black Hellebore (cont'd.)

SAFETY: Contains cardiac glycosides.

INTERACTIONS:

Digoxin/Cardiac glycosides[150] Helleborein/Hellebrin, contained in black hellebore, has cardioactive activity which may be additive with cardiac glycoside drugs.

Quinidine (Quinaglute)[150] Drug may decrease clearance of herb. Theoretical increased toxicity of herb.

Quinine[150] Drug may decrease clearance of herb. Theoretical increased toxicity of herb.

Black Pepper *Piper nigrum* Part of Trikatu, an ayurvedic preparation (see **Trikatu**)

PART USED: Fruit.

CONTRAINDICATIONS: Pregnancy.

SAFETY: GRAS (spice, seasoning, flavoring, oil, extract, oleoresin). AHPA Class: 1.[66]

ADVERSE REACTIONS: Oral irritation. Inhalation has been fatal.

INTERACTIONS:

Drugs metabolized by P450 enzymes[151,152] (see Appendix 38) In research using laboratory animals, CYP2E1 expression was suppressed and CYP2B and CYP1A expression was enhanced. Metabolism of drugs which are substrates of these isozymes may be altered. In research by Atal, piperine was found to be a nonspecific inhibitor of P450 enzymes. Use caution with concurrent use of drugs which are substrates of various P450 isozymes.

Coenzyme Q10[157] Five mg piperine, a component of black pepper, administered for 21 days, increased serum levels of coenzyme Q10.

Black Pepper (cont'd.)

Hexobarbital[151] Piperine, a component of pepper, increased hexobarbital-induced sleep time.

Indomethacin (Indocin)[153] In research using mice, piperine was protective against drug-induced ulcers.

Pentobarbitone[158] Piperine potentiated drug sleep time, possibly due to the inhibition of liver enzymes.

Phenytoin (Dilantin)[155] Piperine may enhance bioavailability of drug.

Propranolol (Inderal)[154] Piperine enhanced systemic availability of drug, possibly resulting in a lower amount of drug needed to reach therapeutic levels.

Theophylline (Uniphyl, Uni-Dur)[154] Piperine enhanced systemic availability of drug, possibly resulting in a lower amount of drug needed to reach therapeutic levels.

Zoxazolamine[151] Piperine, a component of pepper, increased drug-induced sleep time.

Black Seed *Nigella sativa*

PART USED: Seed.

CONTRAINDICATIONS: Bleeding disorders, hypotension, pregnancy. Safety in lactation not established.

SAFETY: GRAS (spice, seasoning, flavoring).

ADVERSE REACTIONS: Contact dermatitis.

INTERACTIONS:

Alcohol[159] In rats, black seed was protective against ethanol-induced ulcers.

Black Seed (cont'd.)

Anticoagulants and drugs that increase the risk of bleeding[164] (see Appendix 8) Methanol soluble portion of black cumin oil inhibits platelet aggregation, which may increase the risk of bleeding if used concurrently with drugs which also increase the risk of bleeding.

Antihypertensives[161] (see Appendix 11) Volatile oil of seeds may lower blood pressure. Theoretically, concurrent use with antihypertensives may be additive.

Cisplatin (Platinol)[160] In animal research, extract was protective against decrease in hemoglobin and leukocytes.

Doxorubicin (Adriamycin, Doxil, Rubex)[228] Thymoquinone (volatile oil of black seed) may suppress drug-induced nephrosis.

Black Walnut *Juglans nigra*

PART USED: Fruit.

CONTRAINDICATIONS: Safety in pregnancy and lactation not established.

SAFETY: Short-term use only. GRAS (flavoring from leaves or green nuts). AHPA Class: 2d—not for extended use.[66] Contains juglone, which may be toxic and carcinogenic.

ADVERSE REACTIONS: Black walnut toxicosis/laminitis.

INTERACTIONS:

Alkaloids (see Appendix 4)[4] High tannin content of herb may cause alkaloids to become insoluble and precipitate, as well as reduce the absorption of other drugs.

Blackberry *Rubus fruticosus*
PART USED: Fruit, leaf.
SAFETY: Safety of root not established. AHPA Class: 1.[66]
INTERACTIONS:
Insulin/Oral hypoglycemic agents[165,173] (see Appendix 24) Possible hypoglycemia or loss of blood glucose control.

Blackthorn Berry *Prunus spinosa*
PART USED: Flower, fruit.
SAFETY: Seeds and fresh flowers contain cyanogenic glycosides, which can release cyanide, which is toxic in large amounts. Not for long-term use. AHPA Class: 2d—do not use excessive doses.[66]

Blazing Star *Aletris farinosa*
PART USED: Root, rhizome.
CONTRAINDICATIONS: Safety in pregnancy and lactation not established. AHPA Class: 2d—may antagonize oxytocin.[66]
INTERACTIONS:
Oxytocin (Pitocin)[66] Herb antagonizes drug.

Blessed Thistle *Cnicus benedictus*
PART USED: Herb.
CONTRAINDICATIONS: Safety in pregnancy and lactation not established.
SAFETY: AHPA Class: 2b.[66]

Blessed Thistle (cont'd.)
    ADVERSE REACTIONS: Allergic response, GI distress, vomiting.
    INTERACTIONS:
       Alkaloids (see Appendix 4)[4] High tannin content of herb may cause alkaloids to become insoluble and precipitate.

Blue Cohosh *Caulophyllum thalictroides*
    PART USED: Root.
    CONTRAINDICATIONS: Pregnancy, lactation.
    SAFETY: AHPA Class: 2b.[66]
    ADVERSE REACTIONS: CHF in newborn (mother ingested in pregnancy), chest pain, dermatitis, diarrhea, GI distress, irritation of mucous membranes, hypertension, hypoglycemia, myocardial infarction in newborn.
    INTERACTIONS:
       Nicotine[166] Herb may increase effects of nicotine.

Blue Flag *Iris versicolor*
    PART USED: Root, rhizome.
    SAFETY: Safety not established. AHPA Class: 2b, 2d—emetic.[66]
    ADVERSE REACTIONS: Headache, irritation of mucous membranes, N&V.

Bogbean *Menyanthes trifoliata*
    PART USED: Leaf.
    CONTRAINDICATIONS: Safety in pregnancy and lactation not established.

Bleeding disorders.

SAFETY: GRAS (flavoring in alcoholic beverage). AHPA Class: 2d—not for use with diarrhea, dysentery or colitis.[66]

ADVERSE REACTIONS: Bleeding, GI distress.

INTERACTIONS:

Anticoagulants and drugs that increase the risk of bleeding[169] (see Appendix 8) Ferulic acid, a component of herb, may prevent and dissolve thromboses. Herb also contains caffeic acid, which may inhibit platelet aggregation.

Boldo Leaf *Peumus boldus*

PART USED: Leaf.

CONTRAINDICATIONS: Bleeding disorders, common bile duct obstruction, gallstones, liver disease. Unsafe in pregnancy and lactation.

SAFETY: GRAS (flavoring in alcoholic beverage). AHPA Class: 2d—not for use with liver disease, obstruction of common bile duct or gallstones.[66]

ADVERSE REACTIONS: Convulsions. Large doses may cause paralysis, respiratory distress and death.

INTERACTIONS:

Drugs metabolized by P450 CYP1A and CYP3A[289] (see Appendix 38) In vitro research shows alkaloid (boldine) in boldo leaf and bark may inhibit CYP1A and CYP3A, which may increase levels of drugs metabolized by these enzymes.

Warfarin[290] Case report of 67 year old female with increased INR after consumption of boldo and fenugreek. Patient had history of HTN and atrial fibrillation

Boldo Leaf (cont'd.)

on metoprolol and warfarin. Supplements taken prior to increased INR included zinc, multivitamin, artichoke extract and vitamin E. INR increased to 3.4 after starting boldo and fenugreek (previously maintained at 2.0-3.0). INRs returned to previous levels with discontinuation of boldo and fenugreek.

Boneset *Eupatorium perfoliatum*

USES: Common cold (H- homeopathic preparation Eupatorium perfoliatum D2).
PART USED: Herb.
CONTRAINDICATIONS: Pregnancy, lactation.
SAFETY: Large amounts unsafe. Contains pyrrolizidine alkaloids, which are hepatotoxic. AHPA Class: 4.[66]
ADVERSE REACTIONS: Allergic reaction, anorexia, constipation, nausea, weakness. Large amounts emetic and cathartic. Long-term use may cause liver impairment and muscle paralysis.

Borage *Borago officinalis*

USES: Atopic eczema (H-oil-equivocal), HTN (A-oil), Rheumatoid arthritis (H-oil).
PART USED: Herb.
CONTRAINDICATIONS: Safety in pregnancy and lactation not established. Bleeding disorder, liver disease.
SAFETY: Leaf and flowers contains pyrrolizidine alkaloids (2-20ppm), which are carcinogenic. Seed oil contains little or no hepatotoxic pyrrolizidine alkaloids.[66] AHPA Class: 2a, 2b, 2c, 2d—not for long-term use.[66]

Borage (cont'd.)

ADVERSE REACTIONS: Bleeding.

INTERACTIONS:

Anticoagulants and drugs that increase the risk of bleeding[212] (see Appendix 8) **and Surgery** High gamma-linolenic acid content of seed oil may inhibit platelet aggregation, which may increase the risk of bleeding.

Hepatotoxic drugs (see Appendix 21) Flower and above ground parts of herb contain pyrrolizidine alkaloids, which may have an additive hepatotoxic effect when combined with drugs that are hepatotoxic.

Tamoxifen (Nolvadex)[223] Concurrent use of gamma linolenic acid (contained in borage seed oil) and tamoxifen caused a faster clinical response in ER+ breast cancer patients than tamoxifen alone.

Brahmi *Bacopa monnieri*

INTERACTIONS:

Pentobarbitone[170] In research using rats and mice, herb prolongs hypnotic effect and may antagonize the haloperidol-induced catalepsy, suggesting an involvement of the GABA-ergic system.

Phenothiazines[189] (see Appendix 28) Herb potentiates drug.

Bromelain *Ananas comosus* part of Phlogenzym®

USES: Breast engorgement (H-bromelain/trypsin complex), post-operative or post-traumatic swelling (H-equivocal), sinusitis (H).

PART USED: Enzyme complex of pineapple plant stem.

Bromelain (cont'd.)

CONTRAINDICATIONS: Bleeding disorders, pineapple allergy. Safety in pregnancy and lactation not established.

ADVERSE REACTIONS: Allergic response, diarrhea, GI disturbance.

Antibiotics[98,177] (see Appendix 7) Increased blood and urine antibiotic levels.

Anticoagulants and drugs that increase the risk of bleeding[98,177] (see Appendix 8) Bromelain decreases thrombus formation, which increases the risk of bleeding. Monitor patients closely.

Chemotherapy such as 5-fluorouracil and vincristine[176] (see Appendix 16) Improved drug efficacy.

Cyclosporine (Neoral)[176] Phlogenzym (bromelain, trypsin, rutin) in combination with cyclosporin inhibited inflammation and destructive arthritis in rats used as models of rheumatoid arthritis.

Tetracyclines[1] (see Appendix 7) Increased blood and urine antibiotic levels.

Buchu *Barosma spp., Agathosma spp.*

PART USED: Leaf.

CONTRAINDICATIONS: Safety in amounts exceeding those found in food has not been established in pregnancy and lactation.

SAFETY: GRAS (flavoring). Pulegone, a component, can be toxic to the liver. AHPA Class: 2b, 2d—not with kidney inflammation.[66]

ADVERSE REACTIONS: GI irritation, increased menstrual flow, kidney irritation, may induce labor.

USES: Constipation (H).

PART USED: Bark, fruit.

CONTRAINDICATIONS: Abdominal pain of unknown origin, age of under 12 years, appendicitis, Crohn's disease, ileus, intestinal inflammation, lactation, pregnancy, ulcerative colitis.

SAFETY: Bark must be aged 1-2 years prior to use. No excessive amounts, extended period of use or use with stimulant laxatives. Use no longer than 1-2 weeks without medical supervision. AHPA Class: 2b, 2c, 2d—not with intestinal obstruction, abdominal pain of unknown origin, inflammatory GI disease (appendicitis, colitis, Crohn's disease, IBS), not for longer than 8-10 days.[66]

ADVERSE REACTIONS: Cramps, altered intestinal motility. Long-term use may lead to cardiac irregularities, electrolyte imbalance, hematuria, hypokalemia, pseudomelanosis coli.

INTERACTIONS:

Herb may reduce intestinal absorption of other drugs.[4]

Corticosteroids[1,175] (see Appendix 18) Chronic use of herb with corticosteroids increases the risk of hypokalemia.

Digoxin/Cardiac glycosides[175] Chronic use of herb with cardiac glycosides increases risk of hypokalemia, which may increase risk of drug toxicity.

Diuretics[1] (see Appendix 11) Diuretics that deplete potassium may lead to hypokalemia when combined with buckthorn, which also depletes potassium.

Bugleweed *Lycopus virginicus*
  PART USED: Herb.
  CONTRAINDICATIONS: Goiter, hyperthyroidism, hypothyroidism, lactation, pregnancy.
  AHPA Class: 2b, 2c, 2d—not with goiter, hypothyroidism or thyroid medications.[66]
  ADVERSE REACTIONS: Large amounts for extended periods may cause thyroid enlargement .
  INTERACTIONS:
    Thyroid replacement therapy[182,183] Herb may interfere with drug. In research using animals, herb inhibited enzymic T_4-5'-deiodination to T_3.
    Thyroidal radioactive isotopes[182,183] Herb interferes with tests using radioactive isotopes. In research using animals, herb inhibited enzymic T_4-5'-deiodination to T_3.

Burdock *Arctium lappa, Arctium spp.*
  PART USED: Root.
  CONTRAINDICATIONS: Safety in pregnancy and lactation not established.
  SAFETY: Contains tannins; avoid high dose for extended period. AHPA Class: 1.[66]
  ADVERSE REACTIONS: Contact dermatitis.
  INTERACTIONS:
    Acetaminophen/Paracetamol[184] In mice, herb decreased hepatotoxicity of acetaminophen.
    Insulin/Oral hypoglycemic agents[105] (see Appendix 24) Possible hypoglycemia or loss of blood glucose control.

Butcher's Broom *Ruscus aculeatus*

USES: Chronic venous insufficiency (H), hemorrhoids, orthostatic hypotension (H).

PART USED: Rhizome, root.

CONTRAINDICATIONS: Safety in pregnancy and lactation not established.

SAFETY: AHPA Class: 1.[66]

ADVERSE REACTIONS: GI disturbance, nausea.

INTERACTIONS:

Alpha-adrenergic agonists[185] (see Appendix 36) Herb has alpha-adrenergic agonist activity, which theoretically could be additive when used concurrently with drugs having similar activity.

Calendula *Calendula officinalis*

USES: Wound healing (A).

PART USED: Flower.

CONTRAINDICATIONS: Pregnancy. Safety in lactation not established.

SAFETY: GRAS (spice, flavoring, seasoning). AHPA Class: 1.[66]

ADVERSE REACTIONS: Allergic reaction, contact dermatitis, delayed gastric emptying, sedation.

INTERACTIONS:

Acyclovir (Zovirax)[186] In patients with herpetic keratitis treated with acyclovir, concurrent use of herbs (*Calendula officinalis, Arctium lappa* and *Geranium robertianum*) resulted in faster healing.

CNS depressants[187] (see Appendix 15) High doses of herb may have a sedative effect. Theoretical increase in sedation with sedating drugs.

Calendula (cont'd.)

Insulin/Oral hypoglycemic agents[188] (see Appendix 24) In research using animals, a hypoglycemic effect was found for herb. Monitor patients with diabetes.

California Poppy *Eschscholzia californica*

PART USED: Whole plant when flowering.

CONTRAINDICATIONS: Safety in pregnancy and lactation not established.

SAFETY: AHPA Class: 2b, 2d—may potentiate MAOIs.[66]

ADVERSE REACTIONS: Sedation.

INTERACTIONS:

Analgesics[190,191] Herb induces peripheral analgesia, which theoretically may be additive with analgesics.

Anxiolytics[190,191] (see Appendix 13) Herb has anxiolytic effect, which theoretically may be additive with drug.

Barbiturates[190,191] (see Appendix 12) Herb may increase the hypnotic effect of barbiturates due to its sedating effect.

Benzodiazepines[190] (see Appendix 13) Herb binds to benzodiazepine receptor, which may alter the effect of concurrent benzodiazepine administration.

CNS depressants[191] (see Appendix 15) Herb has sedative action, which may be additive with drugs which also cause sedation.

MAOIs, and possibly other antidepressants[197] (see Appendix 9) Herb may inhibit enzymatic breakdown of catecholamines, which may potentiate drug.

Pentobarbital (Nembutal)[191] Herb may increase hypnotic effect.

INTERACTIONS:

Herb may reduce intestinal absorption of other drugs.[4] Contains a high amount of pectic substances.

Cascara Sagrada *Rhamnus purshiana*

USES: Constipation.

PART USED: Bark.

CONTRAINDICATIONS: Age less than 12 years, pregnancy, lactation, abdominal pain of unknown origin, appendicitis, Crohn's disease, intestinal obstruction or inflammation, ulcerative colitis.

SAFETY: Bark must be aged 1-2 years before use. Use no longer than 1-2 weeks without medical supervision. There has been a case report of cholestatic hepatitis, complicated by portal hypertension with ingestion of *Cascara sagrada*. GRAS (flavoring). AHPA Class: 2b, 2c, 2d.[66]

ADVERSE REACTIONS: Long-term use or excessive amounts may cause albuminuria, cardiac irregularities, cramps, electrolyte imbalance, hematuria, hypokalemia, pseudomelanosis coli, slowing of intestinal transit. Case report of cholestatic hepatitis complicated by portal hypertension.

INTERACTIONS:

Herb may reduce intestinal absorption of other drugs.[4]

Antiarrhythmics[175] (see Appendix 6) Excessive doses or long-term use of herb may increase the loss of potassium, which may potentiate drug.

Corticosteroids[175] (see Appendix 18) Excessive doses or long-term use of herb

Cascara Sagrada (cont'd.)

may increase the loss of potassium, which may lead to hypokalemia when used with drug.

Digoxin/Cardiac glycosides[175] Chronic use increases risk of hypokalemia, which may increase risk of drug toxicity.

Diuretics[175] (see Appendix 11) Excessive doses or long-term use of herb may increase the loss of potassium, which may be additive and increase risk of hypokalemia.

Cashew Leaf *Anacardium occidentale*
INTERACTIONS:
Insulin/Oral hypoglycemic agents[105,199] (see Appendix 24) In research using rats with chemically induced diabetes, blood glucose levels were decreased with use of herb. Concurrent use with insulin and/or OHA may increase the risk of hypoglycemia.

Castor *Ricinus communis*
USES: Constipation.
PART USED: Seed oil.
CONTRAINDICATIONS: Safety when lactating not established. Use under medical supervision in pregnancy. Abdominal pain of unknown origin, appendicitis, children, Crohn's disease, intestinal obstruction or inflammation, ulcerative colitis.
SAFETY: Seed contains toxin, ricinine, which is not present in oil. GRAS (oil-flavoring). Cathartic colon with extended use. AHPA Class: 2b, 2d—not with GI

Castor (cont'd.)

obstruction or abdominal pain of unknown origin, not for longer than 8-10 days.[66]

ADVERSE REACTIONS: Cramping, GI discomfort, nausea. Ricinine may cause convulsions, gastroenteritis, hepatic damage, renal damage and death. Use of leaf may cause burning mouth and throat, vision changes, renal failure, uremia, death.

INTERACTIONS:

Digoxin/Cardiac glycosides[200] Excessive doses or long-term use of herb may increase the loss of potassium, which may be additive with drug and increase the risk of hypokalemia and drug toxicity.

Castor-Aralia Tree (stem bark) *Kalopanax pictus*

INTERACTIONS:

Insulin/Oral hypoglycemic agents[283] (see Appendix 24) In research using rats, stem bark decreased serum glucose. Kalopanaxsaponin A, a component of castor-aralia, decreased blood glucose the greatest (95%). Therapeutic use of castor-aralia should only be made under the supervision of a health care provider. The effect when combined with diabetes medications is unknown and may require an alteration of drug dosage.

Catnip Leaf *Nepeta cataria*

PART USED: Herb.

SAFETY: AHPA Class: 2b.[66]

INTERACTIONS:

Alcohol[201] Increased sedation.

Catnip Leaf (cont'd.)

CNS depressants[201] (see Appendix 15) Increased sedation.

Hexobarbital[201] Catnip oil increased hexobarbital sleep time.

Cat's Claw *Uncaria tomentosa*

USES: Osteoarthritis (H).

PART USED: Root.

CONTRAINDICATIONS: Age under 3 years, pregnancy, transplant recipients.

SAFETY: Contains tannins and alkaloids. Use no longer than 4 weeks. AHPA Class: 4.[66]

ADVERSE REACTIONS: Case report of acute renal failure in lupus patient.

INTERACTIONS:

Drugs which are substrates of P450 CYP3A4[227] (see Appendix 38) Preliminary in vitro research has shown that cat's claw may alter metabolism and/or effectiveness of drugs which are substrates of CYP3A4 isozymes. Further research is needed to determine if interaction will also occur in humans.

Antihypertensives[206,208] (see Appendix 11) Herb may decrease blood pressure. Concurrent use may theoretically lead to hypotension.

Chemotherapy/Immunosuppressants[203,204] (see Appendix 16 and 23) Herb has immunostimulant activity. In one study using breast cancer cells, herb had an antiproliferative effect. It is not known if herb will interfere with chemotherapeutic effectiveness.

Doxorubicin (Adriamycin, Doxil, Rubex)[204] In research using rats, C-Med-100 (water extract of herb) treatment improved white blood cell parameters.

Cat's Claw (cont'd.)

Indomethacin (Indocin)[202] Herb was protective against indomethacin-induced GI damage.

Pneumococcal vaccine[213] Enhancement of immune function in patients receiving 300 mg bid C-Med-100 (water extract of herb), which improved effectiveness of vaccine

Cayenne *Capsicum annuum, Capsicum frutescens*

USES: Fibromyalgia (topical), neuralgia (topical), osteoarthritis (topical), rheumatoid arthritis (topical).

PART USED: Fruit.

SAFETY: GRAS (extract, oleoresin, spice, seasoning). AHPA Class: 1 (internal).[66]

ADVERSE REACTIONS: GI distress. Topical: contact dermatitis or irritation.

INTERACTIONS:

Herb may inhibit P450 CYP1A1/2, CYP2A2, CYP2C11, CYP2B1, CYP2B2, CYP2C6[351,358,359,360] (see Appendix 38) In in vitro research, herb inhibited drug metabolizing isozymes, which may increase serum level of drugs that are substrates of these isozymes.

ACE inhibitors[352] (see Appendix 11) Concurrent use of drug and topical capsaicin cream may cause coughing.

Alcohol[215] Capsaicin, a component of cayenne, reduced the oxidative damage caused by ethanol.

Antihypertensives[50,357] (see Appendix 11) Cayenne increases catecholamine secretion, which may decrease the effect of antihypertensives.

Cayenne (cont'd.)

Anticoagulants and drugs that increase the risk of bleeding[353] (see Appendix 8) Capsaicin may inhibit platelet aggregation, which may increase bleeding risk.

Aspirin[355,356] Capsaicin, a component of cayenne pepper, reduced gastric injury caused by ASA. In laboratory animals, bioavailability of salicylic acid, a component of aspirin, was reduced.

Barbiturates[354] (see Appendix 12) Cayenne may increase effect of drug.

CNS depressants[354] (see Appendix 15) Cayenne may increase effect of drug.

Ethylmorphine[358,359] Capsaicin inhibited metabolism of ethylmorphine.

Hexobarbital[354] Capsaicin, a component of cayenne pepper, increased hexobarbital sleep time.

Insulin/Oral hypoglycemic agents[214] (see Appendix 24) In dogs, capsaicin had a hypoglycemic effect. Insulin release was increased. Monitor blood glucose of patients with type 2 diabetes.

MAOIs[50,357] (see Appendix 9) Cayenne increases catecholamine secretion, which may increase the risk of adverse effects of drug.

NSAIDs[355] (see Appendix 28) Capsaicin, a component of cayenne pepper, has been shown to decrease gastric injury from aspirin. Based on that observation, the herb may provide a protective effect against NSAID-induced gastric injury if taken prior to NSAIDs administration. However, herb may increase the risk of bleeding.

Pentobarbital[358,359] Capsaicin prolonged pentobarbital sleep time due to altering of hepatic drug metabolizing enzymes.

Theophylline (Uniphyl, Uni-Dur)[16] Herb may increase absorption of drug.

Apium graveolens **Celery**

PART USED: Fruit/seed.

CONTRAINDICATIONS: Bleeding disorders, kidney disease, pregnancy.

SAFETY: Contains psoralens, which are photosensitizing. GRAS (spice, seasoning, flavoring, oil, extract, oleoresin). AHPA Class: 2b, 2d—caution with renal disorders.[66]

ADVERSE REACTIONS: Allergic reactions, anaphylactic shock, increased risk of photoxicity.

INTERACTIONS:

Acetaminophen/Paracetamol[219] Methanolic extract of seeds decreased the hepatotoxicity of drug.

Anticoagulants and drugs that increase the risk of bleeding[221] (see Appendix 8) Apigenin, a component of celery, inhibits platelet aggregation, which increases the risk of bleeding. Concurrent use of herb with drug may further increase the risk of bleeding

Photosensitivity, drugs causing[217] (see Appendix 29) Herb contains psoralens, which may increase photosensitivity. Theoretical increased photosensitivity when used concurrently with drugs that also enhance photosensitivity.

PUVA therapy, drugs used with[218] Response to PUVA therapy may be increased by herb and may increase risk of photoxicity.

Thioacetamine[219] Methanolic extract of seeds decreased hepatotoxicity of drug.

Thyroxine (Levothroid, Levoxyl, Synthroid)[275] 2 Case reports - 1. 55 and 49 year old females on thyroxine had decreased T_4 after consuming celery seed tablets. The Queensland Medication Helpline in Australia has had 10 reports of interaction between thyroxine and celery seed.

Cereus *Selenicereus grandiflorus*
  PART USED: Flower, stem.
  CONTRAINDICATIONS: Cardiac disease, HTN. Safety in pregnancy and lactation not established.
  SAFETY: Contains cactine, which has effect similar to cardiac glycosides.
  ADVERSE REACTIONS: Burning of mouth, diarrhea, GI distress, vomiting. AHPA Class: 1.[66]
  INTERACTIONS:
    Cardiac drugs[138] (see Appendix 14) Herb may increase effect of drug.
    Digoxin/Cardiac glycosides[160] Herb contains cactine, which has a digitalic effect, possibly additive with cardiac glycosides.
    MAOIs[138,250] (see Appendix 9) Theoretical interaction. Hordenine, a component of herb, may inhibit uptake of norepinephrine and liberate norepinephrine from endogenous stores.

Chamomile *Matricaria recutita, Chamomilla recutita*
  USES: Antiinflammatory for stomach and duodenum (H), atopic eczema (H-Kamillosan cream), gastric ulcers (A), irritation of mucous membranes following radiation or systemic chemotherapy for cancer (H- Kamillosan oral rinse-equivocal-No benefit was found in a prospective clinical trial using 5-FU published in 1996[238]), wound healing (H).
  PART USED: Flower.
  CONTRAINDICATIONS: Safety in pregnancy and lactation not established. Bleeding disorders. Allergy to *Asteraceae/Compositae* family.

Chamomile (cont'd.)

SAFETY: GRAS (spice, seasoning, flavoring). AHPA Class: 1.[66]

ADVERSE REACTIONS: Allergic reaction, anaphylaxis, contact dermatitis, emetic (strong hot tea), sedation.

INTERACTIONS:

Drugs metabolized by P450 CYP1A2[313] (see Appendix 38) In liver microsomes or cytosol from rats given chamomile tea, CYP1A2 activity was 15% that in control animals. It is not known if inhibition also occurs in humans. Monitor patients taking chamomile and drugs that are substrates of CYP1A, as serum levels may increase due to inhibition of metabolism.

Drugs which are substrates of P450 CYP3A4 isozymes[227] (see Appendix 38) Preliminary in vitro research has shown that chamomile may alter metabolism and/or effectiveness of that which are substrates of CYP3A4 isozymes. Further research is needed to determine if interaction will also occur in humans.

Anticoagulants and drugs that increase the risk of bleeding[361] (see Appendix 8) Herniarin, a component of German chamomile, may inhibit platelet aggregation, which may increase the risk of bleeding. Theoretically, risk of bleeding may be increased with concurrent use.

Aspirin[323] (-)-Alpha-bisabolol (from chamomile oil) has protective effect against aspirin-induced gastric ulcers.

Benzodiazepines[326] (see Appendix 13) Apigenin, a component of chamomile, binds to benzodiazepine receptors, which may alter effect of drug. Chamomile has an effect similar to benzodiazepines.

CNS depressants[317] (see Appendix 15) Herb has sedative activity, which may be

Chamomile (cont'd.)

additive with sedating drugs.

Iron[269] Chamomile tea decreased absorption of non-heme iron by 47% due to polyphenol content (77 human subjects).

Local radiation and systemic chemotherapy[239] (see Appendix 16) Kamillosan Liquidum (made from flower) increases resolution of mucositis due to radiation of head and neck or to systemic chemotherapy. No control group in this small study published in 1991.

Chan Su From dried skin of Chinese toads

SAFETY: Contains cardioactive substances.

INTERACTIONS:

Digoxin/Cardiac glycosides[235] Moderate amount of bufalin (the cardioactive substance in this Asian medicine) may displace digitoxin from protein-binding site, which may lead to high free serum digitoxin levels.

Chaparral *Larrea tridentata*

PART USED: Leaf.

SAFETY: On FDA's list of herbs associated with illness or injury (liver disease).[178] Several reports of kidney and liver toxicity. May be unsafe for oral use due to pyrrolizidine alkaloid content. Avoid use. AHPA Class: 2d—do not use large amounts with kidney disease and liver conditions—cirrhosis and hepatitis.[66]

ADVERSE REACTIONS: Contact dermatitis, liver dysfunction and liver failure.

Chaparral (cont'd.)

INTERACTIONS:

MAOIs[117] (see Appendix 9) Amino acids, such as phenylalanine, tryptophan and tyrosine, in herb may interfere with drug and increase risk of hypertensive crisis.

Hepatotoxic drugs[262] (see Appendix 21) Herb has exhibited hepatotoxicity. Combining with hepatotoxic drugs may increase the risk of liver damage.

Chard *Beta vulgaris*

INTERACTIONS:

Oral hypoglycemic agents[236] (see Appendix 24) In research using rats, chard increased regeneration of B cells in pancreas. Concurrent use should be supervised by health care personnel. Maximum reduction of blood glucose was after 42 days of administration.

Chaste Tree *Vitex agnus castus*

USES: Acne (H), amenorrhea (H), cyclical mastalgia (H), inadequate flow of breast milk (H), luteal phase insufficiency due to hyperprolactinemia (H), PMS (H-equivocal).

PART USED: Fruit/berry, root bark.

CONTRAINDICATIONS: Safety in pregnancy, lactation and children not established. Hormone-sensitive cancers, in vitro fertilization.

AHPA Class: 2b, 2d—may counteract birth control pills.[66]

ADVERSE REACTIONS: Allergic reaction, diarrhea, GI distress, headache, hypermenorrhea.

INTERACTIONS:

Chaste Tree (cont'd.)

Bromocriptine (Parlodel) and drugs or hormones that affect the pituitary.[363] Herb inhibited prolactin secretion in rats. Theoretical additive effect with drug.

Dopamine-receptor antagonists[364] (see Appendix 19) In research using animals, it was noted that herb had dopaminergic activity, which may interfere with the drugs that bind to dopamine receptors. Theoretical interaction between herb and dopamine-receptor antagonists in humans.

Oral contraceptives/Hormone replacement therapy[365] Herb binded to estrogen receptor in in vitro research. Effect on drugs containing estrogen is not known.

Chicory *Chichorium intybus*

SAFETY: GRAS (oil, extract, oleoresin). AHPA Class: 1.

INTERACTIONS:

Insulin/Oral hypoglycemic agents[302] (see Appendix 24) Water-soluble extract of chicory reduced the uptake of glucose in the perfused jejunum of rats by 21%. Use of herb with insulin should only be made under the supervision of a knowledgeable health care professional.

Chinese Cinnamon *Cinnamomum aromaticum, Cinnamomum cassia*

PART USED: Bark.

CONTRAINDICATIONS: Safety of therapeutic amounts (especially oil) in pregnancy and lactation not established.

SAFETY: GRAS (spice, seasoning, flavoring). AHPA Class: 2b.[66]

ADVERSE REACTIONS: Allergic reaction.

Chinese Cinnamon (cont'd.)

INTERACTIONS:

May alter drug-metabolizing enzymes[367] (see Appendix 38)

Alcohol[366] Herb inhibited ulcers induced by ethanol.

Indomethacin[366] Herb failed to prevent ulcers induced by drug.

Metacycline[91,104] Decreased absorption of drug due to decreased dissolution of gelatin capsule.

Phenylbutazone[366] Herb inhibited ulcers induced by drug.

Tetracycline[66,91,104] (see Appendix 7) Decreased absorption of drug due to decreased dissolution of gelatin capsule in vitro. Clinical significance not established.

Chitosan (derived from crustacean shell)

USES: Chronic renal failure on dialysis (H), hypercholesterolemia (H), periodontitis (H), plastic surgery donor sites (H), weight loss (H-equivocal).

CONTRAINDICATIONS: Safety in pregnancy and lactation not established. Shellfish allergy.

INTERACTIONS:

Lipid-lowering drugs[368] (see Appendix 25) Concurrent use may have an additive effect.

Chondroitin Sulfate (derived from shark and bovine cartilage—often combined with glucosamine)

USES: Osteoarthritis (H).

Chondroitin Sulfate (cont'd.)

CONTRAINDICATIONS: Bleeding disorders, pregnancy, lactation.

ADVERSE REACTIONS: GI distress. Theoretical increased risk of bleeding when combined with anticoagulants has not been confirmed in clinical studies.

INTERACTIONS:

NSAIDs[369,370] (see Appendix 8) Concurrent use may increase treatment efficacy for osteoarthritis.

Sodium hyaluronate (Wydase)[371] With use of sodium hyaluronate there was a decreased intraocular pressure following phacoemulsification cataract extraction with intraocular lens implantation.

Cinchona Bark *Cinchona spp.*

USES: Malaria (H).

PART USED: Bark.

CONTRAINDICATIONS: Bleeding disorders, gastric ulcers.

SAFETY: Not excessive amounts. Contains quinine. GRAS (flavoring--83 mcg alkaloid). AHPA Class: 2b, 2d.[66]

ADVERSE REACTIONS: Abdominal pain, blindness, convulsions, death, delirium, diarrhea, GI distress, headache, loss of hearing, paralysis, tinnitus, vision disturbance.

INTERACTIONS:

Anticoagulants and drugs that increase the risk of bleeding[373] (see Appendix 8) Cinchonine, a component of cinchona, has an antiplatelet effect. The effect on platelets is via inhibition of $Ca2+$ influx and protein kinase c pathways. Theoretical increased risk of bleeding with concurrent use of anticoagulants.

Cinchona Bark (cont'd.)

Digoxin (Lanoxin)[375] Herb may decrease clearance of drug.

Mefloquine (Lariam)[372] Concurrent use may cause cardiac abnormalities.

Neuromuscular blocking agents[374] Effect may be additive.

Cinnamon *Cinnamomum verum*
PART USED: Bark.
CONTRAINDICATIONS: Pregnancy, lactation.
SAFETY: GRAS (spice, seasoning, flavoring, oil, extract, oleoresin).
Contains safrole. AHPA Class: 2b, 2d—no long term or excessive dose.[66]
ADVERSE REACTIONS: Burning sensation when oil used topically or orally. Large doses have caused methemoglobinemia, hematinemia with nephritis and stimulation of the vasomotor center. Dermatitis, oral irritation, stomatitis.

Climbing Groundsel *Senecio scandens*
INTERACTIONS:
HIV therapies[338] In research using rats, herb inhibited erythrocyte hemolysis, decreased lipid peroxidation in brain and kidney, decreased generation of superoxide peroxidation and decreased hydroxyl radicals. This research suggests that antioxidant activity of herb may delay progress of HIV to AIDS

Cloves *Syzygium aromaticum*
PART USED: Bud.
CONTRAINDICATIONS: Bleeding disorders, GERD (essential oil).

Cloves (cont'd.)
SAFETY: Case reports of acute liver toxicity, intravascular coagulation, acidosis, CNS depression and coma. GRAS (oil, seasoning, spice). AHPA Class: 1.[66]
ADVERSE REACTIONS: Dermatitis (oil). Smoking cloves may cause blood in sputum. Hemoptysis and irritation of mucous membranes.
INTERACTIONS:
  Anticoagulants and drugs that increase the risk of bleeding[376] (see Appendix 8) Eugenol and acetyl eugenol in clove oil inhibit platelet aggregation, which may be additive with anticoagulants.

Coccinia *Coccinia grandis*
INTERACTIONS:
  Insulin/Oral hypoglycemic agents[105,377] (see Appendix 24) Pectin from fruit, as well as extract from leaf and roots, of coccinia has a hypoglycemic in laboratory animals. Monitor patients with diabetes.

Cocoa *Theobroma cacao*
PART USED: Fruit.
CONTRAINDICATIONS: Bleeding disorders, GERD, ulcers.
SAFETY: GRAS (oil, extract, oleoresin).
ADVERSE REACTIONS: Allergic reaction, headache.
INTERACTIONS:
  Acetaminophen/Paracetamol[636] Caffeine, a component of cocoa, may increase pain relief.

Cocoa (cont'd.)

Anticoagulants and drugs that increase the risk of bleeding[378] (see Appendix 8) Very high consumption of cocoa may have an effect on hemostasis similar to aspirin. This may be due in part to the flavonoid content of cocoa, which varies considerably depending on processing.

Aspirin[638] Caffeine in cocoa may increase effectiveness of ASA pain relief.

Benzodiazepines[637] (see Appendix 13) Theoretical decrease in sedative and antianxiolytic effects.

Beta-adrenergic agonists[101] (see Appendix 36) Concurrent use may increase the risk of cardiac arrhythmias.

Cimetidine (Tagamet)[658] Drug may decrease clearance of caffeine, a component of cocoa. Theoretically, this may increase serum caffeine, which may result in increased caffeine side effects. Results of research have been equivocal.

Clozapine, and possibly other drugs metabolized by P450 CYP1A2[296,350] (see Appendix 38) Caffeine intakes greater than 400 mg may decrease clearance of clozapine (and possibly induce other drugs metabolized by CYP1A2). In randomized crossover research of 12 males, the AUC of clozapine was increased by 19% and oral clearance of clozapine was decreased 14% with concurrent caffeine intake. Cocoa seeds contain 12,900 ppm of caffeine.

Disulfiram (Antabuse)[654] Drug may decrease metabolism of caffeine, a component of cocoa. Concurrent use may increase serum caffeine and caffeine side effects.

Ephedra/Ephedrine[434] Concurrent use of products containing high amounts of caffeine, a component of cocoa, and stimulants (such as ephedra and ephedrine)

Cocoa (cont'd.)

may have an additive stimulant effect.

Ergotamine (Ergomar)[653] Caffeine, a component of cocoa, may increase serum levels of drug. Caffeine is often added to migraine medications because it enhances vasoconstrictive effect of drugs used for pain relief.

Fluvoxamine (Luvox)[658] Drug decreases metabolism of caffeine, a component of cocoa. This may increase serum caffeine and increase caffeine side effects.

Furafylline[658] Drug inhibits CYP1A2, which decreases the metabolism of caffeine, a component of cocoa. This may increase serum levels of caffeine and increase caffeine side effects.

Grapefruit juice[531] Grapefruit juice inhibits CYP1A2, which decreases the metabolism of caffeine, a component of cocoa, thereby increasing caffeine side effects.

Ibuprofen[650] Concurrent use of both cocoa and drug may enhance pain relief.

Idrocilamide[658] Drug alters caffeine metabolism, which may increase serum levels of caffeine and increase caffeine side effects.

Insulin/Oral hypoglycemic agents[84,651] (see Appendix 24) Caffeine, a component of cocoa, may increase insulin resistance. Monitor patients with diabetes.

Iron[269] Cocoa beverage decreased absorption of non-heme iron by 71% due to polyphenol content in 77 human subjects.

Lithium (Eskalith, Lithobid, Lithonate, Lithotabs)[658] Caffeine, a component of cocoa, increases the renal excretion of lithium, which may decrease serum levels of drug. Discontinuation of cocoa use may likewise increase serum levels of drug.

MAOIs[103] (see Appendix 9) Excessive amounts of cocoa may increase risk of

Cocoa (cont'd.)

hypertension and hypertensive crisis. Cocoa contains tyramine.

Methotrexate (Rheumatrex)[224] Caffeine in cocoa may decrease effectiveness of drug.

Methoxsalen (8-MOP, Oxsoralen)[658] Drug inhibits metabolism of caffeine, a component of cocoa. Increased serum caffeine may increase caffeine side effects.

Mexiletine (Mexitil)[656] Drug delays metabolism of caffeine, a component of cocoa. This may increase side effects of caffeine.

Oral contraceptives[658] Long-term use of oral contraceptives (ethinyl estradiol or estradiol) causes an impaired CYP1A2 clearance of caffeine, a component of cocoa. This may increase serum caffeine and increase caffeine side effects.

Phenylpropanolamine[658] Drug may inhibit the metabolism of caffeine, a component of cocoa, increasing serum levels of caffeine and side effects. On 11/6/00, the FDA released an advisory to remove phenylpropanolamine from all products.[657]

Quinolones (ciprofloxacin, enoxacin, grepafloxacin, norfloxacin, pefloxacin, tosufloxacin)[658] Drugs may decrease clearance of caffeine, a component of cocoa. This may increase the side effects of caffeine, due to increased serum caffeine.

Terbinafine (Lamisil)[658] Drug may inhibit the metabolism of caffeine, a component of cocoa. This may increase serum levels of caffeine and increase caffeine side effects. Research on this interaction has been equivocal.

Theophylline (Uniphyl, Uni-Dur)[658] Concurrent use of theophylline and caffeine, a component of cocoa, may lead to an increase in serum levels of both.

Cocoa (cont'd.)

Verapamil (Calan, Isoptin, Verelan)[658] Drug delays clearance of caffeine, a component of cocòa. This may increase caffeine side effects.

Coenzyme Q10

USES: Cardiomyopathy (H), coronary artery bypass graft (H), CHF (H-equivocal), HTN (H), mitral valve prolapse (H-pediatric), myocardial infarction (H), periodontitis (H), various cardiovascular diseases (H).

CONTRAINDICATIONS: Safety in pregnancy, lactation and children not established.

SAFETY: With severe heart disease consult medical advisor.

ADVERSE REACTIONS: GI distress. Large doses may cause an increase in serum LDH and SGOT levels.

INTERACTIONS:

Anthracyclines[381,390,391,392] (see Antibiotics in Appendix 16) Coenzyme Q10 is protective against cardiotoxicity of drug. It is not known if this action may also decrease drug's effectiveness against cancer cells. This may be true for all chemotherapeutic agents which act by increasing oxidative stress. Since coenzyme Q10 has antioxidant properties, it is theoretically possible that coenzyme Q10 may decrease effectiveness of chemotherapeutic agents.

Anticoagulants and drugs that increase the risk of bleeding[379,387,388,923] (see Appendix 8) Concurrent use may reduce the effectiveness of drug. Coenzyme Q10 may increase excretion or metabolism of warfarin.

Antihypertensives[382,383] (see Appendix 11) Coenzyme Q10 may lower blood pressure. A reduction in antihypertensive medicine may be needed.

Coenzyme Q10 (cont'd.)

Beta blockers[389] (see Appendix 11) (Propranolol and Metoprolol, but not Timolol) Drug therapy may decrease coenzyme Q10 enzymes in myocardium. Further research is needed to determine if supplementation would be helpful to patients taking beta blockers.

Hepatitis B vaccination[380] Supplement increased antibody response to vaccine.

HMG-CoA reductase inhibitors[334,384,385,386] (See Appendix 25) Statin drugs may inhibit the synthesis of mevalonate, which is a precursor of ubiquinone/coenzyme Q10. Some research has shown statin drugs lower coenzyme Q10. One recent study found no decrease in coenzyme Q10, but duration was only 4 weeks. Further research is needed.

Oral hypoglycemic agents[382,389] Some diabetes medications, including acetohexamide, glyburide, phenformin and tolazamide, may inhibit NADH-oxidase, which may decrease coenzyme Q10 levels. Most research has found no alteration in blood glucose when supplemented with coenzyme Q10.

Coffee *Coffea arabica*

USES: Stimulant.

PART USED: Roasted seed kernel.

CONTRAINDICATIONS: Gastric ulcer, glaucoma, children. Limit intake in pregnancy and lactation.

SAFETY: GRAS (oil, extract, oleoresin). Coffee contains 40-140 mg caffeine per cup.[172] AHPA Class: 2b, 2d—not long-term use of excessive amounts.[66]

ADVERSE REACTIONS: Anxiety, arrhythmias, GI distress, HTN, increased intraocular

pressure, nervousness, nausea.
INTERACTIONS:

Herb may reduce intestinal absorption of other drugs due to tannin content.[4]

Alendronate (Fosamax)[918] Coffee decreases bioavailability of drug by about 60%.

Alkaloids (see Appendix 4)[4] High tannin content of seed may cause alkaloids to become insoluble and precipitate.

Acetaminophen/Paracetamol[393,636] Caffeine, a component of coffee, may increase pain relief.

Aspirin[638] Caffeine in coffee increases effectiveness of ASA pain relief.

Benzodiazepines[637] (see Appendix 13) Theoretical decrease in sedative and antianxiolytic effects.

Beta-adrenergic agonists[101] (see Appendix 36) Concurrent use may increase the risk of cardiac arrhythmias.

Cimetidine (Tagamet)[658] Drug may decrease clearance of caffeine, a component of coffee. Theoretically, this may increase serum caffeine and increase caffeine side effects. Results of research have been equivocal.

Clozapine, and possibly other drugs metabolized by P450 CYP1A2[296,350] (see Appendix 38) Caffeine intakes greater than 400 mg may decrease clearance of clozapine (and possibly induce other drugs metabolized by CYP1A2). In randomized crossover research of 12 males, the AUC of clozapine was increased by 19% and oral clearance of clozapine was decreased 14% with concurrent caffeine intake.

Disulfiram (Antabuse)[654] Drug may decrease metabolism of caffeine, a component of coffee. Concurrent use may increase serum caffeine and caffeine side effects.

Ephedra/Ephedrine[434] Concurrent use of high amounts of products containing caffeine and stimulants may have an additive stimulant effect. Ephedrine is a stimulant.

Ergotamine (Ergomar)[653] Caffeine, a component of coffee, increases serum level and efficacy of drug. The drug Wigraine contains both.

Fluvoxamine (Luvox)[658] Drug decreases metabolism of caffeine, a component of coffee. This may increase serum caffeine and increase caffeine side effects.

Furafylline[658] Drug inhibits CYP1A2, which decreases the metabolism of caffeine, a component of coffee. This may increase serum levels of caffeine and increase caffeine side effects.

Grapefruit Juice[531] Grapefruit juice inhibits CYP1A2, which decreases the metabolism of caffeine, a component of coffee, thereby increasing caffeine side effects.

Ibuprofen[650] Concurrent use of both coffee and drug may enhance pain relief.

Idrocilamide[658] Drug alters caffeine metabolism, which increases serum levels of caffeine and increases caffeine side effects.

Insulin/Oral hypoglycemic agents[84, 651] (see Appendix 24) Caffeine, a component of coffee, may increase insulin resistance. Monitor patients with diabetes.

Lithium (Eskalith, Lithobid, Lithonate, Lithotabs)[658] Caffeine, a component of coffee, increases the renal excretion of lithium, which may decrease serum levels of

Coffee (cont'd.)

drug. Discontinuation of herb use may likewise increase serum levels of drug.

MAOIs[109] (see Appendix 9) Excessive amounts of coffee may increase risk of hypertension.

Methotrexate (Rheumatrex)[224] Caffeine in coffee may decrease effectiveness of drug.

Methoxsalen (8-MOP, Oxsoralen)[658] Drug inhibits metabolism of caffeine, a component of coffee. Increased serum caffeine may increase side effects.

Metoprolol (Lopressor, Toprol)[101] Blood pressure may be increased by caffeine in coffee.

Mexiletine (Mexitil)[656] Drug delays metabolism of caffeine, a component of coffee. This may increase side effects of caffeine.

Oral contraceptives[658] Long-term use of oral contraceptives (ethinyl estradiol or estradiol) causes an impaired CYP1A2 clearance of caffeine, a component of coffee. This may increase serum caffeine and increase caffeine side effects.

Phenylpropanolamine[658] Drug may inhibit the metabolism of caffeine, a component of coffee, increasing serum levels of caffeine and side effects. On 11/6/00, the FDA released an advisory to remove phenylpropanolamine from all products.[657]

Propranolol (Inderal)[394] Blood pressure may be increased by caffeine in coffee.

Pseudoephedrine[434] Coffee may increase side effects of drug.

Quinolones (ciprofloxacin, enoxacin, grepafloxacin, norfloxacin, pefloxacin, tosufloxacin)[658] Drug decreases clearance of caffeine, a component of coffee.

Coffee (cont'd.)

This may increase the side effects of caffeine due to increased serum caffeine.

Terbinafine (Lamisil)[658] Drug may inhibit the metabolism of caffeine, a component of coffee. This may increase serum levels of caffeine and increase caffeine side effects. Research on this interaction has been equivocal.

Theophylline (Uniphyl, Uni-Dur)[658] Concurrent use of theophylline and caffeine may lead to an increase in serum levels of both.

Verapamil (Calan, Isoptin, Verelan)[658] Drug delays clearance of caffeine, a component of coffee. This may increase caffeine side effects.

Cola *Cola nitida*

PART USED: Seed.

CONTRAINDICATIONS: HTN, ulcers. Avoid high intake in pregnancy and lactation.

SAFETY: GRAS (oil, extract, oleoresin). AHPA Class: 2b, 2d—no excessive or long-term use.[66]

ADVERSE REACTIONS: GI disturbance, restlessness, sleep disturbance.

INTERACTIONS:

Benzodiazepines[637] (see Appendix 13) Theoretical decrease in sedative and antianxiolytic effects.

Beta-adrenergic agonists[101] (see Appendix 36) Concurrent use may increase the risk of cardiac arrhythmias.

Caffeine-containing medications[1,175] Effects may be additive.

Cimetidine (Tagamet)[658] Drug may decrease clearance of caffeine, a component

Cola (cont'd.)

of cola. Theoretically this may increase serum caffeine, which may result in increased caffeine side effects. Results of research have been equivocal.

Clozapine, and possibly other drugs metabolized by P450 CYP1A2[296,350] (see Appendix 38) Caffeine intakes greater than 400 mg may decrease clearance of clozapine (and possibly induce other drugs metabolized by CYP1A2).

Disulfiram (Antabuse)[653] Drug may decrease metabolism of caffeine, a component of cola. The result may be increased serum caffeine and caffeine side effects.

Ephedra/Ephedrine[434] Concurrent use of high amounts of products containing caffeine and stimulants may have an additive stimulant effect.

Furafylline[658] Drug inhibits CYP1A2, which decreases the metabolism of caffeine, a component of cola. This may increase serum levels of caffeine and increase caffeine side effects.

Grapefruit juice[531] Grapefruit juice inhibits CYP1A2, which decreases the metabolism of caffeine, a component of cola, thereby increasing caffeine side effects.

Ibuprofen[650] Concurrent use of both cola and drug may enhance pain relief.

Idrocilamide[658] Drug alters caffeine metabolism, which increases serum levels of caffeine and increases caffeine side effects.

Insulin/Oral hypoglycemic agents[84, 651] (see Appendix 24) Caffeine, a component of cola, may increase insulin resistance. Monitor patients with diabetes.

Lithium (Eskalith, Lithobid, Lithonate, Lithotabs)[658] Caffeine, a component of cola, increases the renal excretion of lithium, which may decrease serum levels

Cola (cont'd.)

of drug. Discontinuation of herb use may then increase serum levels of drug.

MAOIs[109] (see Appendix 9) Excessive amounts of cola (caffeine) may increase risk of hypertension.

Methotrexate (Rheumatrex)[224] Caffeine in cola may decrease effectiveness of drug

Methoxsalen (8-MOP, Oxsoralen)[658] Drug inhibits metabolism of caffeine, a component of cola, which may increase serum caffeine and caffeine side effects.

Metoprolol (Lopressor, Toprol)[101] Blood pressure may be increased by caffeine in cola.

Mexiletine (Mexitil)[656] Drug delays metabolism of caffeine, a component of cola. This may increase side effects of caffeine.

Oral contraceptives[658] Long-term use of oral contraceptives (ethinyl estradiol or estradiol) causes an impaired CYP1A2 clearance of caffeine, a component of cola. This may increase serum caffeine and caffeine side effects.

Phenylpropanolamine[658] Drug may inhibit the metabolism of caffeine, a component of cola, increasing serum levels of caffeine and caffeine side effects. On 11/6/00, the FDA released an advisory to remove phenylpropanolamine from all products.[657]

Propranolol (Inderal)[394] Blood pressure may be increased by caffeine in cola.

Pseudoephedrine[434] Cola may increase side effects of drug.

Quinolones (ciprofloxacin, enoxacin, grepafloxacin, norfloxacin, pefloxacin, tosufloxacin)[658] Drugs may decrease clearance of caffeine, a component of cola.

Cola (cont'd.)

This may increase the side effects of caffeine due to increased serum caffeine.

Terbinafine (Lamisil)[658] Drug may inhibit the metabolism of caffeine, a component of cola. This may increase serum levels of caffeine and increase caffeine side effects. Research on this interaction has been equivocal.

Theophylline (Uniphyl, Uni-Dur)[658] Concurrent use of theophylline and caffeine may lead to an increase in serum levels of both.

Verapamil (Calan, Isoptin, Verelan)[658] Drug delays clearance of caffeine, a component of cola. This may increase caffeine side effects.

Coleus *Coleus forskohlii*
INTERACTIONS:

Anticoagulants and drugs that increase the risk of bleeding[395] (see Appendix 8) Forskolin, a component of coleus, inhibits platelet aggregation, which increases risk of bleeding.

Insulin/Oral hypoglycemic agents[396] (see Appendix 24) Coleonol, a component of coleus, increases blood glucose. Patients with diabetes should be counseled about use of this herb.

Coltsfoot *Tussilago farfara*
PART USED: Flower, leaf.
SAFETY: Contains pyrrolizidine alkaloids, which are hepatotoxic and hepatocarcinogenic. AHPA Class: 2b, 2c, 2d—no long-term use or in more than recommended amounts.[66] Flower, external use only.

Coltsfoot (cont'd.)

ADVERSE REACTIONS: Allergic reaction, increased blood pressure, anorexia, hepatic veno-occlusive disease in newborn of mother who consumed coltsfoot.

INTERACTIONS:

Alkaloids[4] (see Appendix 4) High tannin content of herb may cause alkaloids to become insoluble and precipitate.

Antihypertensives[398] (see Appendix 11) Tussilagone, a component of coltsfoot, has a cardiostimulant effect, which theoretically may interfere with drug.

Cardiovascular drugs[398] (see Appendix 14) Excessive herb intake may interfere with drug.

Hepatotoxic drugs[397] (see Appendix 21) Herb can cause hepatotoxicity. Concurrent use with drugs that increase hepatotoxicity may result in increased risk of damage to liver.

Comfrey *Symphytum officinale*

PART USED: Leaf, rhizome, root.

SAFETY: On FDA's list of herbs associated with illness or injury (blood flow to liver may be obstructed).[178] Contains pyrrolizidine alkaloids, which are hepatotoxic and hepatocarcinogenic. Avoid oral use unless directed by health care professional. Contraindicated in pregnancy and lactation. AHPA Class: 2a, 2b, 2c.

ADVERSE REACTIONS: Veno-occlusive disease.

INTERACTIONS:

Alkaloids[4] (see Appendix 4) High tannin content of herb may cause alkaloids to become insoluble and precipitate.

Comfrey (cont'd.)

  Hepatotoxic drugs[399] (see Appendix 21) Pyrrolizidine alkaloid content of herb, when used orally, may increase the risk of hepatotoxicity. When combined with drugs that also damage the liver, the effect, theoretically may be additive.

Compound Q *Trichosanthes kirilowii*, tian hua fen (root), gua lou (fruit), gua lou ren (seed)

  PART USED: Fruit, root, seed.

  CONTRAINDICATIONS: Safety in pregnancy and lactation not established. AHPA Class: Fruit: 1; root: 2b; seed: 1.[66]

  ADVERSE REACTIONS: Diarrhea, GI discomfort.

  INTERACTIONS:

  Insulin/Oral hypoglycemic agents[400] (see Appendix 24) In research using mice, blood glucose was decreased by herb. Monitor patients with diabetes to prevent possible hypoglycemia.

Coriander *Coriandrum sativum*

  PART USED: Fruit/seed.

  SAFETY: GRAS (spice, seasoning, flavoring, oil, extract, oleoresin). AHPA Class: 1.[66]

  INTERACTIONS:

  Insulin/Oral hypoglycemic agents[81,401] (see Appendix 24) Possible hypoglycemia or loss of blood glucose control.

Cranberry *Vaccinium spp.*

USES: Odor with urinary incontinence (H), UTI prevention (H-equivocal).
PART USED: Fruit/berry.
CONTRAINDICATIONS: Safety of concentrated cranberry supplements not established in pregnancy and lactation. Patients at risk of nephrolithiasis due to high oxalate content.
ADVERSE REACTIONS: Diarrhea, GI distress, nephrolithiasis (concentrated tablets).
INTERACTIONS
Omeprazole (Prilosec)[402] Concurrent consumption of cranberry juice with omeprazole in elderly patients increased absorption of protein-bound vitamin B12. Omeprazole decreases gastric acid, which leads to malabsorption of vitamin B12.

Creatine

USES: Antineoplastic (A), CHF (H), ergogenic aid in high intensity exercise in younger individuals (H), hepatic guanidinoacetate methyltransferase deficiency (H), hyperornithinemia (H), increased muscle mass/athletic performance (H-equivocal), McArdle disease (H), neuromuscular disease (H).
CONTRAINDICATIONS: Dehydration, impaired renal function. Safety in pregnancy and lactation not established.
SIDE EFFECTS: Electrolyte imbalance, GI distress, N&V, muscle cramps, weight gain.
INTERACTIONS:
Caffeine[403] In one study using healthy male volunteers, ergogenic effect of creatine was eliminated by caffeine.
Cimetidine (Tagamet)[403] Creatinine (some of creatine is metabolized to creatinine)

Creatine (cont'd.)

competes with cimetidine for renal tubular secretion, which may increase the risk of drug side effects.

Crucifer *Brassica spp.* (includes collard greens, cabbage, cauliflower, kale, Brussels sprouts, turnips, broccoli, and kohlrabi)

INTERACTIONS:

Anticoagulants[406] (see Appendix 8) *Brassica spp.* contain variable amounts of vitamin K, which antagonizes the anticoagulant effect of warfarin. Variable intakes may decrease or increase effectiveness of drug. Maintain consistent intake of these vegetables to maintain a constant therapeutic effect of drug .

Drugs that are substrates of P450 CYP1A2[405] (see Appendix 38) *Brassica spp.* decrease the activity of CYP1A2, which may increase serum levels of drugs that are substrates of this isozyme.

Thyroid replacement therapy[112] Many of these vegetables contain glucosinolates which are goitrogenic. Excessive consumption may alter absorption of thyroid hormone in GI tract.

Cumin *Cuminum cyminum*

PART USED: Fruit/seed.

CONTRAINDICATIONS: Safety in pregnancy and lactation not established. Bleeding disorders.

SAFETY: GRAS (spice, seasoning, flavoring, oil, extract, oleoresin). AHPA Class: 1.[66]

ADVERSE REACTIONS: Phototoxicity (oil).

Cumin (cont'd.)

INTERACTIONS:

Anticoagulants and drugs that increase the risk of bleeding[407] (see Appendix 8)
In vivo research showed inhibition of platelet aggregation. Monitor patients on anticoagulants.

Insulin/Oral hypoglycemic agents[75] (see Appendix 24) Possible hypoglycemia or loss of blood glucose control.

Damiana *Turnera diffusa*

PART USED: Leaf.

CONTRAINDICATIONS: Safety in pregnancy and lactation not established.

SAFETY: GRAS (flavoring). AHPA Class: 1.[66]

INTERACTIONS:

Insulin/Oral hypoglycemic agents[55,88] (see Appendix 24) Herb has hypoglycemic activity, which may be additive with diabetes medication. Monitor blood glucose.

Dan Shen *Salvia miltiorrhiza*

PART USED: Root.

CONTRAINDICATIONS: Bleeding disorders. Safety in pregnancy and lactation not established.

SAFETY: AHPA Class: 1.[66]

ADVERSE REACTIONS: Anorexia, gastric distress, pruritus.

INTERACTIONS:

Alcohol[246] Herb decreased alcohol intake by about 50% in laboratory animals.

Dan Shen (cont'd.)

Theoretically, may be beneficial in the treatment of alcoholism.

Anticoagulants and drugs that increase the risk of bleeding[58,62,408] (see Appendix 8) Herb inhibits platelet aggregation, interferes with coagulation and has fibrinolytic activity. Herb should not be used concurrently with drugs which increase the risk of bleeding, as effects may be additive.

Digoxin/Cardiac glycosides[409] Dan shen may interfere with serum measurement of drug. Free serum digoxin should be measured to prevent incorrect results.

Dandelion *Taraxacum officinale*

PART USED: Leaf, root.

CONTRAINDICATIONS: Acute cholecystitis, bile duct obstruction, bleeding disorders, gallstones, ileus. Allergy to *Asteraceae* family.

SAFETY: GRAS (oil, extract, oleoresin). AHPA Class: leaf 1; root 2d—not with bile duct blockage, gallbladder disease or intestinal blockage.[66]

ADVERSE REACTIONS: Allergic reaction, dermatitis, GI distress.

INTERACTIONS:

Drugs metabolized by P450 CYP1A2 and CYP2E[313] (see Appendix 38) In liver microsomes or cytosol from rats given dandelion tea, CYP1A2 activity was 15% and CYP2E was 48% that of control animals. It is not known if inhibition also occurs in humans. Monitor patients taking dandelion and drugs which are substrates of these P450 enzymes, as serum levels may increase due to inhibition of metabolism.

Anticoagulants and drugs that increase the risk of bleeding[410] (see Appendix 8) Herb inhibited ADP-induced platelet aggregation. Theoretical increased risk of

Dandelion (cont'd.)

bleeding with concurrent use.

Ciprofloxacin and other quinolones[233] (see Appendix 7) High mineral content of dandelion may decrease serum levels of drug.

Diuretics[411] (see Appendix 11) Herb has a diuretic effect, which may be additive with diuretic drugs.

Insulin/Oral hypoglycemic agents[105,401] (see Appendix 24) Herb may decrease blood glucose, which may be additive with diabetes medications. Some research using laboratory animals has shown no effect on blood glucose.

Lithium (Eskalith, Lithobid, Lithonate, Lithotabs)[411] Theoretical increase in drug toxicity based on diuretic effect of herb.

Devil's Claw *Harpagophytum procumbens*

USES: Osteoarthritis (H-equivocal).

PART USED: Root, tuber.

CONTRAINDICATIONS: Bleeding disorders, gallstones, gastric and duodenal ulcers.

SAFETY: AHPA Class: 2d—not with gastric or duodenal ulcers.[66]

ADVERSE REACTIONS: Diarrhea, GI distress.

INTERACTIONS:

Antiarrhythmics[413,414] (see Appendix 6) Although no interactions have been reported, the potential exists based on antiarrhythmic action observed in animals.

Anticoagulants and drugs that increase the risk of bleeding[72] (see Appendix 8) In case study, concurrent use of herb and warfarin caused bleeding. Monitor patient.

Antihypertensives[413] (see Appendix 11) Herb had hypotensive effect in laboratory

Devil's Claw (cont'd.)

animals. Effect when combined with antihypertensive drugs is unknown.

Cardiac drugs[413,414] (see Appendix 14) Herb may increase heart rate and contractility, which may alter effect of drug.

Hypotensive therapy[413] In laboratory animals, herb caused a lowering of arterial blood pressure. It is unknown if it interferes with hypotensive therapy.

Diosgenin[322]

Herbs containing diosgenin: *Trigonella foenum-graecum* (fenugreek) – seed 119,000 ppm; *Solanum nigrum* (Black nightshade) – fruit 12,000 ppm; *Daucus carota* (carrot) – root and tissue culture 6,000 ppm; *Dioscorea bulbifera* (air potato, potato yam) – tuber 4,500 ppm.

INTERACTIONS:

Indomethacin (Indocin)[321] Diosgenin (plant-derived sapogenin) decreased subacute indomethacin-induced inflammation in intestines and decreased anti-inflammatory effect of drug. Plasma levels of indomethacin were decreased at 3 and 12 hours. Research used isolated diosgenin in rats. A list of herbs containing diosgenin is provided above.

Dog Bane *Apocynum cannabinum*

PART USED: Root.

SAFETY: Contains cardiac glycosides. AHPA Class: 3.

INTERACTIONS:

Digoxin/Cardiac glycosides[34] Herb contains cardiac glycosides. Theoretical additive effect with concurrent use.

PART USED: Root.

CONTRAINDICATIONS: Bleeding disorders, lactation, pregnancy.

SAFETY: Contains psoralens, which increase photosensitivity and are photocarcinogenic. AHPA Class: 2b.[66]

ADVERSE REACTIONS: Photosensitivity.

INTERACTIONS:

Acetaminophen/Paracetamol[418] Sodium feruluate, a component of dong quai, decreased the hepatotoxicity of drug in mice.

Anticoagulants and drugs that increase the risk of bleeding[79,156,416,417] (see Appendix 8) Herb contains osthole and ferulic acid, which may inhibit platelet aggregation. There has been a case report of increased PT and INR with concurrent use of dong quai with warfarin.

Estrogen replacement therapy/Oral contraceptives[415] In vitro research using dong quai showed antiestrogenic and antiandrogenic effect. Effect on exogenous hormone treatments is not known. Most research has shown no estrogenic effect.

Echinacea *Echinacea angustifolia, Echinacea pallida, Echinacea purpurea*

USES: Decrease duration of colds (H-equivocal), URTI (H).

PART USED: Root, seed.

CONTRAINDICATIONS: Safety in pregnancy and lactation not established. Allergy to *Asteraceae/Compositae* family. Herb is generally considered contraindicated for progressive systemic disease (AIDS/HIV, autoimmune disease, collagenosis, leukosis, MS, TB). There is inadequate research to assess safety in these patients.

Echinacea (cont'd.)

SAFETY: Acute toxicity reported only with parenteral administration, not oral. German Commission E guidelines suggest limiting use to 8 weeks, based on research using injection (not oral) administration in a small number of subjects. In research using HIV patients, oral echinacea for 12 weeks did not result in immune system toxicity. It was noted that viral load decreased during the 12 week phase I trial.[113] No research clearly supports a limitation of use to 8 weeks. AHPA Class: 1.[66]

ADVERSE REACTIONS: Allergic response, chills, fever, N&V. IV administration may cause shivers and fever.

INTERACTIONS:

Drugs which are substrates of P450 CYP3A4 isozymes[227] (see Appendix 38) Preliminary in vitro research has shown that echinacea may alter metabolism and/or effectiveness of drugs which are substrates of CYP3A4 isozymes (*Echinacea angustifolia* and *Echinacea purpurea*). Further research is needed to determine if this interaction occurs in humans.

Chemotherapy[419,420] (see Appendix 16) May enhance chemotherapy, but there is insufficient research on humans to recommend it yet.

Econazole nitrate cream[113] Women with recurrent vaginal infections (*Candida albicans*) were treated with parenteral or topical echinacia (Echinacin) and topical econazole cream. Recurrence rates were lower in patients receiving Echinacin in either form than in patients not receiving Echinacin.

Immunosuppressants[117] (see Appendix 23) Theoretical decrease in immunosuppressant effect. More research is needed to determine effect when combined with immunosuppressant therapy.

Elder *Sambucus nigra*

USES: Flu (H).

PART USED: Flower, ripe cooked fruit.

SAFETY: Fruit (raw and ripe), bark and leaf contain sambunigrin, which is a cyanogenic glycoside. Consumption may cause vomiting and diarrhea. GRAS (leaf as flavoring in alcoholic beverages/flower as spice, seasoning, flavoring). AHPA Class: 1, 66.

ADVERSE REACTIONS: Diarrhea.

INTERACTIONS:

Insulin/Oral hypoglycemic agents[421] (see Appendix 24) In vitro research, water-soluble components of elder flowers enhanced insulin secretion and uptake of glucose by muscle tissue. Monitor patients taking diabetes medications to avoid potential hypoglycemia.

Elder, American *Sambucus canadensis*

PART USED: Flower, ripe fruit.

SAFETY: Contains cyanogenic glycosides. GRAS (flower as spice, seasoning, flavoring).

INTERACTIONS:

Drugs which are substrates of P450 CYP3A4 isozymes[227] (see Appendix 38) Preliminary in vitro research has shown that elder root may alter metabolism and/or effectiveness of drugs which are substrates of CYP3A4 isozymes. Further research is needed to determine if interaction will also occur in humans.

Ephedra *Ephedra sinica*

USES: Asthma (H), weight loss (H-equivocal).

PART USED: Herb.

CONTRAINDICATIONS: Anxiety, BPH, cardiac disease, cerebral insufficiency, children, glaucoma, heart disease, HTN, insomnia, lactation, pheochromocytoma, pregnancy, prostate adenoma, restlessness, thyroid disease.

SAFETY: Numerous reports of adverse effects, including at least 10 deaths. Safety in pregnancy, lactation and children has not been established. On FDA's list of herbs associated with illness or injury (hypertension, heartbeat irregularities, nerve damage, insomnia, tremors, headaches, seizures, heart attack, stroke, and possible death).[178] The FDA has received over 800 adverse event reports related to ephedrine alkaloids. For further information go to http://www.cfsan.fda.gov/~dms/ds-ephed.html. Health Canada requested a recall of certain products containing ephedra/ephedrine on 2/9/02. For further information go to http://www.hc-sc.gc.ca/english/protection/warn ings/ 2002/2002_01e.htm. AHPA Class: 2b, 2c, 2d—not with anorexia, bulimia, glaucoma, MAOIs; no long-term or excessive amounts.[66]

ADVERSE REACTIONS: Anxiety, cardiac arrhythmia, chest pain, death, dizziness, ephedra dependency, flushing, GI distress, headache, hepatitis, HTN, insomnia, irritability, myocardial infarction, N&V, nervousness, palpitations, psychosis, restlessness, seizures, stroke, tachycardia, tingling, tremor, urination difficulty.

INTERACTIONS:

Amitriptyline (Elavil)[425] Drug may decrease hypertensive effect of ephedrine, a component of ephedra.

Anticonvulsants[429] (see Appendix 10) Herb has sympathomimetic effects

Ephedra (cont'd.)

which may interfere with drug.

Antihypertensives[434] (see Appendix 11) Herb may decrease effectiveness of drug due to its stimulant effect.

Antacids[423] (see Appendix 1) Alkaline urine, caused by antacids, may increase the excretion of pseudoephedrine, a component of the herb.

Beta blockers[209] (see Appendix 11) Herb may decrease antihypertensive effect of drug.

Bromocriptine (Parlodel)[427] Case report of 19 year old female developing postpartum psychosis following administration of bromocriptine and pseudoephedrine, a component of ephedra. Possible cardiac arrhythmias.

Bupropion (Wellbutrin, Zyban)[431] Case report of acute MI in a 21 year old male after concurrent administration of bupropion, pseudoephedrine (ephedra contains pseudoephedrine). Ephedra should not be used concurrently with drugs also having sympathomimetic action.

Caffeine[434] Case report of 22 year old male with seizure and unresponsiveness after use of Hydroxycut, which contains ephedra alkaloids and caffeine. Concurrent use of caffeine and ephedra results in a synergistic stimulant effect.

Corticosteroids[426] (see Appendix 18) Ephedrine, in herb, increases the metabolism of drug.

Dexamethasone (Decadron)[432] Ephedrine, a component of ephedra, increased clearance of dexamethasone in humans.

Digoxin/Cardiac glycosides[434] Theoretical altered heart rhythm/arrhythmias.

Ephedra (cont'd.)

Herb may sensitize myocardium to effect of drug.

Diuretics[299] (see Appendix 11) Drug may decrease arterial response to pressor agents such as ephedrine.

Drugs causing alkaline urine[423] Pseudoephedrine reabsorption in distal renal tubules may be increased when combined with drugs causing alkaline urine, possibly increasing sympathomimetic effect of pseudoephedrine.

Entacapone (Comtan)[429] Case report of severe hypertension following consumption of entacapone and ephedrine, a component of ephedra.

Epinephrine[299] Both ephedra and epinephrine elicit pressor response; concurrent use of both theoretically may be additive.

Ergot derivatives[116] Possible increased risk of hypertension.

General anesthetics[299] (see Appendix 20) Concurrent use may result in arrhythmias.

Guanethidine (Ismelin)[502] Herb may displace guanethidine from adrenergic neurons, thereby reducing antihypertensive effect of drug.

Insulin/Oral hypoglycemic agents[105,173] (see Appendix 24) Possible hyperglycemia with concurrent use.

Linezolid (Zyvox)[430] Concurrent administration of linezolid and pseudoephedrine has been shown to increase blood pressure.

MAOIs[428] (see Appendix 9) Potentiation of sympathomimetic effect of ephedrine, a component of ephedra.

Methyldopa (Aldoril)[299] Drug decreases the pressor response of ephedrine,   **100**

which is a component of ephedra.

Methylphenidate (Ritalin)[909] Herb may displace methylphenidate from adrenergic neurons. Theoretically, this may decrease effectiveness of drug.

Methylxanthines including theophylline (Uniphyl, Uni-Dur) and caffeine[434] Stimulant effect may be additive. There has been a case report of seizures with concurrent use of caffeine and ephedra.

Morphine (MSIR, MS Contin, Oramorph, Roxanol)[433] Ephedra increased anal-gesic effect of morphine in animals and humans.

Oxytocin (Pitocin)[1] Possible hypertension.

Pseudoephedrine[299] Herb contains pseudoephedrine. With concurrent use, effects may be additive.

Reserpine (Enduronyl)[299] Drug may decrease the pressor response of ephedrine, which is a component of ephedra.

Sibutramine (Meridia)[422] Possible hypertension with concurrent use.

Sympathomimetics[424] (see Appendix 36) Increased risk of side effects with concurrent use.

Stimulants[434] Possible hypertension.

Surgery, drugs used during[307] It has been recommended that herb be discontinued at least 24 hours prior to surgery. Herb may cause increased heart rate and blood pressure.

Theophylline See **Methylxanthines**, above.

Thyroid replacement therapy[435] There has been a case report of thyroid storm following the use of pseudoephedrine, a component of ephedra, in a patient with

Ephedra (cont'd.)
    Grave's disease.
    Tricyclic antidepressants See **Amitriptyline**, above.

Essaic Formula
    PART USED: Formula of burdock root (*Arctium lappa*), rhubarb *root (Rheum offici-nale)*, sorrel leaf (*Rumex acetosa*) and slippery elm bark (*Ulvus rubra* or *Ulvus fulva*). The mixture is a proprietary secret and may also contain kelp, red clover, blessed this-tle and watercress. See individual herb monographs.

Eucalyptus *Eucalyptus globulus*
    PART USED: Leaf, leaf oil.
    CONTRAINDICATIONS: Leaf and oil—bile duct obstruction or inflammation, children, gastrointestinal inflammation, liver disease. Safety of therapeutic amounts in pregnancy and lactation not established.
    SAFETY: Contains tannins; avoid high dose for extended period. GRAS (flavoring). AHPA Class: 2d—inflammation of bile duct and GI tract, liver disease, not on face of children.[66]
    ADVERSE REACTIONS: Leaf and oil—diarrhea, GI disturbance, N&V.
    INTERACTIONS:
    Weakens or shortens effects of other drugs[436] due to alteration of drug metabolizing enzymes (see Appendix 38) In research on rat liver cells, 1,8-cineole (a component of eucalyptus) may induce drug metabolizing enzymes, such as CYP2B1. In one study, P450 enzymes were increased. This may decrease

Eucalyptus (cont'd.)

serum levels of drugs which are substrates of this isozyme.

Insulin/Oral hypoglycemic agents[57,401] In mice, aqueous extract of herb had hypoglycemic effect. It is not known if effect may be additive with diabetes medications. Monitor patient.

Evening Primrose Oil (EPO) *Oenothera biennis* Contains gamma-linolenic acid (GLA).

USES: Atopic eczema (H), cyclic mastalgia (H), diabetic peripheral neuropathy (H), hypercholesterolemia (H), rheumatoid arthritis (H-equivocal).

PART USED: Seed oil. AHPA Class 1.

CONTRAINDICATIONS: Allergy to herb, bleeding disorders, epilepsy, mania.

ADVERSE REACTIONS: Diarrhea, GI distress, headache, nausea.

INTERACTIONS:

Anticoagulants and drugs that increase the risk of bleeding[234] (see Appendix 8) EPO (3 mg/kg/day) increased bleeding after 4 months of administration in rats. Patients should be monitored for signs of increased bleeding and serum coagulation changes.

General anesthetics[72] (see Appendix 20) Possible seizures. Significance of one case report not established due to administration with other drugs.

Phenothiazines[72] (see Appendix 28) Seizures have been reported in patients with schizophrenia administered phenothiazines and evening primrose oil.

Tamoxifen (Nolvadex)[223] Concurrent use of GLA (contained in evening primrose oil) and tamoxifen caused a faster clinical response (reduction in ER expression) in ER+ breast cancer than tamoxifen alone.

Fennel *Foeniculum vulgare*

PART USED: Fruit/seed, oil.

CONTRAINDICATIONS: Safety in pregnancy, lactation and children not established. Allergy to *Apiaceae* family. Hypotension.

SAFETY: Not for long-term use. Genotoxicity in animals. Psoralens/estragole are carcinogenic. GRAS (spice, seasoning, flavoring, oil, extract, oleoresin). Poison hemlock has been misidentified as fennel. AHPA Class: 1.[66]

ADVERSE REACTIONS: Contact dermatitis, photodermatitis, photosensitivity. Oil: allergic reaction, hallucinations, N&V, pulmonary edema, seizures.

INTERACTIONS:

ACE inhibitors[293] (see Appendix 11) Case report of 60 year old male with HTN and CHF taking enalapril, which induced coughing. Patient was free from cough after chewing fennel fruit on a regular basis.

Antihypertensives[437] (see Appendix 11) In research using rats, boiled aqueous extract of herb leaf lowered arterial blood pressure. It is not known if this effect is additive when combined with antihypertensive agents.

Ciprofloxacin (Cipro)[438] In research using rats, the absorption, distribution and elimination of the drug were decreased by fennel extract.

Diuretics[439] (see Appendix 11) Herb has diuretic activity. It is not known if effect may be additive with drugs that have a diuretic effect.

USES: Loss of appetite, type 1 and type 2 diabetes (H), skin injury or irritation (external).

PART USED: Seed.

CONTRAINDICATIONS: Safety in pregnancy and lactation not established.

SAFETY: GRAS (spice, seasoning, flavoring, oil, extract, oleoresin). AHPA Class: 2b.[66]

ADVERSE REACTIONS: Allergic response, gastroenteritis in newborn, hypoglycemia, myositis, peritonitis, skin reactions (long-term topical).

INTERACTIONS:

Herb may reduce intestinal absorption of other drugs.[4] High mucilage content.

Anticoagulants and drugs that increase the risk of bleeding[290] (see Appendix 8) Case report of 67 year old female with increased INR after consumption of boldo and fenugreek. Patient had history of HTN and atrial fibrillation on metoprolol and warfarin. Supplements taken prior to increased INR included zinc, multivitamin, artichoke extract and vitamin E. INR increased to 3.4 (previously maintained at 2.0-3.0) after starting boldo and fenugreek. INRs returned to previous levels with discontinuation of boldo and fenugreek. Clinical significance not established.

Insulin/Oral hypoglycemic agents[53,55,105,130,162,167,171,173,441] (see Appendix 24) Possible hypoglycemia or loss of blood glucose control. Blood glucose lowering effect not as effective in severe type 2 diabetes. Blood glucose was lowered in type 2 diabetes and type 1 diabetes, an effect related to fiber content of herb.

Lipid-lowering drugs[440] In human research, fenugreek decreased total cholesterol and LDLs. It is not known if this effect may be additive with lipid-lowering drugs. Monitor patient.

Feverfew *Tanacetum parthenium*
   USES: Migraine prophylaxis (H).
   PART USED: Herb.
   CONTRAINDICATIONS: Allergy to *Compositae* family, bleeding disorders, pregnancy. Safety in children or when lactating not established.
   SAFETY: AHPA Class: 2b.[66]
   ADVERSE REACTIONS: Allergic response, decreased taste, dermatitis, increased heart rate, lip swelling, oral ulceration. Discontinuation may cause post-feverfew syndrome: anxiety, muscle aches, rebound migraine, sleep disturbances.
   INTERACTIONS:
      Anticoagulants and drugs that increase the risk of bleeding and surgery[442] (see Appendix 8) Increased risk of bleeding. Herb inhibits platelet aggregation.
      Paclitaxel (Taxol)[259] Parthenolide (from feverfew) may decrease NF-κB DNA binding and may increase sensitivity of breast cancer cells to paclitaxel.

Figwort *Scrophularia nodosa*
   PART USED: Herb, root.
   CONTRAINDICATIONS: Safety in pregnancy and lactation not established. Ventricular tachycardia.
   AHPA Class: 2d—not with ventricular tachycardia.[66]
   INTERACTIONS:
      Digoxin/Cardiac glycosides[34] Herb has cardioactive effect, which may increase side effects of drug.

USES: Atherosclerosis (H), cancer prevention (lignan precursor secoisolariciresinol diglycoside most effective during initiation of cancer cells, seed oil is more
effective after tumor has been established) (H), chronic renal disease (H), constipation,
delay onset of diabetes (secoisolariciresinol diglucoside isolated from flaxseed-A),
hypercholesterolemia (H), lupus nephritis (H).

PART USED: Seed, seed oil.

CONTRAINDICATIONS: Abdominal pain of unknown origin, bleeding disorders, bowel
obstruction, elevated prolactin, hypokalemia, ileus. Do not use large doses during
pregnancy or lactation.

SAFETY: Store in the refrigerator or freezer to prevent oxidation of oils. Seeds
contains variable amounts of cyanide, which is released as hydrogen cyanide when
exposed to water (when homogenized and processed in a laboratory 124 to
196 micrograms/g of cyanide were found, no cyanide was detected when boiled).
AHPA Class: 2d—take with at least 6 oz liquid.[66]

ADVERSE REACTIONS: Flaxseed and defatted flaxseed meal may decrease zinc
status, as shown by decreased alkaline phosphatase.[229] Defatted flaxseed may
increase serum triglycerides. Allergic response, flatulence, increased frequency of
bowel movements.

INTERACTIONS:

Mucilage content of herb may decrease absorption of other drugs.[4]

Anticoagulants and drugs that increase the risk of bleeding[445,446] (see
Appendix 8) Flaxseed oil may decrease platelet aggregation, which may increase
the risk of bleeding.

Flaxseed (cont'd.)

Hormone replacement therapy/Oral hypoglycemic agents[443] Flaxseed has been shown to alter metabolism of endogenous hormone as well as increase serum prolactin in postmenopausal women. Effect on exogenous hormones and clinical significance are not known.

Insulin/Oral hypoglycemic agents[444] (see Appendix 24) Flaxseed decreased postprandial blood glucose by 27% in one study. Monitor blood glucose.

Foxglove *Digitalis purpurea* (purple*), Digitalis lanata* (yellow)

PART USED: Leaf.

SAFETY: Safety of herb cannot be established due to variable amounts of cardiac glycosides, which have a narrow margin of safety. Symptoms of poisoning include: blurred vision, confusion, contracted pupils, convulsions, death, decreased pulse rate, fatigue, increased urination, muscle weakness, N&V, stupor, tremors. Chronic use may cause green urine. Digitalis glycosides are excreted slowly, and serum levels may increase over time. AHPA class: 3.[66]

INTERACTIONS:

Albuterol (Proventil, Ventolin)[910] Drug decreased serum digoxin, which is a drug derived from foxglove.

Amiodarone[911] Amiodarone reduces clearance and increases bioavailability of digoxin, a drug derived from foxglove.

Aminoglycosides[912] Aminoglycosides decrease absorption of digoxin in the GI tract. Digoxin is derived from foxglove.

Amphotericin B (Amphocin, Fungizone)[912] Drug increases the risk of hypokalemia, which would increase the toxicity of foxglove. Based on

Antacids[911] (see Appendix 1) Magnesium and aluminum salts bind to digoxin in the GI tract, decreasing absorption. Digoxin is derived from foxglove.

Anticoagulants and drugs that increase the risk of bleeding[449] (see Appendix 8) Herb may interfere with action of drug.

Antiarrhythmics[912] (see Appendix 6) Possible synergistic or additive effect. Based on interactions with digoxin, a drug derived from foxglove.

Bleomycin (Blenoxane)[915] Use of drug with digoxin may decrease effectiveness of digoxin. Digoxin is derived from foxglove.

Calcium channel blockers[911] (see Appendix 11) Drug inhibits renal clearance of digoxin, which is derived from foxglove.

Carmustine (BiCNU)[912] Use of drug with digoxin has decreased effectiveness of digoxin. Digoxin is derived from foxglove.

Cholestyramine (Questran)[911] Drug decreases absorption of digoxin, a drug derived from foxglove.

Colestipol (Colestid)[911] Drug decreases absorption of digoxin, a drug derived from foxglove

Cyclophosphamide (Cytoxan, Neosar)[912] Use of drug with digoxin has decreased effectiveness of digoxin. Digoxin is derived from foxglove.

Cyclosporine (Neoral)[912] Drug has been found to increase toxicity of digoxin. Digoxin is derived from foxglove.

Cytarabine (Cytosar-U)[914] Use of drug with digoxin has decreased effectiveness of

Foxglove (cont'd.)

digoxin. Digoxin is derived from foxglove.

Digoxin/Cardiac glycosides[34] Herb contains digitoxin, a cardiac glycoside similar to digoxin. Effects may be additive.

Diuretics[34,911] (see Appendix 11) Herb contains cardiac glycosides which may increase potassium loss; possibly additive with potassium-depleting diuretics.

Doxorubicin (Adriamycin)[913] Use of drug with digoxin may decrease binding of doxorubicin to heart muscle cells, as seen with digoxin. Digoxin is derived from foxglove.

Erythromycin (E-mycin, ERYC, Ery-Tab)[911] Drug may increase serum cardiac glycosides (including foxglove/digitalis) by increasing bioavailability, which may increase risk of side effects. Digoxin is derived from foxglove.

Flecainide (Tambocor)[912] Drug increases clearance of digoxin. Digoxin is derived from foxglove.

Hydroxychloroquine (Plaquenil)[912] Drug has been found to decrease clearance of digoxin. Digoxin is derived from foxglove.

Ibuprofen[912] Drug increases serum digoxin. Digoxin is derived from foxglove.

Indomethacin (Indocin)[912] Drug increases serum digoxin. Digoxin is derived from foxglove.

Itraconazole (Sporanox)[911] Drug may increase serum digoxin levels thereby increasing toxicity of digoxin. Digoxin is derived from foxglove.

Macrolide antibiotics and tetracycline[912] (see Appendix 7) Drug may increase serum cardiac glycosides (including foxglove/digitalis) by increasing bioavailability, which may increase risk of side effects.

110

Foxglove (cont'd.)

Nefazodone (Serzone)[448] Nefazodone increases serum digoxin, but clinical significance has not been established. Digoxin is derived from foxglove.

Penicillamine (Cuprimine)[911] Drug may decrease serum levels of digoxin. Digoxin is derived from foxglove.

Phenytoin (Dilantin)[912] Drug has been found to decrease serum levels of digoxin. Digoxin is derived from foxglove.

Procarbazine (Matulane)[912] Use of drug with digoxin has decreased effectiveness of digoxin. Digoxin is derived from foxglove.

Propafenone (Rythmol)[911] Drug increases clearance of digoxin. Digoxin is derived from foxglove.

Quinidine (Quinaglute)/Quinine[911] Drug may decrease clearance of digoxin, which may increase toxicity of digoxin. Digoxin is derived from foxglove.

Sulphasalazine[915] Drug has been found to decrease absorption of digoxin. Digoxin is derived from foxglove.

Stimulant laxatives Excessive use of laxatives increases the risk of hypokalemia, which may increase toxicity of cardiac glycoside in herb.

Trazodone (Desyrel)[912] Drug may increase serum levels of digoxin. Digoxin is derived from foxglove.

Verapamil (Calan, Verelan)[911] Drug decreases clearance of digoxin. Digoxin is derived from foxglove.

Vincristine (Oncovin, Vincasar)[912] Use of drug with digoxin has decreased effectiveness of digoxin. Digoxin is derived from foxglove.

Frangipani *Plumeria rubra*
SAFETY: Contains cardiac glycosides, which have a narrow margin of safety.
INTERACTIONS:
Digoxin/Cardiac glycosides[34] Herb may increase risk of digoxin toxicity.

Fucus *Fucus vesiculosus, Fucus spp.*
PART USED: Thallus.
CONTRAINDICATIONS: Bleeding disorders, hyperthyroidism, hypothyroidism. Safety in pregnancy, lactation and children (heavy metal content).
SAFETY: Contains high amounts of iodine and bioaccumulates heavy metals from environment. AHPA Class: 2b, 2c, 2d—not with hyperthyroidism, not long-term.[66]
ADVERSE REACTIONS: Allergic reactions, hyperthyroidism.
INTERACTIONS:
Decreased absorption of other drugs due to mucilage content.[4] Fucus is 22%-65% mucilage.
Anticoagulants and drugs that increase the risk of bleeding[450,923] (see Appendix 8) Fucoidan FF7/3, a component of fucus, has anticoagulant and fibrinolytic activity. Patients taking drugs that increase the risk of bleeding concurrently with fucus need to be monitored closely.
Diuretics[916] (see Appendix 11) Fucus has a high sodium content (56,100 ppm) and may reduce effectiveness of diuretics.
Hyperthyroid medications[451] Herb contains high amounts of iodine, which may alter effectiveness of drug.

Fucus (cont'd.) 113

Iodine-containing drugs[451] Herb contains high amounts of iodine, which may alter effect of drugs containing iodine.

Lithium (Eskalith, Lithobid, Lithonate, Lithotabs)[451] High intakes of iodine, as seen in herb, may increase the risk of drug-induced hypothyroidism.

Thyroid replacement therapy[916] Herb contains high amounts of iodine, which may alter effectiveness of drug.

Gamma-linolenic Acid (GLA)

USES: Atopic dermatitis (H), diabetic neuropathy (H), RA (H).

PART USED: Seed oils, such as evening primrose oil and borage seed oil.

CONTRAINDICATIONS: Bleeding disorders.

ADVERSE REACTIONS: Excessive bleeding.

INTERACTIONS:

Anticoagulants and drugs that increase the risk of bleeding[453] (see Appendix 8) 12 Hyperlipidemic patients consumed 3 g GLA and linoleic acid/day. Bleeding time increased 40%, TG decreased by 48% and HDL was increased 22%.

Paclitaxel (Taxol)[337] In research using human breast cancer cells, GLA was synergistic with paclitaxel. Preincubation of cells for 24 hours with GLA produced an additive effect when paclitaxel was added to breast cancer cells.

Tamoxifen (Nolvadex)[452] GLA enhanced tamoxifen-induced ER down-regulation in breast cancer patients.

Garlic Cloves *Allium sativum*

USES: Angina pectoris (H-IV garlicin), atherosclerosis prevention, common cold prevention (H), hypercholesterolemia (H-equivocal), mild HTN (H-equivocal), tinea pedis (H).

PART USED: Bulb.

CONTRAINDICATIONS: Allergy to *Liliaceae* family, bleeding disorders, gastric ulcer, thyroid disease.

SAFETY: GRAS (oil, extract, oleoresin). AHPA Class: 2c.[66]

ADVERSE REACTIONS: Allergic response, contact dermatitis, dizziness, garlic body odor, GI distress, headache, increased bleeding, nausea, burning of mouth-esophagus-stomach, lightheadedness, N&V, sweating.

INTERACTIONS:

Drugs metabolized by P450 CYP3A, CYP2B1, CYP2C, CYP2D and CYP2E1[270, 330,454,456,462,463] (see Appendix 38) Rats fed garlic oil had increased CYP2B1 activity in a dose dependent manner. In vitro studies have shown an increase in the metabolism of substrates of CYP2A6, CYP2C, CYP2D and CYP3A isozymes, and possibly CYP2E1.

Acetaminophen/Paracetamol[270] In mice, garlic decreased the risk of acetaminophen-induced hepatotoxicity, most likely through inhibition of P450 CYP2E1.

Antacids[455] (see Appendix 1) Garlic, in large doses, may be irritating to the gastric mucosa, which may decrease effectiveness of antacids.

Anticoagulants and drugs that increase the risk of bleeding[328,464,465,467] (see Appendix 8) Garlic may decrease platelet aggregation. Results of research have been equivocal. Effect appears to be more potent with high intakes and raw, fresh garlic. Thiosulfinates in fresh cut garlic are probably responsible for antiplatelet activity, as seen in this research using human platelets. In one study, allicin, a component of garlic, inhibited aggregation more potently than aspirin.

Antihypertensives[468] (see Appendix 11) Garlic has hypotensive activity. It is not known if this effect is cumulative with drugs which also lower blood pressure.

Doxorubicin (Adriamycin, Doxil, Rubex)[450] In mice, S-allylcysteine (component of garlic) decreased some of the adverse effects of drug.

Insulin/Oral hypoglycemic agents[458,460,461,466] (see Appendix 24) Garlic may have a hypoglycemic effect. In one study of nondiabetic subjects, blood glucose decreased in men but increased in women. Results of research have been equivocal. Urge patient with diabetes to monitor blood glucose.

Isoprenaline[457] In research using dogs, garlic dialysate decreased both chronotropic and positive inotropic effects of drug.

Saquinavir (Fortovase, Invirase)[260] In one study, garlic decreased serum levels of drug. Mean saquinavir AUC decreased 51%. Garlic may induce CYP3A4 (see Appendix 38) and lower serum level of drugs which are substrates of this isozyme.

Surgery, drugs used during[307,328,464,465,467] Review of herbs discusses the need to discontinue herb at least 7 days prior to surgery. May inhibit platelet aggregation, which may increase risk of bleeding.

Genipap / Jagua *Genipa americana*
  INTERACTIONS:
    Clozapine, and possibly other drugs metabolized by P450[296,350] (see Appendix 38) Genipap seed contains 0-22,500 ppm of caffeine. Caffeine intakes greater than 400 mg may decrease clearance of clozapine (and possibly induce other drugs metabolized by CYP1A2). In randomized crossover research of 12 males, the AUC of clozapine was increased by 19% and oral clearance of clozapine was decreased 14% with concurrent caffeine intake.

Germander *Teucrium chamaedrys*
PART USED: Herb.

SAFETY: On FDA's list of herbs associated with illness or injury (liver disease)[178] GRAS (flavoring in alcoholic beverages). Contains hepatotoxic pyrrolizidine alkaloids. AHPA Class: 3.[66]

Ginger *Zingiber officinale*
  USES: Arthritis (H), chemotherapy related nausea (H), hyperemesis gravidarum (H), morning sickness (H), motion sickness (H), N&V (H), postoperative nausea and vomiting (H-not to exceed 4g-equivocal), vertigo (H).
  PART USED: Rhizome, root.
  CONTRAINDICATIONS:, Bleeding conditions, gallstones, ulcers. Safety of large doses in pregnancy has not been established.
  SAFETY: GRAS (spices, seasoning, flavoring, oil, extract, oleoresin). AHPA Class: Fresh root 1; dried root 2b, 2d—not with gallstones.[66]

Ginger (cont'd.)

ADVERSE REACTIONS: Contact dermatitis, GI distress, heartburn, increased bleeding.

INTERACTIONS:

Alcohol[469] In research using rats, ginger was cytoprotective and protective against ethanol-induced ulcers.

Anticoagulants and drugs that increase the risk of bleeding (see Appendix 8) **and surgery**[473,474] In humans, a dose of 2 g or 4 g daily did not affect platelet aggregation, but 5 g and 10 g of powdered ginger did decrease platelet aggregation. There are no reports of bleeding with less than 5 g per day, and form (raw vs. dried) may influence ability to alter platelet function. It is not known if concurrent use with drugs may increase bleeding.

Aspirin[469] In research using rats, ginger was cytoprotective and protective against drug-induced ulcers.

Chemotherapy[470,476] (see Appendix 16) Ginger may reduce nausea side effect of chemotherapy.

Cisplatin (Platinol)[475] Ginger significantly reversed delay in gastric emptying caused by drug.

Hexobarbital[471] Oral (6)-gingerol and (6)-shogaol at doses of 70-140 mg/kg prolonged drug sleep time in laboratory animals. These doses exceed those therapeutically used in humans.

Indomethacin (Indocin)[469] In research using rats, ginger was cytoprotective and protective against drug-induced ulcers.

Insulin/Oral hypoglycemic agents[105,472,477] (see Appendix 24) In research using

Ginger (cont'd.)

laboratory animals, blood glucose was lowered. In one study, there was no effect on blood sugar in patients with type 2 diabetes administered up to 10 g powdered ginger. Monitor blood glucose with large doses of ginger.

NSAIDs[469] (see Appendix 8) In research using rats, ginger was cytoprotective and protective against drug-induced ulcers.

SSRIs[230] (see Appendix 9) Ginger root may decrease disequilibrium and nausea resulting from the discontinuation of SSRIs.

Ginkgo *Ginkgo biloba*

USES: ADHD (H-preliminary research, concurrently with American ginseng), age-related memory loss (H), altitude sickness (H), Alzheimer's disease (H), dementia (H), intermittent claudication (H), macular degeneration (H), mental performance (H-equivocal), peripheral arterial occlusive disease (H), PMS (H), tinnitus (H-equivocal), vertigo (H).

PART USED: Leaf.

CONTRAINDICATIONS: Allergy to poison ivy. Bleeding disorders, epilepsy (raw nuts).

SAFETY: Raw nut/seed contains 4-O-methylpyridoxine, which is toxic. No more than 8-10 cooked nuts should be consumed in one day, not for long-term use. Consumption of raw seeds has caused deaths in children. One study found colchicine in cord blood from pregnant women taking herbs. Ginkgo sold in area tested positive for colchicine, but ginkgo is not known to contain colchicine. AHPA Class: 2d—not with MAOIs.[66]

ADVERSE REACTIONS: Allergic reaction, cheilitis, dermatitis, dizziness, GI distress, headache, hyphema, increased bleeding, palpitations, subdural hematoma.

Ginkgo (cont'd.)

INTERACTIONS:

5-FU/Fluorouracil (Adrucil)[347] In a phase II study of 44 patients with advanced progressive colorectal cancer, subjects were first administered conventional 5-FU. They were then administered GBE 761 (a ginkgo extract) days 1-6, followed by concurrent administration of 5-FU on days 2-6. This process was repeated every 3 weeks. 32 Patients were evaluated (12 not evaluated due to death). A partial remission was found in 2 patients, and 8 patients remained stable for at least 2 therapy cycles. Disease progressed in 22 patients. This treatment may be beneficial in patients with drug resistance and to aid in decreasing side effects. Further research is needed to determine overall benefits to cancer patients. In phase II trial, concurrent use of GBE 761 with 5-FU for pancreatic cancer had an overall response rate of 9.4%.[492]

Drugs which are substrates of P450 CYP3A4 isozyme[227] (see Appendix 38) Preliminary in vitro research has shown that ginkgo may alter metabolism and/or effectiveness of drugs which are substrates of CYP3A4 isozymes. Further research is needed to determine if interaction will also occur in humans.

Drugs which are substrates of P450 CYP2D6 isozyme[479] (see Appendix 38) Ginkgo decreased CYP2D6 activity, which may alter serum levels of drugs which are substrates of this isozyme.

Alcohol[294] Rats were pretreated with ginkgo prior to administration of ethanol. Ginkgo was protective against ethanol-induced ulcers (decreased intensity of lesions and decreased hemorrhage).

Anticoagulants and drugs that increase the risk of bleeding[25,28,110,273,344,486]

Ginkgo (cont'd.)

(see Appendix 8) Increased risk of bleeding. Drug inhibits platelet aggregation. In 18 subjects without diabetes, 120 mg ginkgo for 3 months significantly delayed collagen-induced platelet aggregation, which may have inhibited formation of platelet TXA_2.

Anticonvulsants[480] (see Appendix 10) There have been case reports of seizures, likely due to consumption of nut, not leaf. Leaf contains very little of the toxin which is responsible for seizures.

Cyclosporine (Neoral)[484,485] In research using human patients with asthma, ginkgolide B (component of ginkgo) concurrently used with cyclosporine was found to have an additive effect. In research using microsomes, ginkgo extract was found to prevent free radical damage to cell membranes.

Doxorubicin (Adriamycin)[483] In laboratory mice, ginkgo decreased the cardiotoxic effect of drug.

Fluoxetine (Prozac)[487,488,490] Herb may reverse sexual dysfunction side effect of drug.

General anesthetics[491] (see Appendix 20) In research using mice, aqueous ginkgo extract decreased sleep time induced by anesthetics. Theoretically, ginkgo may also alter heart rate or blood pressure.

Gentamicin (Garamycin)[349] Ginkgo extract 2 days prior to and 8 days concurrently with gentamicin decreased drug-induced nephrotoxicity in rats.

Haloperidol (Haldol)[272] In a study using 82 patients with chronic refractory schizophrenia, ginkgo extract enhanced efficacy and decreased side effects of haloperidol. Enhancement may be due to the antioxidant effect of ginkgo. **120**

Insulin/Oral hypoglycemic agents[482] (see Appendix 24) **and OGTT**[264] After 3 months consuming ginkgo, there was a significant increase in fasting insulin and C-peptide levels in human subjects without diabetes, as well as an increase in the AUC for insulin and C-peptide during an OGTT. Also of interest was an increase in triglycerides (as much as 1.5 to 2-fold) during the first month of consumption, returning to normal by the end of the 3rd month. Blood pressure was significantly lower at the end of the 3rd month. Ginkgo may alter the results of OGTT. In normal subjects, ginkgo may increase fasting insulin during an OGTT. It is unknown what impact long-term ginkgo use may have on patients with diabetes.

MAOIs[210,481] (see Appendix 9) Kaempferol, a component of ginkgo, was shown to have MAO-inhibiting effect in in vitro research. Effect in humans not known.

Meclofenoxate[478] In rats, ginkgo improved effectiveness of drug.

Nifedipine and other drugs metabolized by P450 CYP3A4[278] (see Appendix 38) Research on 22 healthy human subjects showed a 53% increase in mean plasma levels of nifedipine, which suggests inhibition of CYP3A4.

SSRIs[487,488,490] (see Appendix 9) Herb may reverse sexual dysfunction side effect of drug. All reports found a reversal of sexual dysfunction with concurrent use of ginkgo with SSRIs, except for one case report of 22 patients who did not to experience a reversal of sexual dysfunction with the use of ginkgo.

Surgery[273,307] Increased postoperative bleeding. Case report of 34 year old male with postoperative bleeding following laparoscopic cholecystectomy. No medications were taken prior to surgery. Review of herbs discusses the need to discontinue herb at least 36 hours prior to surgery. May inhibit platelet-activating factor, which

Ginkgo (cont'd.)

may increase risk of bleeding. Ginkgo may alter heart rate or blood pressure.

Thiazide diuretics[72] (see Appendix 11) Potential increase in blood pressure.

Trazodone (Desyrel)[231] One case report of coma with concurrent use.

Trimipramine (Surmontil)[489] Concurrent administration of ginkgo extract improved sleep continuity and enhanced non-REM sleep in patients with major depression treated with trimipramine.

Ginseng, American *Panax quinquefolius*

USES: ADHD (H-preliminary research, concurrently with ginkgo).

PART USED: Root.

CONTRAINDICATIONS: Safety in pregnancy and lactation not established. Bleeding disorders.

SAFETY: Use no longer than 3 months at a time. AHPA Class: 1.[66]

ADVERSE REACTIONS: Diarrhea, edema, headache, hyperpyrexia, insomnia, N&V, palpitations, pruritus, vertigo.

INTERACTIONS: Also see Ginseng, Panax. Both contain similar chemicals, so interactions for Ginseng, Panax may also be applicable to Ginseng, American.

Cyclophosphamide (Cytoxan)[216] In in vitro research, herb synergistically inhibited breast cancer cell growth.

Doxorubicin (Adriamycin, Doxil, Rubex)[216] In in vitro research, herb synergistically inhibited breast cancer cell growth.

Insulin/Oral hypoglycemic agents[248,249] (see Appendix 24) Herb had hypoglycemic effect. Herb administered 40 minutes prior to and with a test meal

Ginseng, American (cont'd.)

of 25 g glucose resulted in a lower postprandial blood glucose. Doses greater than 3 g did not lower blood glucose further. Monitor glucose patients with diabetes.

Methotrexate (Rheumatrex)[216] In in vitro research, herb synergistically inhibited breast cancer cell growth.

Morphine (MSIR,MS Contin, Oramorph, Roxanol)[493] Pseudoginsenoside-F1, isolated from herb, antagonized the behavioral effect of morphine in hamsters.

Oral contraceptives/Hormone replacement therapy[216] Theoretically, herb may alter effectiveness of exogenous hormones.

Paclitaxel (Taxol)[216] In in vitro research, herb synergistically inhibited breast cancer cell growth.

Surgery, drugs used during[307] It has been recommended that herb be discontinued at least 7 days prior to surgery. Risk of hypoglycemia and risk of bleeding.

Tamoxifen (Nolvadex)[216] In in vitro research, herb synergistically inhibited breast cancer cell growth.

Ginseng, Panax or Asian *Panax ginseng*

USES: Erectile dysfunction (H-red ginseng), cognitive function (H), improve immunity (H).

PART USED: Root.

CONTRAINDICATIONS: Safety in pregnancy, lactation and children not established. Bleeding disorders, HTN.

SAFETY: Red ginseng (steamed ginseng) may potentiate caffeine and other stimulants. AHPA Class: 2d—not with HTN, not longer than 3 months.[66]

ADVERSE REACTIONS: Bleeding disorders, diarrhea, diffuse mammary nodularity, edema, headache, hyperpyrexia, menstrual abnormalities, N&V, nervous excitation, palpitations, pruritus, rose spots, vertigo. Large doses over an extended period of time may cause diarrhea, estrogenic effect, HTN, hypertony, decreased libido, insomnia, menstruation in menopausal women and nervousness.

INTERACTIONS:

Drugs metabolized by P450 CYP2D6[505] (see Appendix 38) Ginseng decreased CYP2D6 by 6%. May not be of clinical significance.

Alcohol[196,246] Herb may decrease alcohol absorption, which may be useful (hypothesized) in the treatment of alcoholism.

Anticoagulants and drugs that increase the risk of bleeding[263,501] (see Appendix 8) No change in pharmacokinetics or pharmacodynamics of warfarin in concurrent administration with *Panax ginseng* was noted in this study using rats. It is important to note that herb-drug interactions in rats may differ from interactions in man. In another study, the lipophilic fraction of ginseng had an antithrombotic effect. One case report showed a decline in INR with the use of ginseng. Monitor labs closely.

Antihypertensives[495] (see Appendix 11) In patients with essential hypertension, red ginseng lowered blood pressure, which may be additive with antihypertensive medications.

Anxiolytics[494] (see Appendix 13) In mice, white and red ginseng had effect similar to diazepam. Theoretical additive effect with anxiolytic drugs.

Caffeine[66] Red ginseng (steamed) has stimulant effect, which may be additive **124**

with other stimulants.

Digoxin/Cardiac glycosides[503] Concurrent use of red ginseng enhanced effect of drug in treatment of CHF patients.

Immunosuppressants[497] (see Appendix 23) Ginseng has immunostimulant activity and should not be used with immunosuppressants until more research has been conducted to determine potential interactions.

Influenza vaccination[315,345] Research on 227 volunteers over 12 weeks, using 100 mg Ginsana G115, showed a decrease in frequency of the common cold and influenza. Findings include significantly higher NK activity and antibody titers in the G115 group at 8 weeks and 12 weeks. 9 Cases of insomnia, nausea, epigastralgia and anxiety were reported. In a randomized, double-blind, placebo-controlled trial, 175 humans received the vaccination one month after the initiation of 100 mg ginseng bid. There was an enhanced IgM and IgA antibody response in those receiving ginseng.

Insulin/Oral hypoglycemic agents[291,500] (see Appendix 24) In research on healthy subjects, doses up to 3 g did not affect postprandial glucose. It is possible that panax ginseng alters blood glucose control, as seen in laboratory animals. Those taking oral hypoglycemic agents and insulin should consult a health care professional prior to using ginseng.

Kanamycin (Kantrex)[504] Concurrent administration of herb with drug increased effectiveness of antibiotic treatment for dysentery and *proteus* infection in children.

MAOIs[27] (see Appendix 9) Herb potentiated phenelzine, causing manic symptoms.

Monomycin[504] Concurrent administration of herb with drug increased effectiveness

Ginseng, Panax or Asian (cont'd.)

of antibiotic treatment for dysentery and *proteus* infection in children.

Morphine (MSIR, MS Contin, Oramorph, Roxanol)[499] Concurrent use of ginseng total saponin partially blocked morphine-induced apoptosis of thymocytes.

Phenelzine see MAOIs, above.

Stimulants[66] Red ginseng (steamed) has stimulant effect, which may be additive with other stimulants.

Surgery, drugs used during[307] It has been recommended that herb be discontinued at least 7 days prior to surgery. Risk of hypoglycemia and risk of bleeding.

Zidovudine (Retrovir)[498] Korean red ginseng combined with zidovudine maintained CD4+ count, perhaps due to delay in development of resistance to drug.

Globularia *Globularia alypum*
INTERACTIONS:

Insulin/Oral hypoglycemic agents[329] (see Appendix 24) In rats given .7g/kg of herb infusion, hypoglycemic effect was seen in normal and hypoglycemic rats. Mechanism of action is believed to be an increased peripheral metabolism of glucose and an increase in insulin release. Water-soluble extract of *globularia* reduced the uptake of glucose in the perfused jejunum of rats by 21%. Use of herb with insulin should only be made under the supervision of a knowledgeable health care professional.

Glucosamine cartilage (often combined with chondroitin)

USES: Osteoarthritis (H)

CONTRAINDICATIONS: Pregnancy, lactation, children, peptic ulcer, shellfish allergy.

ADVERSE REACTIONS: Constipation, diarrhea, drowsiness, GI distress, headache, rash.

INTERACTIONS:

Insulin/Oral hypoglycemic agents[506,507] (see Appendix 24)   In research using rats, glucosamine increased plasma glucose, but this has not been found to be true in humans.   Therapeutic amounts have not been found to cause insulin resistance.

Goat's Rue *Galega officinalis*

PART USED: Herb.

SAFETY: Insufficient data available to evaluate safety.   Animals grazing on large amounts of herb have been fatally poisoned.

INTERACTIONS:

Anticoagulants and drugs that increase the risk of bleeding[508] (see Appendix 8)   In in vitro research, herb inhibited platelet aggregation.   Effect in humans not known.

Insulin/Oral hypoglycemic agents[1,105,173] (see Appendix 24)   Herb contains galegin, which has a hypoglycemic effect.

Goldenrod *Solidago virgaurea*

PART USED: Herb.

CONTRAINDICATIONS: CHF, edema, kidney disease.   Safety in pregnancy and lactation not established.

SAFETY: AHPA Class: 2d—not with kidney disorders without medical supervision.[66]

ADVERSE REACTIONS: Allergic reactions, contact dermatitis.

INTERACTIONS:

Diuretics[509] (see Appendix 11) Herb may decrease excretion of sodium, which may interfere with effect of diuretics.

Lithium (Eskalith, Lithobid, Lithonate, Lithotabs)[510] Goldenrod increases the excretion of water, which may increase the toxicity of lithium.

Goldenseal *Hydrastis canadensis*

PART USED: Rhizome, root.

CONTRAINDICATIONS: Cardiovascular disease, bleeding disorders, hyperbilirubinemia, jaundice. Safety in pregnancy, lactation and children not established.

SAFETY: Contains berberine, which has a hypotensive effect. AHPA Class: 2b.[66]

ADVERSE REACTIONS: Anxiety, depression, hallucinations, increased bilirubin, N&V, paralysis, seizures. Photosensitivity with topical application. Caution is urged with use of other herbs containing berberine (Amur cork tree, barberry, celandine, goldthread, Oregon grape).

INTERACTIONS:

Drugs which are substrates of P450 CYP3A4 isozymes[121,227] (see Appendix 38) Preliminary in vitro research has shown that goldenseal may alter metabolism and/or effectiveness of drugs which are substrates of CYP3A4 isozymes. Further research is needed to determine if interaction will also occur in humans.

Acetaminophen/Paracetamol[121] Berberine, a component of goldenseal,

Goldenseal (cont'd.)

decreased hepatic damage of acetaminophen.

Alpha-adrenergic agonist[122,123] (see Appendix 36) Berberine, a component of herb, blocked contraction by phenylephrine, norepinephrine and caffeine.

Anticoagulants and drugs that increase the risk of bleeding[133] (see Appendix 8) Berberine, a component of herb, may inhibit platelet aggregation, which may increase bleeding.

Antiarrhythmics[130] (see Appendix 6) Herb has antiarrhythmic activity, which theoretically may have an additive effect with drug.

Antihypertensives[130] (see Appendix 11) Herb may have calcium channel blocking activity, which may have an additive effect when used concurrently with calcium channel blockers.

CNS depressants[129] (see Appendix 15) Components of goldenseal (berberine, hydrastine) have a sedative effect, which theoretically may be additive with drugs causing sedation.

Cyclophosphamide (Cytoxan, Neosar)[124,128] Berberine, a component of herb, decreased urotoxicity of drug in rats. In another study, berberine decreased retention of chemotherapeutic agents. Concurrent use is not suggested.

Digoxin/Cardiac glycosides[130] Berberine, a component of herb, may have an additive effect with cardiac glycosides.

General anesthetics[130] (see Appendix 20) Berberine, a component of herb, may potentiate hypotensive action of anesthetics.

Highly protein-bound drugs[131] (see Appendix 30) Herb may displace highly protein-bound drugs.

Isoprenaline[135] In research using isolated guinea pig trachea, goldenseal potentiated the relaxation effect of drug.

MAOIs[134] (see Appendix 9) Berberine, a component of herb, competitively inhibited MAO-A in rat brain mitochondria. Avoid concurrent use.

Paclitaxel (Taxol)[124,132] In research using cancer cells, berberine, a component of herb, decreased the effectiveness of drug. Berberine altered expression and function of PGP-170, and may have the same effect on other drugs.

Pentobarbital (Nembutal)[121] Berberine, a component of herb, increased pentobarbital-induced sleep time.

Photosensitivity, drugs causing[127] (see Appendix 29) Preliminary research revealed a potential increase in photosensitivity with use of berberine (a component of herb), which theoretically may be additive with drugs that also increase photosensitivity. Avoid concurrent use.

Pyrimethamine (Daraprim, Fansidar)[126] Berberine, a component of herb, combined with pyrimethamine was more effective than combinations with other antibiotics in treating chloroquine-resistant malaria.

Tetracycline[511] (see Appendix 7) In humans, berberine, a component of herb, when used in combination with tetracycline, reduced drug's effectiveness.

Goldthread /Coptis/*Coptidis rhizoma* Coptis spp. : *Coptis chinensis (huang lian)*
  PART USED: Rhizome.
  CONTRAINDICATIONS: Safety in pregnancy, lactation and children not established. Bleeding disorders.

Goldthread (cont'd.)

SAFETY: Contains berberine, which has a hypotensive effect. AHPA Class: 2b.[66]

ADVERSE REACTIONS: Increased bilirubin, increased bleeding, N&V. Caution is urged with concurrent use of other herbs containing berberine (Amur cork tree, celandine, goldenseal, Oregon grape). Berberine may increase risk of photosensitivity.

INTERACTIONS: SEE INTERACTIONS UNDER GOLDENSEAL FOR BERBERINE.

Esophageal cancer therapies[250] Herb may be a useful antichachetic agent and adjunct to conventional therapies. Berberine in herb may down-regulate tumor IL-6 production.

HIV therapies[338] Suggests that antioxidant activity of herb (*Coptis chinensis*) may delay progress of HIV to AIDS. In rats, the herb inhibited erythrocyte hemolysis, decreased lipid peroxidation in brain and kidney, decreased generation of superoxide peroxidation and decreased hydroxyl radicals.

MAOIs[134] (see Appendix 9) Herb has MAOI activity, which may be additive with MAOIs.

Paclitaxel (Taxol)[512] In research using cancer cells, berberine, a component of herb, decreased the effect of drug. Berberine altered expression and function of PGP170, and may have the same effect on other drugs.

Gossypol *Gossypium spp.*

USES: Male contraceptive (H).

PART USED: Seed extract.

CONTRAINDICATIONS: Hypokalemia, urogenital irritation/inflammation. Safety in pregnancy and lactation not established.

Gossypol (cont'd.)

SAFETY: Chronic use in males may cause sterility.

ADVERSE REACTIONS: Decreased sperm counts, diarrhea, hair discoloration, heart failure, hypokalemia, inhibited spermatogenesis, malnutrition, weakness. Long-term use may cause sterility.

INTERACTIONS:

Drugs metabolized by P450 enzymes[516] (see Appendix 38) Gossypol decreased P450 levels, which may alter the metabolism of drugs that are substrates of P450 isozymes.

Alcohol[514] In research using mice, gossypol caused an aversion to alcohol.

Alkylating agents[513] (see Appendix 16) Gossypol may have a synergistic effect when combined with alkylating agents. Further research in humans is needed.

Digoxin/Cardiac glycosides and antiarrhythmics[518,519] (see Appendix 6) Gossypol delayed the onset of digoxin-induced antiarrhythmias in in vitro research. Gossypol increases the loss of potassium, which may increase the toxicity of cardiac glycosides.

Diuretics[519] (see Appendix 6) Gossypol increases the excretion of potassium, which may be additive with diuretics. Risk of hypokalemia is increased.

Isoproterenol[518] Gossypol decreased the inotropic effect of drug.

Pentobarbital (Nembutal)[515] In rats, gossypol acetic acid increased drug-induced sleep time.

Stimulant laxatives[519] Potassium loss from laxative and gossypol may be additive. Avoid concurrent use.

Thyroid hormone replacement therapy[517] In research using rats, gossypol

Gossypol (cont'd.)

decreased serum thyroid hormone concentration. Concurrent use with thyroid replacement therapy may require an increase in dosage of drug.

Gotu Kola Centella asiatica

USES: Venous insufficiency (H), varicose veins (H), wound healing (A).

PART USED: Herb.

CONTRAINDICATIONS: Safety in pregnancy, lactation and children not established.

SAFETY: AHPA Class: 1.[66]

ADVERSE REACTIONS: Allergic reaction, contact dermatitis. Large doses may be sedating.

INTERACTIONS:

Alcohol[515] In research using rats, herb had a protective effect against alcohol-induced ulcers.

Aspirin[515] In research using rats, herb had a protective effect against aspirin-induced ulcers.

CNS depressants[916] (see Appendix 15) Brahmoside and brahminoside, components of gotu kola, have a sedative effect, which theoretically may be additive with sedative drugs.

Insulin/Oral hypoglycemic agents[50-excessive doses] (see Appendix 24) Herb contains asiaticosides, which have a hyperglycemic effect. Monitor patients with diabetes for elevated blood glucose.

Grape *Vitis vinifera*

USES: Atherosclerosis (H), edema due to injury (H), night vision (H), post surgery edema (H), venous insufficiency (H).

PART USED: Seed (oligomeric proanthocyanidin extract).

CONTRAINDICATIONS: Safety in pregnancy, lactation and children not established.

ADVERSE REACTIONS: Allergic reaction, GI distress.

INTERACTIONS:

Drugs metabolized by P450 enzymes[520] (see Appendix 38) Procyanidolic oligomer (extracted from grape seeds) may inhibit the metabolism of drugs which are substrates of CYP1A2 and CYP3A4.

Acetaminophen/Paracetamol[295] Proanthocyanidin IH636 grape seed extract decreased hepatotoxicity of acetaminophen in mice.

Alcohol[318] In research using rats, grape polyphenols extracted from skin and seeds decreased hepatic injury from alcohol, but had no effect on ethanol-induced lipid changes.

Anticoagulants and drugs that increase the risk of bleeding[336] (see Appendix 8) Flavonoids from purple grape juice decreased platelet aggregation and increased platelet-derived nitric oxide release and superoxide production. Research was in vitro and in vivo, using 20 humans. Increased risk of bleeding with high doses.

Idarubicin[348] In human non-malignant cultured cells, IH636 grape seed proanthocyanidin extract decreased toxicity of drug to cells through its ability to protect against free radicals. There was a decrease in the number of cells which underwent apoptosis.

4-hydroxyperoxycyclophosphamide[348] In human non-malignant cultured

Grape (cont'd.)

cells, IH636 grape seed proanthocyanidin extract decreased toxicity of drug to cells through its ability to protect against free radicals. There was a decrease in the number of cells which underwent apoptosis.

Gravel Root *Eupatorium purpureum*
PART USED: Herb, rhizome, root.
CONTRAINDICATIONS: Do not use in pregnancy, lactation or children.
SAFETY: Contains pyrrolizidine alkaloids, which are carcinogenic. External use only. AHPA Class: 2a, 2b, 2c, 2d—not long-term.[66]
ADVERSE REACTIONS: Potential veno-occlusive disease.
INTERACTIONS:
Hepatotoxic drugs[521] (see Appendix 21) Due to pyrrolizidine alkaloid content of herb, drugs which are hepatotoxic should not be used concurrently.

Greater Celandine *Chelidonium majus*
PART USED: Herb.
CONTRAINDICATIONS: Safety in pregnancy, lactation and children not established. Biliary tract disease, gallbladder disease, hepatitis and other liver diseases.
SAFETY: Cases of acute hepatitis have been reported. AHPA Class: 2b, 2d—not for children.[66]
ADVERSE REACTIONS: Contact dermatitis, hemolytic anemia, hepatitis.
INTERACTIONS:
Gamma-irradiation[522] (thiophosphate-modified alkaloids) (Ukrain) a component of

Greater Celandine (cont'd.)

greater celandine, minimized radiation impact on endocrine system / normalized intracellular glucocorticoid-receptor system in animals.

Guar Gum *Cyamopsis tetragonolobus*

USES: Diabetes (H), constipation, dumping syndrome (H), hypercholesterolemia (H).
PART USED: Seed.
CONTRAINDICATIONS: GI obstruction, ileus.
SAFETY: AHPA Class: 2d—take with 8 oz liquid, not with bowel obstruction.[66]
ADVERSE REACTIONS: Abdominal distension, bowel obstruction, diarrhea, flatulence, GI distress, nausea.
INTERACTIONS:

Herb may reduce intestinal absorption of other drugs.[526]
Acetaminophen/Paracetamol[526,527] Guar gum slows absorption of drug, and may affect amount absorbed.
Cimetidine (Tagamet)[526] In research animals, guar gum delayed drug absorption.
Digoxin/Cardiac glycosides[80] Digoxin levels decreased during early absorption, but 24-hour urine drug was similar whether consuming or not consuming guar gum.
Enteral nutrition support[523] The addition of partially hydrolyzed guar gum (20 g sunfiber/ 1000 ml) to enteral feedings decreased the incidence of diarrhea.
Ethinyl estradiol[528] In research using rabbits, amount of drug absorbed was decreased.
Hydrochlorothiazide[526] In research using animals, guar gum delayed and decreased absorption of drug.

Insulin/Oral hypoglycemic agents[49,86,525,529] (see Appendix 24) Herb delays absorption of carbohydrates, which may lower blood glucose levels.

Nitrofurantoin (Macrobid, Macrodantin)[524] Guar gum delayed absorption of drug.

Penicillin[80] Guar gum decreased AUC and peak concentration of drug.

Guarana *Paullinia cupana*

USES: Weight loss (H-equivocal).

PART USED: Seed.

CONTRAINDICATIONS: Safety in pregnancy, lactation and children not established. Anxiety, bleeding disorders, cardiovascular disease, HTN, kidney disease, ulcers.

SAFETY: 2.6%-7% caffeine (2x amount in coffee). GRAS (flavoring). AHPA Class: 2d—not long-term or excessive amounts.[66]

ADVERSE REACTIONS: Anxiety, arrhythmias, GI distress, headache, HTN, insomnia, N&V, nervousness, palpitations, restlessness, tremors.

INTERACTIONS:

Acetaminophen/Paracetamol[636] Caffeine, a component of guarana, increases the analgesic effect of acetaminophen.

Alkaloids (see Appendix 4)[4] High tannin content of seed may cause alkaloids to become insoluble and precipitate.

Anticoagulants and drugs that increase the risk of bleeding[530] (see Appendix 8) In research animals, herb decreased thromboxane synthesis, which is responsible for antiaggregatory effect.

Aspirin[638] Caffeine in guarana increases effectiveness of ASA pain relief.

Guarana (cont'd.)

Benzodiazepines[637] (see Appendix 13) Theoretical decrease in sedative and antianxiolytic effects, due to stimulant effect of guarana.

Beta-adrenergic agonists[101] (see Appendix 36) Concurrent use may increase the risk of cardiac arrhythmias.

Cimetidine (Tagamet)[658] Drug may decrease clearance of caffeine, a component of guarana. Theoretically, this may increase serum caffeine and increase caffeine side effects. Results of research have been equivocal.

Clozapine, and possibly other drugs metabolized by P450 CYP1A2[296,350,531] (see Appendix 38) Caffeine intakes greater than 400 mg may decrease clearance of clozapine (and possibly induce other drugs metabolized by CYP1A2). In randomized crossover research of 12 males, the AUC of clozapine was increased by 19% and oral clearance of clozapine was decreased 14% with concurrent caffeine intake. Guarana leaf contains 76,000 ppm of caffeine.

Disulfiram (Antabuse)[654] Drug may decrease metabolism of caffeine, a component of guarana. The result may be increased serum caffeine and caffeine side effects.

Ephedra/Ephedrine[434] Concurrent use of high amounts of products containing caffeine (such as guarana) and stimulants may have an additive stimulant effect.

Ergotamine (Ergomar)[653] Caffeine, a component of herb, increases serum level and efficacy of drug. The drug Wigraine contains both.

Fluvoxamine (Luvox)[658] Drug decreases metabolism of caffeine, a component of guarana. This may increase serum caffeine and increase caffeine side effects

Furafylline[658] Drug inhibits CYP1A2, which decreases the metabolism of caffeine, a component of guarana. This may increase serum levels of caffeine and increase caffeine side effects.

Grapefruit Juice[531] Grapefruit juice inhibits CYP1A2, which decreases the metabolism of caffeine, a component of guarana, thereby increasing caffeine side effects.

Ibuprofen[650] Concurrent use of guarana and drug may enhance pain relief.

Idroclamide[658] Drug alters caffeine metabolism, which increases serum levels of caffeine and increases caffeine side effects.

Insulin/Oral hypoglycemic agents[84,651] (see Appendix 24) Caffeine, a component of coffee, may increase insulin resistance. Monitor patients with diabetes.

Lithium (Eskalith, Lithobid, Lithonate, Lithotabs)[658] Caffeine, a component of guarana, increases the renal excretion of lithium, which may decrease serum levels of drug. Discontinuation of herb use may likewise increase serum levels of drug.

MAOIs[109] (see Appendix 9) Excessive amounts of guarana may increase risk of hypertension.

Methotrexate (Rheumatrex)[224] Caffeine in guarana may decrease effectiveness of drug.

Methoxsalen (8-MOP, Oxsoralen)[658] Drug inhibits metabolism of caffeine, a component of guarana. Increased serum caffeine may increase side effects.

Mexiletine (Mexitil)[656] Drug delays metabolism of caffeine, a component of guarana. This may increase side effects of caffeine.

Oral contraceptives[658] Long-term use of oral contraceptives (ethinyl estradiol or

Guarana (cont'd.)

estradiol) causes an impaired CYP1A2 clearance of caffeine, a component of guarana. This may increase serum caffeine and increase caffeine side effects.

Phenylpropanolamine[658] Drug may inhibit the metabolism of caffeine, a component of guarana, increasing serum levels of caffeine and side effects. On 11/6/00, the FDA released an advisory to remove phenylpropanolamine from all products.[657]

Propranolol (Inderal)[394] Blood pressure may be increased by caffeine in guarana.

Quinolones (ciprofloxacin, enoxacin, grepafloxacin, norfloxacin, pefloxacin, tosufloxacin)[658] Drug may decrease clearance of caffeine, a component of guarana. This may increase the side effects of caffeine due to increased serum caffeine.

Terbinafine (Lamisil)[658] Drug may inhibit the metabolism of caffeine, a component of guarana. This may increase serum levels of caffeine and increase caffeine side effects. Research on this interaction has been equivocal.

Theophylline (Uniphyl, Uni-Dur)[658] Concurrent use of theophylline and caffeine may lead to an increase in serum levels of both.

Verapamil (Calan, Isoptin, Verelan)[658] Drug delays clearance of caffeine, a component of guarana. This may increase caffeine side effects.

Guava *Psidium guajava, Psidium spp.*

INTERACTIONS:

Alkaloids (see Appendix 4)[4] High tannin content of bark may cause alkaloids to become insoluble and precipitate.

Oral hypoglycemic agents[277] (see Appendix 24) In research using rats and humans, guava juice was found to be hypoglycemic. Juice may be helpful in regulating blood sugar in type 2 diabetes and syndrome X. Monitor blood glucose.

Guggul *Commiphora mukul*

USES: Hypercholesterolemia (H), Nodulocystic acne (H).

PART USED: Gum resin.

CONTRAINDICATIONS: Hypothyroidism, hyperthyroidism, pregnancy.

SAFETY: AHPA Class: 2b.[66]

ADVERSE REACTIONS: GI distress, nausea.

INTERACTIONS:

Diltiazem (Cardizem)[241] Gugulipid (oleoresin similar to resin in colestipol and cholestyramine) decreased peak serum concentration and area under the curve of diltiazem.

Propranolol (Inderal)[241] Guguilipid (oleoresin similar to resin in colestipol and cholestyramine) decreased peak serum concentration and area under the curve of propranolol.

Thyroid replacement therapy[243] Z-Guggulsterone (ketosteroid from oleoresin in guggul) may increase uptake of iodine by thyroid gland and increase oxygen uptake in liver and bicep tissues.

Gulancha Plant *Tinospora cordifolia*
  INTERACTIONS:
   Insulin/Oral hypoglycemic agents[53,105,309] (see Appendix 24) In research using rats, gulancha plant decreased blood glucose in mild to moderate diabetes, which may be dependent on amount of beta cell function. Maximum effect of aqueous extract was found at 400 mg/kg/d and at 3rd week of administration. Monitor blood glucose in patients with diabetes.

Gymnema *Gymnema sylvestre*
  PART USED: Leaf.
  ADVERSE REACTIONS: Decreased ability to taste sweetness.
  INTERACTIONS:
   Insulin/Oral hypoglycemic agents[532,533] (see Appendix 24) Herb has hypoglycemic action. Herb may decrease sucrose absorption and enhance beta cell function.

Hawthorn *Crataegus oxyacantha*
  USES: CHF (H), hyperlipidemia (A).
  PART USED: Leaf, flower, fruit.
  CONTRAINDICATIONS: Bleeding disorders, chest pain, low blood pressure.
  ADVERSE REACTIONS: Allergic response, fatigue. Large doses may cause hypotension and sedation.
  INTERACTIONS:

Anticoagulants and drugs that increase the risk of bleeding[538] (see Appendix 8)
Herb inhibits biosynthesis of thromboxane A2, which may increase bleeding risk.

Antihypertensives[537] (see Appendix 11) Herb may relax vascular tone, which may increase the effect of antihypertensives.

Cardiac drugs[535] (see Appendix 14) Herb may interfere with therapeutic effect of drug.

CNS depressants[536] (see Appendix 15) In research using mice, herb had sedative activity, which may be additive when combined with CNS depressants.

Digoxin/Cardiac glycosides[534,535] Concurrent use of herb with drug may alter effects of drug. Arrhythmias occurred sooner in one study using rats administered this herb, but in other study arrhythmias were decreased. More research is needed before concurrent use.

Vasodilators[537] (see Appendix 14) Herb may relax vascular tone, which may be additive when used with vasodilators.

Heal-All *Prunella vulgaris*

PART USED: Herb

SAFETY: AHPA Class: 1.[66]

INTERACTIONS:

HIV therapies[338] (see Appendix 22) Antioxidant activity of herb may delay the progression of HIV to AIDS. In rats, the herb inhibited erythrocyte hemolysis, decreased lipid peroxidation in brain and kidney and decreased generation of superoxide peroxidation and hydroxyl radicals.

Hellebore, American *Veratrum viride*
   PART USED: Root.
   CONTRAINDICATIONS: Safety in pregnancy and lactation not established. Cardiac disease.
   SAFETY: Atropine has been used in acute poisonings. AHPA Class: 3.[66]
   ADVERSE REACTIONS: Bradycardia. Large doses: bradycardia, decreased mental status, heart block, hypotension, nausea, substernal chest pain, vomiting.
   INTERACTIONS:
      Antihypertensives[539] (see Appendix 11) Herb may further lower blood pressure.

Hemlock *Conium maculatum*
   SAFETY: All parts of plant are poisonous and should not be consumed.
   ADVERSE REACTIONS Death, incoordination, initial central nervous system stimulation, muscular weakness, neuromuscular blockage, trembling. Use during pregnancy leads to malformations.

Henbane *Hyoscyamus niger*
   PART USED: Leaf.
   CONTRAINDICATIONS: Pregnancy, arrhythmias, GI stenosis, ileus, narrow-angle glaucoma, megacolon, prostate adenoma, pulmonary edema, tachycardia.
   SAFETY: Contains hyoscyamine and scopolamine alkaloids, which have anticholinergic activity.
   ADVERSE REACTIONS: Blurred vision, difficulty urinating, mydriasis, prostate adenoma, sedation, tachycardia, xerostomia. Overdoses have caused death.

INTERACTIONS:
Anticholinergic drugs[540] (see Appendix 5) Herb contains hyoscyamine and scopolamine alkaloids, which may have an additive effect with anticholinergic drugs.

Hops *Humulus lupulus*

PART USED: Strobiles.
CONTRAINDICATIONS: Depression, estrogen-sensitive cancers.
SAFETY: GRAS (oil, extract, oleoresin). AHPA Class: 2d—not with depression.[66]
ADVERSE REACTIONS: Allergic reaction, contact dermatitis.
INTERACTIONS:
Drugs metabolized by P450 CYP2B isozymes[262] (see Appendix 38) ß-Myrcene (acyclic monoterpene in essential oil of hops) may induce CYP2B isozymes, which may decrease serum level of drugs (including barbiturates and cyclophophamide) metabolized by these enzymes. This research was conducted on rat hepatic microsomes. Further research is needed to determine if serum levels of drugs metabolized by P450 enzymes are altered in humans by ß-Myrcene. Health care providers need to be aware of potential for alteration in serum level of drugs metabolized by CYP2B isozymes.
Drugs metabolized by P450 CYP1A isozymes[266] (see Appendix 38) In this in vitro (liver microsomes) study, CYP1A1 and CYP1A2 were inhibited by flavonoids in hops. Further research is needed using human subjects to determine if these enzymes are inhibited. Patients who are taking drugs which are substrates of these enzymes should be monitored.

Hops (cont'd.)

Alcohol[542] Herb has sedative activity, which may have an additive sedative effect when combined with alcohol.

CNS depressants[542] (see Appendix 15) Herb has sedative activity, which may be additive when combined with drugs with sedative activity.

Hormone replacement therapy/Oral contraceptives[541,543] In research using human cells, hops bound competitively to estrogen receptors, possibly affecting estrogenic activity. Component of hops with estrogenic activity is 8-prenylnaringen. Effect on hormone replacement therapy or oral contraceptives not known.

Horehound *Marrubium vulgare*

PART USED: Herb.

CONTRAINDICATIONS: Safety in pregnancy not established.

SAFETY: GRAS (spice, seasoning, flavoring, oil, extract, oleoresin). AHPA Class: 2b.

ADVERSE REACTIONS: High doses may cause cardiac irregularities.

INTERACTIONS:

Antihypertensives[544] (see Appendix 11) In research using rats, herb had a hypotensive effect, which may be additive with antihypertensive drugs.

Insulin/Oral hypoglycemic agents[545] (see Appendix 24) In research using rats, herb had hypoglycemic activity, which may be additive when combined with diabetes medications. Monitor blood glucose.

Horse Chestnut *Aesculus hippocastanum*

USES: Post-operative or post-traumatic swelling (H), varicose veins (H), chronic venous insufficiency (CVI) (H), hypercholesterolemia (A), diuretic (A-aesculin).

PART USED: Seed.

CONTRAINDICATIONS: Bleeding disorders, open wounds on skin, liver disease. Safety in pregnancy and lactation not established.

SAFETY: Consumption of large quantity of seeds has led to death. Use only products that have had esculin removed.

ADVERSE REACTIONS: Allergic response, anaphylaxis, bleeding, cholestatic liver disease (after IM extract), depression, diarrhea, dilated pupils, GI distress, hepatic injury, incoordination, muscle twitching, muscle weakness, N&V, nephropathy, paralysis, pruritus, stupor, urticaria.

INTERACTIONS:

Alcohol[550] Aescine, a component of horse chestnut, is protective against ethanol-induced gastric ulcers.

Anticoagulants and drugs that increase the risk of bleeding[549] (see Appendix 8) Esculetin, a component of horse chestnut, inhibits platelet aggregation, which may increase the risk of bleeding.

Diuretics[551] (see Appendix 11) Aesculine, a component of horse chestnut, has diuretic activity. The renal excretion of sodium, chloride and potassium is increased.

Insulin/Oral hypoglycemic agents[546,547,548] (see Appendix 24) Escins Ia, Ib, IIa, and IIb, components of horse chestnut, have hypoglycemic activity. It is not known if effect is additive with medications used for diabetes. Components of herb may delay gastric emptying and decrease intestinal absorption of sucrose.

Horseradish *Armoracia rusticana*
   PART USED: Rhizome, root.
   CONTRAINDICATIONS: Pregnancy, children, hypothyroidism, hyperthyroidism, renal inflammation or renal disease, gastric or duodenal ulcers.
   SAFETY: GRAS (spice, seasoning, flavoring). AHPA Class: 2d—not with gastric or kidney irritation.[66]
   ADVERSE REACTIONS: Diarrhea, GI distress, irritated mucous membranes, vomiting.
   INTERACTIONS:
      Thyroid replacement therapy[552] Kaempferol, a component of horseradish, inhibits thyroid peroxidase, which is involved in the biosynthesis of thyroid hormone.

Horsetail *Equisetum arvense*
   PART USED: Herb.
   CONTRAINDICATIONS: Children should not consume powdered herb. Safety in pregnancy and lactation not established. CHF, kidney disease.
   SAFETY: Enzyme in horsetail destroys thiamine (heating destroys enzyme). Plant concentrates may contain heavy metals, especially zinc. AHPA Class: 2d—not with cardiac or renal dysfunction.[66]
   ADVERSE REACTIONS: Dermatitis, hypokalemia, thiamine deficiency.
   INTERACTIONS:
      Digoxin/Cardiac glycosides[1] Herb has diuretic effect, which may increase the risk of hypokalemia and drug toxicity.
      Diuretics[1] (see Appendix 11) Herb has diuretic effect, which may be additive with drugs having a diuretic action.

149

Horsetail (cont'd.)

Lithium (Eskalith, Lithobid, Lithotabs)[1] Herb has diuretic effect, which may increase the toxicity of lithium.

Huperzine A

USES: Alzheimer's disease (H-equivocal), memory enhancement (H).

PART USED: Alkaloid from Chinese club moss (*Huperzia serrata*).

CONTRAINDICATIONS: HTN, kidney disease. Safety in pregnancy and lactation not established.

SAFETY: Inhibits acetylcholinesterase, which breaks down acetylcholine, leading to an increase in acetylcholine.

INTERACTIONS:

Anticholinergic drugs[553] (see Appendix 5) Herb has anticholinesterase activity, which may interfere with drug therapy.

Cholinergic drugs[553] (see Appendix 17) Herb has anticholinesterase activity, which may interfere with drug therapy.

Hydrophila *Asteracanthus longifolia*

INTERACTIONS:

Oral hypoglycemic agents[335] (see Appendix 24) Aqueous extract decreased fasting glucose and improved glucose tolerance in rats. The maximum effect was found with 10 ml/kg (5 g/kg plant material). Suggests a mechanism of action similar to sulfonylureas. Monitor blood glucose.

Iboga *Tabernanthe iboga*

PART USED: Root.

ADVERSE REACTIONS: Anxiety, apprehension, convulsions, euphoria, hallucinations, hypotension, paralysis, respiratory arrest.

INTERACTIONS:

Alcohol[246] Ibogaine, a component of herb, reduced alcohol intake in alcohol-preferring laboratory animals. Hypothetically, this may be helpful in treating alcoholism.

Cocaine[554,555] Herb decreased craving for drug in a patient being treated for drug dependency. A safer congener of ibogaine, 18-methoxycoronaridine, has been developed without the side effects of ibogaine.

Drugs altering serotonin levels in brain[555] (see Appendix 33 & 34) Ibogaine, an indole alkaloid from iboga, increases serotonin levels in the brain, which may alter the effect of drugs altering serotonin levels.

Heroin[554,555] Herb decreased craving for drug in a patient being treated for drug dependency. A safer congener of ibogaine, 18-methoxycoronaridine, has been developed without the side effects of ibogaine. 18-Methoxycoronaridine has the potential to be developed as a drug.

Morphine[555] Ibogaine, a component of iboga, decreased craving for drug. A safer congener of ibogaine, 18-methoxycoronaridine, has been developed without the side effects of ibogaine.

Iceland Moss *Cetraria islandica*

USES: Oral or pharyngeal inflammation and dryness (H).

PART USED: Thallus.

CONTRAINDICATIONS: Gastric or duodenal ulcers. Safety in pregnancy and lactation not established.

SAFETY: Possible heavy metal contamination due to plant's ability to bioconcentrate metals. Contains potentially toxic lichen acids. GRAS (Flavoring in alcoholic beverage). AHPA Class: 1—decoction or infusion (tea); 2d—not with gastric or duodenal ulcers.[66]

ADVERSE REACTIONS: GI irritant.

INTERACTIONS:

Herb may reduce intestinal absorption of other drugs.[4]

Indian Snakeroot *Rauwolfia serpentina*

USES: Mild essential HTN (H).

PART USED: Root.

CONTRAINDICATIONS: Safety in pregnancy and lactation not established. Bleeding disorders, depression, gastric or duodenal ulcers, pheochromocytoma.

SAFETY: Should only be used under supervision of a qualified health care professional.

ADVERSE REACTIONS: May slow motor responses. Bradyarrhythmia (homeopathic dose), decreased sexual potency, depression, fatigue, GI distress, nasal congestion.

INTERACTIONS:

Indian Snakeroot (cont'd.)

Drugs that are substrates of PGP[559] (see Appendix 38) Reserpine, a component of herb inhibits PGP. Serum level of drugs that are transported by PGP may be increased by concurrent herb use.

Alcohol[116] Concurrent use may cause additive sedation.

Anticoagulants and drugs that increase the risk of bleeding[556] (see Appendix 8) In preliminary research, raubasine, a component of herb, reduced platelet aggregation. Effect of concurrent use with anticoagulants is not known.

Antihypertensives[116] (see Appendix 11) Herb may potentiate drug (risk of hypotension).

Appetite suppressants[1] Herb potentiates drug (may increase blood pressure).

Barbiturates[1] (see Appendix 12) Concurrent use may cause additive sedation.

Benzodiazepines[558] (see Appendix 13) Raubasine, a component of herb, has benzodiazepine agonist-type activity.

CNS depressants[116] (see Appendix 15) Potentially additive sedative effects.

Cough and cold medicines[1] Herb may potentiate drug and increase blood pressure.

Digoxin/Cardiac glycosides[1,116] Concurrent use may increase risk of arrhythmias or bradycardia.

Diuretics[557] (see Appendix 11) Herb used concurrently with diuretic for mild HTN was more effective than the diuretic alone. Concurrent treatment should not be undertaken unless under medical supervision.

General anesthetics[116] (see Appendix 20) Possible blood pressure decrease.

Levodopa (Lodosyn)[1],[116] Decreased drug effectiveness and possible increase in extrapyramidal symptoms.

MAOIs[116] (see Appendix 9) Concurrent use may lead to excitation and hypertension.

Neuroleptics[1] Mutual potentiation.

Quinidine (Quinaglute)[116] Concurrent use may increase cardiac depression.

Sympathomimetics[1],[116] (see Appendix 36) Herb potentiates drug (may increase blood pressure).

Tricyclic antidepressants[116] (see Appendix 9) Herb adds to beta-adrenoceptor blocking activity of drug.

Inulin linear beta (2-1)-fructan

INTERACTIONS:

5-Fluorouracil[274] Research using mice showed additive effect of 5-fluorouracil and inulin (15% of diet) combination.

Cyclophosphamide (Cytoxan, Neosar)[274] Research using mice showed synergistic effect of cyclophosphamide and inulin (15% of diet) combination.

Cytarabine (Cytosar-U)[274] Research using mice showed synergistic effect of cytarabine and inulin (15% of diet) combination.

Doxorubicin (Adriamycin)[274] Research using mice showed additive effect of doxorubicin and inulin (15% of diet) combination.

Methotrexate (Rheumatrex)[274] Research using mice showed synergistic effect of methotrexate and inulin (15% of diet) combination.

Inulin (cont'd.)

Vincristine (Oncovin, Vincasar)[274] Research using mice showed additive effect of vincristine and inulin (15% of diet) combination.

Isothiocyanates and diallyl sulfide In garlic (*Allium sativum*) and cruciferous vegetables – cabbage, broccoli, Brussels sprouts
INTERACTIONS:
Drugs metabolized by P450 CYP1A2, CYP2B1, CYP2E1 and CYP3A4[325] (see Appendix 38) Organosulfur-containing herbs containing isothiocyanates may alter the metabolism of drugs. These changes in enzymes also enhance the excretion of environmental chemicals.

Ivy *Hedera helix*
PART USED: Leaf.
CONTRAINDICATIONS: Safety in pregnancy and lactation not established. Bleeding disorders.
ADVERSE REACTIONS: Allergic and contact dermatitis.
INTERACTIONS:
Anticoagulants and drugs that increase the risk of bleeding[563] (see Appendix 8) In vitro research showed that methylene chloride extract and methanol extract of *Hedera helix* had antithrombin activity. It is not known if herb has antithrombic activity in humans and whether bleeding risk increases with concurrent use of drugs that also increase bleeding.

Ivy Gourd *Coccinia indica*

INTERACTIONS:

Insulin/Oral hypoglycemic agents[560,561,562] (see Appendix 24) Extract of herb has hypoglycemic effect due to its pectin content. Patients on diabetes medication should be monitored to prevent hypoglycemia.

Jamaica Dogwood Bark *Piscidia erythrina*

SAFETY: Safety of use in humans not established.

INTERACTIONS:

CNS depressants[563] (see Appendix 15) In research using mice, herb had sedative activity. It is not known if herb has sedative activity in humans or if sedation is additive when combined with drugs with sedating effect.

Japanese Honeysuckle *Lonicera japonica* jin yin hua (flowers) ren dong teng (stem)

PART USED: Flowers, stem.

SAFETY: AHPA Class: 1.[66]

INTERACTIONS:

Anticoagulants and drugs that increase the risk of bleeding[565] (see Appendix 8) Methyl caffeate, 3,4-di-O-caffeoylquinic acid and methyl 3,4-di-O-caffeoylquinate inhibited platelet aggregation in cell cultures. It is not known if herb has antiplatelet aggregation effect in humans, but caution is urged in patients taking drugs which increase the risk of bleeding.

Java Brucea *Brucea javanica*

SAFETY: Herb contains bruceoside A and B and yadanzioside F, which have been found to be toxic in mice.

INTERACTIONS:

Chloroquine[566] Dihydrobruceajavanin A and bruceacanthinoside were found to have activity against quinine-resistant malaria. Potential synergism has not been studied yet.

Java Plum *Eugenia jambolana*

INTERACTIONS:

Insulin/Oral hypoglycemic agents[304,309] (see Appendix 24) In research using rats, java plum decreased blood glucose in mild to moderate diabetes, which may be dependent on beta cell function. Maximum effect was found with 200 mg/kg/d of lyophilized powder at the 6th week of administration. Herb may be useful in treatment of those with syndrome X, polycystic ovary disease and those at high risk of developing diabetes. Monitor patients with diabetes.

Java Tea *Orthosiphon spicatus, Orthosiphon stamineus*

PART USED: Leaf.

CONTRAINDICATIONS: Safety in pregnancy and lactation not established. CHF, edema, kidney disease.

INTERACTIONS:

Diuretics[567] (see Appendix 11) Herb was found to have a diuretic effect in rats. Concurrent use with diuretic drugs may lead to loss of diuresis control.

INTERACTIONS:

Cisplatin (Platinol)[341] In research using rats, medicinal herbs decreased the nephrotoxicity of cisplatin.

Cisplatinum[340] Abstract states that 49 out of 95 patients were given Chinese medicinal herb decoction concurrently with cisplatinum. In patients receiving herbs, there was a decrease in nephrotoxicity of cisplatinum.

Jimsonweed *Datura stramonium*

PART USED: Leaf, seed.

SAFETY: Jimsonweed contains toxic anticholinergic alkaloids, and fatal poisonings have been reported. Most poisonings have been effectively treated with gastrointestinal decontamination, supportive care and physostigmine.

ADVERSE REACTIONS: Symptoms of poisoning include agitation, blurred vision, coma, difficulty urinating, dilated pupils, disorientation, hallucinations, mydriasis, tachycardia, seizures and xerostomia.

INTERACTIONS:

Anticholinergic drugs[568] (see Appendix 5) Herb has anticholinergic activity. Herb's effect may be additive with drugs that also have anticholinergic effect.

Juniper *Juniperus spp*

PART USED: Fruit/berry.

CONTRAINDICATIONS: Safety in pregnancy not established. Kidney disease

SAFETY: Not for long-term use. Potentially carcinogenic--causes DNA damage. GRAS (oil, extract, oleoresin). AHPA Class: 2b, 2d—not greater than 4-6 weeks, not

Juniper (cont'd.)

with inflammatory kidney disease.[66]

ADVERSE REACTIONS: Allergic response, kidney inflammation, skin irritation. Overdose or prolonged use may cause kidney damage.

INTERACTIONS:

Anticoagulants, including warfarin (Coumadin), not heparin[719] (see Appendix 8) Herb may contain variable amounts of vitamin K, which antagonizes the anticoagulant effect of warfarin.

Insulin/Oral hypoglycemic agents[173,401,569] (see Appendix 24) In research using rats, herb had hypoglycemic action, in part from the potentiation of insulin release from the pancreas and an increase in peripheral glucose uptake. Patients taking diabetes medication with herb should be monitored to prevent possible hypoglycemia.

Kava *Piper methysticum*

USES: Anxiety (H).

PART USED: Rhizome, root.

CONTRAINDICATIONS: Bile duct obstruction, bleeding disorders, depression, pregnancy, lactation, liver disease. Safety in pregnancy and lactation not established.

SAFETY: Not when driving vehicle. Do not use for extended periods of time unless directed by health care professional. MONITOR LIVER FUNCTION. Several countries have or are considering placing a ban on the use of kava. The American Botanical Association has drafted guidelines for the safe use of kava until case reports of liver damage from kava use can be fully examined. These guidelines are:

(1) Persons with liver disease, those who use drugs that may damage the liver and those who consume alcohol on a regular basis should not use kava. (2) Limit use to 4 weeks or less. (3) Discontinue if symptoms of jaundice occur. (4) Consult a health care professional prior to use of kava if there was prior liver disease or the suspicion of prior liver disease.[920] Germany may ban kava due to numerous cases of liver disease. AHPA Class: 2b, 2c, 2d—not excessive dose.[66]

ADVERSE REACTIONS: Allergic response, extrapyramidal effects, GI distress, hepatitis, kava dermopathy, ocular accomodation disturbance, red eyes, scaly rash, yellowing of skin.

INTERACTIONS:

Alcohol[573,575,576] In research using WS 1490 (kava extract), no significant difference was noted on battery of performance tests with blood alcohol level of 0.05%. In research on mice, the concurrent use of alcohol and a lipid-soluble extract of kava increased hypnotic action. Sedating effect due to lipid-soluble components of kava. In light of reports of hepatotoxicity, consumption of alcohol concurrently with kava is not recommended.

Alprazolam (Xanax)[22] Excessive sedation—lethargy, not coma.

Anticoagulants and drugs that increase the risk of bleeding[572] (see Appendix 8) Kavain, a component of kava, inhibits platelet aggregation, which may increase the risk of bleeding.

Antipsychotics[220] Herb may decrease extrapyramidal side effects of drug.

Barbiturates[570] (see Appendix 12) Kava administered concurrently with pentobarbital had an additive effect (GABA-A receptor binding).

Kava (cont'd.)

Benzodiazepines (see Appendix 13) See case report for **Alprazolam**, above.

CNS depressants[570] (see Appendix 15) Herb may cause excessive sedation via action on GABA-A receptor binding.

Estrogen replacement therapy[571] Kava was successfully administered successfully with estrogen replacement therapy for menopausal-related anxiety. There was a reduction in HAM-A score.

Hepatotoxic drugs (see Appendix 21) Numerous reports of liver toxicity. Kava should not be used concurrently with hepatotoxic drugs.

Levodopa (Lodosyn)[577] Herb decreases effectiveness of drug.

Psychopharmacological agents[1] (see Appendix 9) Herb potentiates drug.

Surgery, drugs used during[307] It has been recommended that herb be discontinued at least 24 hours prior to surgery. Herb may increase sedative effect of anesthetics.

Kelp Various spp.

CONTRAINDICATIONS: Bleeding disorders, hypothyroidism, hyperthyroidism, thyroid disease.

SAFETY: Allergic reaction. Kelp may contain variable amounts of arsenic. Contains high amounts of iodine; not for long-term use. Safety in pregnancy and lactation not established.

ADVERSE REACTIONS: Autoimmune thrombocytopenia, dyserythropoiesis.

INTERACTIONS:

Anticoagulants and drugs that increase the risk of bleeding[574] (see

Kelp (cont'd.)

Appendix 8) Fucoidan fraction of kelp has anticoagulant activity, which theoretically may be additive with anticoagulant drugs.

Iodine-containing drugs[38] High iodine content of kelp may interfere with drug.

Lithium[578] High iodine intake may increase the risk of lithium-induced hypothyroidism

Thyroid replacement therapy[38] Herb may interfere with drug.

Khat *Catha edulis*

PART USED: Leaf.

CONTRAINDICATIONS: Hypothyroidism, hyperthyroidism, pregnancy, lactation, children.

SAFETY: Khat has been found to cause genetic damage in humans. Contains the stimulant cathinone, which is similar in structure and pharmacology to amphetamines.

ADVERSE REACTIONS: Anorexia, brown pigmentation of gingiva, cerebral hemorrhage, constipation, decreased sex drive, decreased rate of urine flow, delayed gastric emptying, hepatic cirrhosis, impotency, increased heart rate and blood pressure, low birth weight, khat addiction, migraine, myocardial infarction, optic atrophy, oral cancer, pulmonary edema.

INTERACTIONS:

Amoxicillin (Amoxil)[583] Take medication no sooner than 2 hours after khat chewing to prevent a decrease in the bioavailability of drug.

Amphetamines[579,580] Cathinone, a component of khat, has action similar to amphetamines. Effects are thought to be additive.

Khat (cont'd.)

Ampicillin[583] Take medication no sooner than 2 hours after khat chewing to prevent a decrease in the bioavailability of drug.

Furazolidone (Furoxone)[579] Drug has MAOI activity. Herb may increase pressor sensitivity.

Guanethidine (Ismelin)[579] Herb may displace guanethidine from adrenergic neurons, thereby reducing antihypertensive effect of drug.

Indoramin[581] Drug prevented the decrease in urine flow in males using khat.

MAOIs[579] (see Appendix 9) Catecholamines stored by MAOIs may be released by khat, thereby increasing sympathomimetic effect.

Sympathomimetics[579] (see Appendix 36) Theoretical additive sympathomimetic effect of concurrent use.

Thyroid replacement therapy[582] Cathinone and N-formylnorephedrine, components of khat, increase serum T4 and T3 (at higher doses) in rats. Theoretically, concurrent use may cause a thyroid storm.

Kidney Bean *Phaseolus vulgaris*
PART USED: Cooked bean.
SAFETY: Raw bean contain lectins, which are destroyed when cooked.
ADVERSE REACTIONS: Flatulence, GI distress.
INTERACTIONS:

Insulin/Oral hypoglycemic agents[592] (see Appendix 24) Kidney beans can aid in the lowering of blood glucose, most likely due to its chromium, trigonelline and fiber content. Monitor patients with diabetes to prevent hypoglycemia.

King's Crown *Calotropis procera*

SAFETY: Contains cardiac glycosides.

ADVERSE REACTIONS: Allergic contact dermatitis, sedation. Can alter menstrual cycle and temporarily inhibit ovulation. Large doses: convulsions, death, diarrhea.

INTERACTIONS:

Digoxin/Cardiac glycosides[34] Herb contains cardiac glycosides, which may be additive when combined with drug.

Konjac *Amorphophallus konjac*

USES: Hypercholesterolemia (H), weight loss (H).

PART USED: Glucomannan (from tuber).

CONTRAINDICATIONS: Ileus, obstruction of esophagus or intestines, swallowing difficulty.

INTERACTIONS:

Insulin/Oral hypoglycemic agents[173,593] (see Appendix 24) Glucomannan, a polysaccharide fiber from konjac, has been found to have hypoglycemic action. In one study, it decreased the absorption of glibenclamide (glyburide), but blood glucose was lowered. Glucomannan may be helpful in the management of insulin resistance. Patients on diabetes medication should be monitored to prevent hypoglycemia.

Kudzu *Pueraria lobata*
  PART USED: Root.
  CONTRAINDICATIONS: Safety in pregnancy and lactation not established.
  SAFETY: Has been found to remove heavy metals from soil. AHPA Class: 1.[66]
  INTERACTIONS:
  May alter metabolism of drugs metabolized by P450 enzymes[261] (see Appendix 38) In vitro study of puerarin (flavonoid of kudzu) showed induction of CYP2A1, CYP1A1/2, CYP3A1, CYP2C11 and inactivation of CYP3A, CYP2E1 and CYP2B1. Ge-gen (*Radix Puerariae the* root of *P. lobata)* induced CYP1A2, CYP3A1, CYP2B1 and inactivation of CYP3A, CYP2E1 and CYP2B1. Further research is needed to determine if serum level of drugs metabolized by P450 enzymes are altered in humans by kudzu or its flavonoid. Health care providers need to be aware of potential for alterations in serum level of drugs metabolized by P450 enzymes with kudzu consumption.
  Alcohol[246] Herb decreased alcohol intake by 50% in laboratory animals and may be beneficial (hypothesized) in the treatment of alcoholism. It was hypothesized that kudzu may delay gastric emptying.

Lagerstroemia *Lagerstroemia speciosa*
  PART USED: Leaf, ripe fruit.
  INTERACTIONS:
  Insulin/Oral hypoglycemic agents[594] (see Appendix 24) In research using mice, serum glucose and insulin were reduced. Monitor patients on diabetes medications to prevent hypoglycemia.

Lavender *Lavandula spp.*

USES: Anxiety (H-equivocal), mood improvement (H), sleep disturbances (H-equivocal).

PART USED: Flower, essential oil.

CONTRAINDICATIONS: Pregnancy. Safety not established in lactation and children. Allergy to *Labiatae* family.

SAFETY: Caution with internal use of essential oil. GRAS (Spice, seasoning, flavoring, oil, extract, oleoresin). AHPA Class: 1.[66]

ADVERSE REACTIONS: Allergic reaction, dermatitis.

INTERACTIONS:

Alkaloids[4] (see Appendix 4) High tannin content of plant may cause alkaloids to become insoluble and precipitate.

Barbiturates[595] (see Appendix 12) Essential oil increased drug-induced sleep time in mice.

CNS depressants[595,596] (see Appendix 15) In research using mice, essential oil of lavender increased drug-induced sleep time. Theoretical additive sedation with drugs causing sedation.

Pentobarbital (Nembutal)[595,596] In research using mice, essential oil of lavender increased drug-induced sleep time. Effect was not seen after 5 days of administration.

Lemon Balm *Melissa officinalis*

USES: Gastric ulcers (A), hyperthyroidism (A), loss of appetite, recurrent herpes labialis (H).

Lemon Balm (cont'd.)
  PART USED: Leaf.
  CONTRAINDICATIONS: Hypothyroidism, hyperthyroidism (only under medical supervision), thyroid disease. Safety in pregnancy, lactation and children not established.
  SAFETY: Not for use in excess of 14 days. GRAS (oil, spice, flavoring, oleoresin). AHPA Class: 1.[66]
  INTERACTIONS:

    Barbiturates[597] (see Appendix 12) Based on herb's ability to increase sedation of pentobarbital.

    CNS depressants[597] (see Appendix 15) Based on herb's ability to increase sedation of pentobarbital. Theoretical additive effect.

    Hexobarbital[597] Based on herb's ability to increase sedation of pentobarbital.

    Pentobarbital (Nembutal)[597] Herb potentiated drug in laboratory animals.

    Thyroid replacement therapy[598] In research using animals, herb inhibited enzymic T_4-5'-deiodination to T_3.

Lemongrass *Cymbopogon citratus*
  PART USED: Herb.
  CONTRAINDICATIONS: Pregnancy.
  SAFETY: GRAS (oil, extract, oleoresin).   AHPA Class: 2b.[66]
  ADVERSE REACTIONS: Allergic reaction, alveolitis (inhalation). Slight elevation of direct bilirubin and amylase.
  INTERACTIONS:

Lemongrass (cont'd.)

Drugs metabolized by P450 CYP2B[262] (see Appendix 38) ß-Myrcene (acyclic monoterpene in essential oil of lemon grass) may induce CYP2B isozymes, which may decrease serum levels of drugs metabolized by these enzymes.

Leuca-F-1
INTERACTIONS:
Chemotherapy[342] (see Appendix 16) Pancreatic cancer patients taking herbal granules for 3 days prior to receiving chemotherapy had increased appetite and decreased GI disturbances. Significant effect on WBC, ANC and platelet count.

Li Ren *Semen litchi*
INTERACTIONS:
Insulin/Oral hypoglycemic agents[599] (see Appendix 24) In research using 45 patients with type 2 diabetes, 80% had improvement in blood glucose levels.

Licorice *Glycyrrhiza glabra*
USES: Gastric ulcers (A), chronic hepatitis C (H-glycyrrhizin decreased ALT), chronic hepatitis B (H-glycyrrhizinic acid), prostate cancer (H-part of PC-SPES).
PART USED: Root.
CONTRAINDICATIONS: Bleeding disorders, CHF, cardiovascular disease, cholestatic liver disease, cirrhosis, diabetes (on insulin), edema, hypertonia, HTN, hypokalemia, impotence, kidney disease, male infertility, myoglobinuria, pregnancy, renal insufficiency.
SAFETY: GRAS (spice, seasoning, flavoring, oil, extract, oleoresin). AHPA Class: 2b.

Licorice (cont'd.)

2c, 2d—not excessive dose or extended period unless under medical supervision.[66]

ADVERSE REACTIONS: Prolonged or excessive use may deplete potassium and increase retention of sodium, which may lead to HTN, decreased testosterone in males, edema, flaccid weakness, fluid retention, headache, hypokalemia, inhibition of renin-angiotensin system, mineralocorticoid effects, myoglobinuria, vertigo. Deglycyrrhizinated licorice use is usually free of adverse reactions.

INTERACTIONS:

Drugs metabolized by P450 CYP1A2, CYP2B and CYP3A4 isoenzymes[262,611] (see Appendix 38) ß-Myrcene may induce CYP2B isozymes, which may decrease serum levels of drugs (including barbiturates and cyclophosphamide) metabolized by these enzymes. This research was conducted on rat hepatic microsomes. High doses of extract induced CYP1A2 and CYP3A4 in rats. Further research is needed to determine if serum levels of drugs metabolized by P450 enzymes are altered in humans by ß-myrcene. Health care providers need to be aware of potential for alteration in serum level of drugs metabolized by these isozymes.

Acetaminophen/Paracetamol[606,607] Glycyrrhizin, 18-alpha-glycyrrhetinic acid and 18-beta-glycyrrhetinic acid, components of licorice, decreased acetaminophen-induced liver injury. In research using rats, methanol extract of herb activated glucuronidation of acetaminophen, which decreases serum levels of drug.

Alcohol[604] Potenlini (injectable glycyrrhizin isolated from licorice), was protective against carbon tetrachloride and ethanol-induced liver cirrhosis.

Amiloride (Midamor)[620] Amiloride decreased metabolic side effects and ulcer healing activity of carbenoxolone sodium (component of licorice).

Amphotericin B (Amphocin, Fungizone)[619] Glycyrrhizinate increased dissolution and bioavailability of amphotericin B suppositories in rabbits.

Anticoagulants and drugs that increase the risk of bleeding[527,628] (see Appendix 8) GU-7 (a 3 arylcoumarin from licorice) has antiplatelet activity. Monitor labs if used concurrently with drugs which increase the risk of bleeding.

Antihypertensives[612,615] (see Appendix 11) Licorice increases blood pressure (most likely due to retention of sodium), which may decrease the effectiveness of antihypertensives. Licorice decreases serum potassium, which theoretically may be additive with antihypertensives that also deplete potassium.

Aspirin[626] Herb may protect against gastric ulcer induced by aspirin (100-500 mg deglycyrrhizinated licorice).

Cimetidine (Tagamet)[616] Use of cimetidine and licorice together provides greater protection against gastric erosion.

Corticosteroids[612,613] (see Appendix 18) Synergistic potentiation of potassium loss and possible hypokalemia.

Cortisol[608] Glycyrrhizin and glycyrrhetinic acid, components of licorice, inhibit the enzymes which convert cortisol to cortisone, dihydrocortisol and tetrahydrocortisol. This may result in a decreased clearance of cortisol and increased half-life of cortisol.

Cyclophosphamide (Cytoxan, Neosar)[605] In mice, extract of licorice potentiated antitumor and antimetastatic effects of drug.

Digoxin/Cardiac glycosides[612,613] Synergistic potentiation of potassium loss and possible hypokalemia.

Licorice (cont'd.)

Diuretics[624] (see Appendix 11) Case reports of hypokalemic myopathy with concurrent use of licorice and diuretics. Concurrent use may increase the excretion of potassium.

Estrogen replacement therapy/Oral contraceptives[603] In one study, concurrent use of glycyrrhizin with oral contraceptives led to hypertension, hypokalemia and peripheral edema. Estrogen may increase sensitivity to glycyrrhizin acid in licorice. More research is needed to determine safety of concurrent use.

Hydrocortisone (Cortef, Hydrocortone)[621] Hydrocortisone was potentiated on skin by glycerrhetinic acid, a component of licorice.

Ibuprofen[618] Ibuprofen caused a release of albumin-bound glycyrrhetic acid.

Insulin/Oral hypoglycemic agents[601,602] (see Appendix 24) Insulin may be synergistic with glycyrrhizin and may cause electrolyte imbalance and suppression of renin and aldosterone. In one study using rats, glycyrrhizin, a component of licorice, had an antidiabetic effect on type 2 diabetes rat model. More research is needed to determine safety in patients with diabetes.

Interferon[609,610] Glycyrrhizin, a component of herb, was found to increase effectiveness of drug in the treatment of hepatitis.

MAOIs[600,623] (see Appendix 9) In vitro research of several compounds from licorice showed an inhibition of MAO. Herb may increase risk of drug side effects such as potential hypertensive crisis.

Midazolam (Versed)[267] Licorice was administered for 7 days. On the 8th day midazolam was administered. There was no significant difference in serum levels of midazolam with concurrent use of licorice. Suggests licorice induces CYP3A4. **170**

Licorice (cont'd.)

Nitrofurantoin (Macrobid, Macrodantin)[614] In humans, excretion of drug was increased by concurrent use of deglycyrrhizinated licorice.

Prednisolone[622] Glycyrrhizin increased serum levels of drug by decreasing drug metabolism.

Spironolactone (Aldactone)[617] Spironolactone was antagonistic toward carbenoxolone (derived from licorice) used for treatment of gastric ulcer.

Stimulant laxatives[66,177,612] Increased risk of hypokalemia.

Sympathomimetics[600] (see Appendix 36) In vitro research with several compounds from licorice showed an inhibition of MAO. Herb may increase risk of sympathomimetics' side effects such as potential hypertensive crisis.

Thiazide diuretics[625] (see Appendix 11) Long term use of licorice reduces sodium and water excretion, which reduces effectiveness of drug and may increase risk of hypokalemia. In one case report of concurrent use, the adverse reaction included respiratory and kidney failure, somnolence, flaccid paralysis, paralysis of extremities, arterial hypertension, edema, severe hypokalemia and rhabdomyolysis.

Lily of the Valley *Convallaria majalis*

PART USED: Whole plant.

CONTRAINDICATIONS: Hypercalcemia, hypokalemia. Safety in pregnancy and lactation not established.

SAFETY: Contains cardiac glycosides. AHPA Class: 3.[66]

ADVERSE REACTIONS: Arrhythmias, N&V.

INTERACTIONS:

Lily of the Valley (cont'd.)

Calcium[1] Increased effectiveness.

Corticosteroids[1] (see Appendix 18) Extended use of herb may increase side effects of drug.

Digoxin/Cardiac glycosides[34] Herb contains cardiac glycosides, which may be additive with drugs that contain cardiac glycosides.

Quinidine (Quinaglute)[1] Herb increases effectiveness and side effects of drug.

Saluretics[1] Herb increases effectiveness and side effects of drug.

Stimulant laxatives[1] Herb increases effectiveness and side effects of drug.

Linden Flower *Tilia cordata*

PART USED: Flower.

SAFETY: GRAS (flower--spice, seasoning, flavoring, oil, extract, oleoresin, leaves-- flavoring in alcoholic beverages).

ADVERSE REACTIONS: Allergic response.

INTERACTIONS:

Iron[269] In a study with 77 human subjects, linden flower tea decreased absorption of non-heme iron by 52% due to polyphenol content.

LIV.100 Ayurvedic formulation of *Cichorium intybus, Solanum nigrum, Phyllanthus amarus, Picrorhiza kurroa, Embelica officinalis*

INTERACTIONS:

Isoniazid (Nydrazid)[311] In male rats, the hepatotoxicity of the drug was decreased by LIV.100.

172

Pyrazinamide (Rifater)[311] In male rats, the hepatotoxicity of the drug was decreased by LIV.100.

Rifampicin[311] In male rats, the hepatotoxicity of the drug was decreased by LIV.100.

Lobelia *Lobelia inflata*

PART USED: Herb.

SAFETY: On FDA's list of herbs associated with illness or injury (difficulty breathing, sweating, tachycardia, decreased blood pressure, possible coma or death).[178] AHPA Class: 2b, 2d—not large doses.[66]

ADVERSE REACTIONS: Abdominal pain, anxiety, arrhythmias, bradycardia, decreased respiratory rate, dermatitis, diaphoresis, diarrhea, dizziness, euphoria, headache, HTN, muscle spasms and weakness, N&V, paresthesias, seizures, tremors.

Long Pepper *Piper longum* Part of Trikatu, an ayurvedic preparation (see Trikatu)

PART USED: Fruit.

CONTRAINDICATIONS: Pregnancy.

ADVERSE REACTIONS: Herb contains piperine, which inhibits gastric emptying and GI transit.

INTERACTIONS:

Drugs metabolized by P450 enzymes[151,152] (see Appendix 38) In research using laboratory animals, CYP2E1 expression was suppressed and CYP2B and CYP1A

Long Pepper (cont'd.)

expression was enhanced. Metabolism of drugs which are substrates of these isozymes may be altered. In research by Atal, piperine was found to be a nonspecific inhibitor of P450 enzymes. Use caution with concurrent use of drugs which are substrates of various P450 isozymes.

Aspirin[629] In mice, water decoction of herb was protective against aspirin-induced ulcers.

Coenzyme Q10[157] Five mg of piperine, a component of long pepper, administered for 21 days, increased serum levels of coenzyme Q10.

Hexobarbital[151] Piperine, a component of pepper, increased drug-induced sleep time.

Indomethacin (Indocin)[153] In research using mice, piperine was protective against drug-induced ulcers.

Pentobarbitone[158] Piperine potentiated drug-induced sleep time, possibly due to the inhibition of liver enzymes.

Phenytoin (Dilantin)[151] Piperine may enhance bioavailability of drug.

Propranolol (Inderal)[154] Piperine enhanced systemic availability of drug, which may result in a lower amount of drug needed to reach therapeutic levels.

Theophylline (Uniphyl, Uni-Dur)[114,154] Piperine enhanced systemic availability of drug, which may result in a lower amount of drug needed to reach therapeutic levels.

Zoxazolamine[151] Piperine, a component of pepper, increased drug-induced sleep time.

Loosestrife *Lythrum salicaria*
PART USED: Herb.
SAFETY: Contains tannins; not for long-term use.
INTERACTIONS:
Alkaloids (see Appendix 4)[4] High tannin content of flower may cause alkaloids to become insoluble and precipitate.
Insulin/Oral hypoglycemic agents[162,173,630,631] (see Appendix 24) In rats, herb decreased blood glucose levels. Mice without diabetes also had a decrease in blood glucose. Patients using loosestrife should be monitored to prevent possible hypoglycemia.

Lovage *Levisticum officinale*
PART USED: Root.
CONTRAINDICATIONS: Safety in pregnancy and lactation not established. Bleeding disorders, CHF, edema, HTN, kidney disease.
SAFETY: GRAS (flavoring). AHPA Class: 2b, 2d—not with kidney impairment or inflammation.[66]
ADVERSE REACTIONS: Possible photosensitivity with long-term use.
INTERACTIONS:
Anticoagulants and drugs that increase the risk of bleeding[632] (see Appendix 8) Herb contains bergapten and imperatorin, which inhibited platelet aggregation in vitro.

Lycium *Lycium barbarum*
    USES: Adjunct to cancer therapy (H-polysaccharides).
    PART USED: Berry, root bark.
    CONTRAINDICATIONS: Bleeding disorders, hypoglycemia, pregnancy.
    SAFETY: AHPA Class: 2b.[66]
    INTERACTIONS:
        Anticoagulants and drugs that increase the risk of bleeding[633] (see Appendix 8) Case report of increased INR with concurrent use of warfarin and consumption of *Lycium barbarum* tea.

Madagascar Periwinkle *Catharanthus roseus*
    PART USED: Herb.
    CONTRAINDICATIONS: Pregnancy.
    SAFETY: Source of vinblastine and vincristine, which are chemotherapeutic agents used to treat some cancers. Only under care of health care provider. AHPA Class: 3[66]
    INTERACTIONS:
        Insulin/Oral hypoglycemic agents[105,634] (see Appendix 24) Possible hypoglycemia or loss of blood glucose control.
        Digoxin (Lanoxin)[727] High dose chemotherapeutic agents have been found to decrease absorption of digoxin tablet (not capsule). It is possible that high doses of herb will also decrease absorption of digoxin, due to the alkaloids with chemotherapeutic action contained in herb.
        Vincristine/Vinblastine[726] Drug is an alkaloid derivative of herb. Effect would most likely be additive.

Magnolia-Stephania preparation

SAFETY: On FDA's list of herbs associated with illness or injury (kidney disease).[178]

Maitake Mushroom *Grifola frondosa*

USES: Hypercholesterolemia (A--fiber extracted from mushroom), HTN (A).

PART USED: Fruiting bodies, mycelium.

SAFETY: AHPA Class: 1.[66]

INTERACTIONS:

Insulin/Oral hypoglycemic agents[635] (see Appendix 24) In research using rats with experimental diabetes, insulin levels were increased and glucose levels were decreased. No changes were noted in normal rats. Patients taking diabetes medications should be monitored to prevent possible hypoglycemia.

Marshmallow *Althaea officinalis*

PART USED: Root, leaf, flower.

SAFETY: AHPA Class: 1.[66]

INTERACTIONS:

May delay absorption of other drugs due to high mucilage content.[1]

Matarique *Pasacalium decompositum*

INTERACTIONS:

Oral hypoglycemic agents[258] (see Appendix 24) Water extract of herb decreased serum glucose in healthy mice and mice with mild diabetes, but not in mice with severe diabetes. Suggests beta cell function needed for glucose lowering effect.

Maté *Ilex paraguariensis*

PART USED: Leaf.

CONTRAINDICATIONS: Safety in pregnancy, lactation and children not established. Cardiovascular disease, diabetes, HTN, ulcers.

SAFETY: Contains caffeine (2,000-20,000 ppm), tannins (40,000-160,000 ppm), theobromine (960-5,000 ppm), theophylline (500 ppm). No high dose for extended period. Increased incidence of esophageal cancer with long-term use. GRAS (oil, extract, oleoresin). AHPA Class: 2d—not excessive or long-term.[66]

ADVERSE REACTIONS: Anxiety, blurred vision, diarrhea, dizziness, GI distress, headache, HTN, hyperglycemia, increased urination, increased risk of cancer (esophagus, kidney, larynx, lung, mouth), increased bile flow, insomnia, irritability, N&V, nervousness, palpitations, restlessness.

INTERACTIONS:

Alkaloids[4] (see Appendix 4) High tannin content of herb may cause alkaloids to become insoluble and precipitate.

Acetaminophen/Paracetamol[636] Caffeine, a component of herb, may increase pain relief.

Aspirin[638] Caffeine in herb increases effectiveness of ASA pain relief.

Benzodiazepines[637] (see Appendix 13) Theoretical decrease in sedative and antianxiolytic effect.

Beta-adrenergic agonists[101] (see Appendix 36) Concurrent use may increase the risk of cardiac arrhythmias.

Cimetidine (Tagamet)[658] Drug may decrease clearance of caffeine, a component of maté. Theoretically, this may increase serum caffeine and increase caffeine side effects. Results of research have been equivocal.

Clozapine (Clozaril) and possibly other drugs metabolized by P450
CYP1A2[296,350] (see Appendix 38) Caffeine intakes greater than 400 mg may decrease clearance of clozapine (and possibly increase serum levels of other drugs metabolized by CYP1A2). In randomized crossover research on 12 males, the AUC of clozapine was increased by 19% and oral clearance of clozapine was decreased 14% with concurrent caffeine intake. Maté leaf contains up to 20,000 ppm of caffeine.

Disulfiram (Antabuse)[654] Drug may decrease metabolism of caffeine, a component of herb. The result may be increased serum caffeine and caffeine side effects.

Ephedra/Ephedrine[434] Concurrent use of high amounts of products containing caffeine and stimulants may have an additive stimulant effect.

Ergotamine (Ergomar)[653] Caffeine, a component of herb, increases serum level and efficacy of drug. The drug Wigraine contains both ergotamine and caffeine.

Estrogen[658] Ethinyl estradiol and estradiol inhibits CYP2A2 metabolism of caffeine, which increases caffeine's side effects.

Fluvoxamine (Luvox)[658] Drug decreases metabolism of caffeine, a component of the herb. This may increase caffeine serum levels and increase caffeine side effects.

Furafylline[658] Drug inhibits CYP1A2, which decreases the metabolism of caffeine, a component of herb. This may increase serum levels of caffeine and increase caffeine side effects.

Grapefruit juice[531] Grapefruit juice inhibits CYP1A2, which decreases the metabolism of caffeine, a component of maté, may increase caffeine side effects.

Maté (cont'd.)

Ibuprofen[650] Concurrent use of both herb and drug may enhance pain relief.

Idrocilamide[658] Drug alters caffeine (a component of herb) metabolism, increasing serum levels of caffeine and caffeine side effects.

Insulin/Oral hypoglycemic agents[84,651] (see Appendix 24) Caffeine, a component of herb, may increase insulin resistance. Monitor patients with diabetes.

Lithium (Eskalith, Lithobid, Lithonate, Lithotabs)[658] Caffeine, a component of herb, increases the renal excretion of lithium, which may decrease serum levels of drug. Discontinuation of herb use may likewise increase serum levels of drug.

MAOIs[103] (see Appendix 9) Excessive amounts of coffee may increase risk of hypertension.

Methotrexate (Rheumatrex)[224] Caffeine in maté may decrease effectiveness of drug.

Methoxsalen (8-MOP, Oxsoralen)[658] Drug inhibits metabolism of caffeine, a component of herb. Increased serum caffeine may increase side effects.

Mexiletine (Mexitil)[656] Drug delays metabolism of caffeine, a component of herb. This may increase side effects of caffeine.

Oral contraceptives[658] Long-term use of oral contraceptives (ethinyl estradiol or estradiol) causes an inhibition of CYP1A2 metabolism of caffeine. This may increase serum caffeine and increase caffeine side effects.

Phenylpropanolamine[658] Drug may inhibit caffeine metabolism (herb component), increasing serum levels of caffeine and caffeine side effects. On 11/6/00, the FDA released advisory to remove phenylpropanolamine from all products.[657]

Quinolones (ciprofloxacin, enoxacin, grepafloxacin, norfloxacin, pefloxacin, tosufloxacin)[658] Drugs may decrease clearance of caffeine, a component of herb. This may increase the side effects of caffeine due to increased serum caffeine.

Terbinafine (Lamisil)[658] Drug may inhibit the metabolism of caffeine, a component of herb. This may increase serum levels of caffeine and increase caffeine side effects. Research on this interaction has been equivocal.

Theophylline (Uniphyl, Uni-Dur)[658] Concurrent use of theophylline and caffeine may lead to an increase in serum levels of both.

Verapamil (Calan, Isoptin, Verelan)[658] Drug delays clearance of caffeine, a component of herb. This may increase caffeine side effects.

Meadowsweet *Filipendula ulmaria*

PART USED: Herb.

CONTRAINDICATIONS: Asthma, bleeding disorders, lactation, pregnancy, salicylate sensitivity.

SAFETY: Contains salicylates. AHPA Class: 1.[66]

ADVERSE REACTIONS: Bronchospasm.

INTERACTIONS:

Anticoagulants and drugs that increase the risk of bleeding[412,642] (see Appendix 8) Herb contains heparin-like substance, which may increase the risk of bleeding. Salicylate content of herb doesn't inhibit platelet aggregation like aspirin.

Melatonin

USES: Insomnia (H), jet lag (H), pediatric epilepsy (H-preliminary), presurgical anxiety (H).

CONTRAINDICATIONS: Pregnancy, lactation, children, autoimmune disease, depression, hepatic disease.

SAFETY: Safety of long-term use not established.

ADVERSE REACTIONS: Depression, drowsiness, fatigue, GI distress, headache.

INTERACTIONS:

Drugs that inhibit or induce P450 CYP1A2[669] (see Appendix 38) In vitro research has shown melatonin to be metabolized by CYP1A2. Drugs that inhibit or induce CYP1A2 may alter metabolism and serum levels of melatonin.

Alcohol[327] In rats, ethanol-induced gastric injury was reduced with concurrent administration of melatonin. Lesion area was 3x smaller with herb. Antioxidant action responsible for protective effect.

Antidepressants[938] (see Appendix 6) Fluoxetine decreases serum melatonin. Tricyclic antidepressants and fluvoxamine increase serum melatonin.

Barbiturates[659] (see Appendix 12) Melatonin, at low doses, prolonged barbiturate narcosis, but at high doses decreased duration of drug-induced narcosis.

Beta blockers[931,932,933] (see Appendix 11) In human research, beta blockers (S enantiomers) decreased release of melatonin, measured by a decrease in urinary melatonin metabolite excretion. The decrease in melatonin may be responsible for beta blocker-induced sleep disturbances. In another study using humans, serum nocturnal melatonin was lowered in a dose-dependent manner by the beta blocker atenolol. In a study using males, who were administered exogenous melatonin,

182

atenolol-induced sleep disturbances were reduced.

Chemotherapy[664,666,668] (see Appendix 16) Sensitivity to cis-diamminedichloroplatinum (CDDP) was enhanced by administration of melatonin to ovarian cancer cells. Melatonin decreased oxidative damage induced by adriamycin in rats. Melatonin was protective against doxorubicin-induced cardiotoxicity in rats.

Diazepam (Valium)[660] Concurrent use in mice exposed to pain produced a synergistic analgesic effect.

Echinacea (Echinacea purpurea)[662] When melatonin was combined with echinacea in mice, myelopoiesis was disturbed.

Estradiol[665] When rats were injected with melatonin and estradiol, melatonin exerted an antioxidant effect.

Fluvoxamine (Luvox)[935,936,937] Fluvoxamine increases serum melatonin. In research using 5 healthy males, bioavailability of exogenous melatonin was increased with coadministration of fluvoxamine. AUC of melatonin was increased 17-fold. Effect may be due to decreased hepatic metabolism of melatonin. In a study of patients with major depression taking fluvoxamine, sleep disturbances were decreased by melatonin.

Indomethacin (Indocin)[667] Melatonin was protective against indomethacin-induced oxidative damage in rat gastric mucosa and testis.

Isoniazid (Nydrazid)[934] In in vitro research, melatonin increased efficacy of isoniazid three-fold.

Methamphetamine[655] Coadministration with melatonin enhanced the monoaminergic effects of drug.

Melatonin (cont'd.)

Morphine (MSIR, MS Contin, Oramorph, Roxanol)[660] Concurrent use in mice exposed to pain produced a synergistic analgesic effect.

Nifedipine, and possibly other calcium channel blockers[671] (see Appendix 11) Melatonin may counteract the antihypertensive effect of drug. HS melatonin in human subjects taking nifedipine increased both BP and heart rate.

Para-chloroamphetamine[661] Concurrent administration in rats caused an increase in serum adrenocorticotropic hormone, corticosterone and serotonin, which suggests possible adverse peripheral effects.

Reserpine (Enduronyl)[663] In rats, administration of melatonin decreased severity of reserpine-induced dyskinesia—most likely due to an enhancement of GABA-ergic activity through effect on peripheral benzodiazepine receptors.

Succinylcholine (Anectine, Quelicin)[642] In in vitro research, melatonin potentiated muscle blocking effect of drug. Melatonin may have calcium channel blocking effect.

Thyroid replacement therapy[645] Coadministration caused an increase in serum thyroxine, possibly caused by melatonin's effect on TSH.

Milk Thistle *Silybum marianum*

USES: Alcoholic liver disease/cirrhosis (H-silymarin, Legalon), *Amanita phalloides* poisoning (H-silybin), cirrhosis (H), gastric ulcers (A), hypercholesterolemia (H), liver disease (H), occupational exposures to chemicals (H), viral hepatitis (H).
PART USED: Seed.
CONTRAINDICATIONS: Safety in pregnancy, lactation and children not established.

SAFETY: AHPA Class: 1.[66]

ADVERSE REACTIONS: Allergic reaction, GI distress, laxative effect, urticaria.

INTERACTIONS:

Drugs metabolized by cytochrome P450 CYP3A4 and CYP2C9 isozymes and transported by PGP[227,232,251,674,679,680] (see Appendix 38) Silibinin, silybin and silymarin, components of herb may increase serum levels of drugs metabolized by CYP3A4 and CYP2C9 by inhibiting both enzymes. Melatonin enhances PGP transport of drugs. Further research is needed to determine if interaction occurs in humans.

Acetaminophen/Paracetamol[670,675] In in vitro research, silymarin, a component of milk thistle, was protective against acetaminophen-induced toxicity. Silibinin, a component of milk thistle, decreased drug-induced nephrotoxicity to in vitro kidney cells from laboratory animals.

Aspirin[677] Silymarin, a component of milk thistle, improved metabolism and disposition of ASA in animals with cirrhosis.

Butyrophenones[14] Herb reduces risk of liver damage from long-term use of drug.

Cisplatin (Platinol)[306,675,683] Silibinin, a component of milk thistle, was protective against nephrotoxicity of drug. In vitro research using human ovarian carcinoma cells and human breast cancer cells treated with silybin (main flavolignan of milk thistle) showed a dose-dependent synergistic inhibition of cell growth with concurrent use of cisplatin. In in vitro research using kidney cells from animals, silibinin, a component of milk thistle, decreased drug-induced nephrotoxicity.

Cyclosporine (Neoral)[674] Silibinin, a component of milk thistle, decreased cyclosporine-induced lipid peroxidation, but didn't protect against cyclosporine-induced increase in GFR in rats.

Doxorubicin (Adriamycin, Doxil, Rubex)[306] In vitro research using human ovarian carcinoma cells and human breast cancer cells treated with silybin (main flavolignan of milk thistle) showed a dose-dependent synergistic inhibition of cell growth with concurrent use of doxorubicin.

General anesthetics See **Halothane**, below (also see Appendix 20).

Halothane[676] Silybine, a component of milk thistle, was protective against hepatic injury from halothane.

Insulin/Oral hypoglycemic agents[678,681,682] (see Appendix 24) Silymarin, a component of milk thistle, decreases insulin resistance in patients with diabetes and cirrhosis. Fasting insulin, HbA1c and blood glucose were lowered. Research suggest that silymarin plays a protective role against damage to the pancreas.

Oral contraceptives[673] Milk thistle may decrease the effectiveness of oral contraceptives.

Phenothiazines[14] (see Appendix 28) Herb reduces risk of liver damage from long-term use of drug.

Tacrine (Cognex)[672] Silymarin, a component of milk thistle, may decrease GI disturbances and cholinergic side effects of drug.

Vincristine (Oncovin, Vincasar)[675] Silibinin, a component of milk thistle, decreased drug-induced nephrotoxicity to in vitro kidney cells from laboratory animals.

Mint *Mentha arvensis*

PART USED: Essential oil.
CONTRAINDICATIONS: Bile duct obstruction, external use of oil on face of children, gallbladder disease, GERD, liver disease.
ADVERSE REACTIONS: Allergic response, contact dermatitis, GI distress, temporary male infertility, urticaria.

Mistletoe *Viscum album*

USES: Cancer (H-Iscador/lectin-I, which are formulas prepared from mistletoe: Research equivocal, but mostly positive).
PART USED: Leaf, fruit/berry, herb.
CONTRAINDICATIONS: Safety in pregnancy, lactation and children not established. HIV, chronic progressive infections, TB.
SAFETY: Fatalities have been reported. Plant contains toxic substances. To be used only under supervision of health care professional. AHPA Class: 2d.[66]
ADVERSE REACTIONS: Allergic reaction, anaphylaxis, angina, bradycardia, cardiac arrest, chills, diarrhea, fever, gastritis, GI distress, gingivitis, headache, hepatitis, hypotension, hypertension, hypereosinophilia, increased BUN and creatinine, leukocytosis, mydriasis, myosis, orthostatic circulatory disturbances.
INTERACTIONS:
Chemotherapy[254,685,686] (see Appendix 16) Iscador (lectin from mistletoe) has been found to enhance chemotherapy in most cases and is used extensively in Germany. One study found that a lectin from mistletoe had no effect on interleukin 2 immunotherapy and when used alone stimulated tumor growth.

Mistletoe (cont'd.)

MAOIs[810,916] (see Appendix 9) Mistletoe contains tyramine. Advise not to take large amounts of herb with drug.

Radiotherapy and surgery or surgery alone[254] Mistletoe lectin-1 was used as adjunctive therapy for 477 patients receiving radiotherapy and surgery or surgery alone for head and neck squamous cell carcinoma. No improvement in cellular immune reaction, survival time or quality of life was found.

Motherwort *Leonurus cardiaca*

PART USED: Herb.

CONTRAINDICATIONS: Pregnancy, bleeding disorders, breast cancer or a family history of breast cancer. Safety in lactation and children not established.

SAFETY: AHPA Class: 2b.[66]

ADVERSE REACTIONS: Allergic reaction, GI distress.

INTERACTIONS:

Alkaloids[4] (see Appendix 4) High tannin content of herb may cause alkaloids to become insoluble and precipitate.

Anticoagulants[687] (see Appendix 8) Herb has antiplatelet activity, which theoretically may be additive with drugs that increase the risk of bleeding.

CNS depressants[916] (see Appendix 15) Herb contains several components with sedative effect (alpha pinene, benzaldehyde, caryophyllene, limonene and oleanolic acid). Theoretical additive sedation.

Digoxin/Cardiac glycosides[117] Herb contains marrubiin, which is cardioactive, and may theoretically increase toxicity of drug.

Mulberry Leaf *Morus spp*
PART USED: Fruit, leaf, root bark, twig.
SAFETY: AHPA Class: 1.[66]
ADVERSE REACTIONS: Contact urticaria.
INTERACTIONS:
Insulin/Oral hypoglycemic agents[105,688] (see Appendix 24) Extracts of herb decreased blood glucose in a mouse model of diabetes. Monitor patients with diabetes.

Myrrh *Commiphora molmol*
PART USED: Gum resin.
CONTRAINDICATIONS: Pregnancy.
SAFETY: GRAS (flavoring). AHPA Class: 2b, 2d—not with excessive uterine bleeding.[66]
ADVERSE REACTIONS: Allergic reaction, contact dermatitis.
INTERACTIONS:
Alcohol[689] Aqueous suspension of herb decreased ethanol-induced ulcer.
Cyclophosphamide[690] Coadministration of myrrh to mice did not affect cytological or biochemical effects of drug.
Indomethacin[689] Aqueous suspension of herb decreased drug-induced ulcer.

Myrtle *Myrtus communis*
  SAFETY: GRAS (flavoring in alcoholic beverage).
  INTERACTIONS:
    Insulin/Oral hypoglycemic agents[691] (see Appendix 24) In research using mice, extract of myrtle decreased the hyperglycemia of chemically induced diabetes.

N-Acetylcysteine (NAC / N-acetyl L-cysteine)
  USES: Acetaminophen overdose (H), mucolytic (H).
  CONTRAINDICATIONS: Asthma, coma, pregnancy, vomiting (oral).
  SAFETY: Classified as prescription drug (Mucomyst, Mucosil) by FDA. Hepatotoxicity with high doses in animals. NAC has interfered with urine ketone testing.
  ADVERSE REACTIONS: Anaphylaxis, asthma attack, diarrhea, hypotension, N&V, tracheal ciliostasis.
  INTERACTIONS:
    5-FU[698] In research using mice, NAC improved drug treatment of colorectal cancer. Human studies are needed to determine effect in humans.
    Ace inhibitors[693] (see Appendix 11) In research using spontaneously hypertensive mice, the coadministration of NAC enhanced the blood pressure-lowering effect of drugs.
    Acetaminophen/Paracetamol[700] IV N-acetylcysteine (Mucomyst) may be administered in cases of acetaminophen overdose.
    Alkylating agents[699] (see Appendix 16) Aortic infusion of NAC may decrease myelosuppression and organ toxicity, without interfering with intracarotid administration of alkylating agents to CNS.

Contrast media [692] Administration of acetylcysteine and hydration to patients with renal insufficiency reduced effect of radiograph-contrast agents on renal function.

Cyclosporin [695] In research using rats, coadministration of NAC decreased nephrotoxicity of drug.

Doxorubicin (Adriamycin) [694] In research using mice, concurrent administration of NAC decreased cardiotoxicity, myelogenotoxicity as well as alopecia.

Interferon [697] In patients with hepatitis C, concurrent NAC improved treatment response.

Isoniazid (Nydrazid) [696] In research using rats, concurrent administration of NAC reduced drug-induced oxidative hepatic injury.

Nitroglycerin [702] NAC potentiates effect of nitroglycerin in unstable angina patients. Concurrent use may cause hypotension and headaches.

Oral hypoglycemic agents [701] (see Appendix 24) In research animals, NAC decreased blood glucose. Monitor patients with diabetes.

Rifampicin [696] In research using rats, concurrent administration of NAC reduced drug-induced oxidative hepatic injury.

Neem *Azadirachta indica*
PART USED: Various.
CONTRAINDICATIONS: Safety in lactation, pregnancy and children not established.
Male infertility.
SAFETY: Possible damage to chromosomes. Neem oil has caused mitochondrial injury in mice. Poisonous in high doses.

Neem(cont'd.)

ADVERSE REACTIONS: Large amounts may cause convulsions, diarrhea, inactivity, respiratory distress and stupor. Toxic amounts may cause coma, death, drowsiness, loss of consciousness, metabolic acidosis, seizures.

INTERACTIONS:

Insulin/Oral hypoglycemic agents[703,704] (see Appendix 24) In laboratory animals, leaf extract or seed oil had a hypoglycemic effect.

Glyburide/Glibenclamide[298] In research using rats, neem seed kernel powder further reduced blood glucose and lipids. An increase in liver hexokinase was noted. Concurrent use should only be made under the care of a health care professional, as OHA and neem may result in hypoglycemia.

Thyroid replacement therapy[280] In research using mice, leaf extract decreased T_3 and T_4. It may inhibit T_3 production at high doses.

Nettle/Stinging Nettle *Urtica dioica*

USES: BPH (H-combined with saw palmetto).

PART USED: Leaf, root.

CONTRAINDICATIONS: CHF, edema, kidney disease, pregnancy, lactation.

SAFETY: AHPA Class: 1.[66]

ADVERSE REACTIONS: Allergic reaction, diuresis, edema, GI distress, natriuresis, oliguria, sedation, urticaria.

INTERACTIONS:

Antihypertensives[706] (see Appendix 11) In research using rats, herb was found to have a diuretic and hypotensive effect, which theoretically may be additive. **192**

Anticoagulants and drugs that increase the risk of bleeding[705] (see Appendix 8)
Herb contains serotonin, which has coagulant activity. Concurrent use of herb may decrease effectiveness of drugs. Herb also contains vitamin K, which antagonizes the anticoagulant effect of warfarin.

CNS depressants[117] (see Appendix 15) Herb has sedative activity, which theoretically may be additive with sedating drugs.

Diuretics[706] (see Appendix 11) In research using rats, herb was found to have diuretic and hypotensive effects, which theoretically may be additive.

Insulin/Oral hypoglycemic agents[105] (see Appendix 24) Possible hypoglycemia or loss of blood glucose control.

Niauli Oil *Melaleuca viridiflora*
PART USED: Oil.
CONTRAINDICATIONS: Gallbladder inflammation, GI inflammation, liver disease.
Should not be used on facial area of children.
ADVERSE REACTIONS: Diarrhea, N&V.
INTERACTIONS:
May reduce or shorten effect of other drugs[1] Increased liver detoxification.

Noni *Morinda spp.*
PART USED: Juice.
CONTRAINDICATIONS: Renal disease patients needing potassium restriction (contains as much potassium as orange juice). Safety in pregnancy and lactation not

Noni (cont'd.)

established. Hyperkalemia.

ADVERSE REACTIONS: Case report of chronic renal insufficiency with hyperkalemia following use of noni juice.

INTERACTIONS:

Oral hypoglycemic agents[279] (see Appendix 24) Research using streptozotocin-induced hyperglycemic rats showed significant hypoglycemic activity after 3 days of continuous administration of 400 mg/kg. Herb may stimulate beta cells of pancreas to increase release of insulin. Therapeutic use of noni juice should only be made under the supervision of a health care provider. The effect when combined with diabetes medications is unknown and may require an alteration of drug dosage.

Nutmeg *Myristica fragrans*

PART USED: Aril, seed.

CONTRAINDICATIONS: Pregnancy.

SAFETY: Contains myristicin (methoxysafrole), which has been found to be carcinogenic and mutagenic. Greater than 5 g may cause changes in consciousness and hallucinations. Greater than 9 g may have effects similar to atropine. Large doses have caused death. AHPA Class: 2b, 3.[66]

ADVERSE REACTIONS: High amounts may cause abortion, alterations in pulse, anticholinergic hyperstimulation, disorientation, hallucinations, fear of impending death, feeling of pressure on chest and abdomen, giddiness, hypothermia, N&V, palpitations, psychosis.

INTERACTIONS:

Drugs that are metabolized by P450 isozymes CYP1A1/2, CYP2B1/2 and CYP2E1[708] In research using rats, myristicin, a component of nutmeg, induced the above isozymes, which may decrease serum levels of drugs that are substrates of these isozymes.

Flunitrazepam (Rohypnol)[707] Case report (55 year old female) of death, most likely due to toxic interaction between nutmeg and drug.

MAOIs[916] (see Appendix 9) Myristicin, a component of herb, inhibits MAO, and theoretically may have an additive effect.

Oak *Quercus petraea, Quercus robur*

PART USED: Bark.

CONTRAINDICATIONS: Cardiac insufficiency, hypertonia, infectious disease, external use on broken skin.

SAFETY: Contains tannins; avoid high dose for extended period. AHPA Class: 2d— not with extensive open wounds, fever and infectious disease, cardiac deficiency stage III & hypotonia stage IV.[66]

INTERACTIONS:

Reduces or inhibits absorption of alkaline drugs.[1,175]

Alkaloids[4] (see Appendix 4) High tannin content of herb may cause alkaloids to become insoluble and precipitate.

Atropine[4] Tannins in herb may interfere with absorption of drug.

Codeine[4] Tannins in herb may interfere with absorption of drug.

Oak (cont'd.)

    Ephedrine[4] Tannins in herb may interfere with absorption of drug.

    Iron[4] Tannins in herb cause iron to precipitate.

    Pseudoephedrine[4] Tannins in herb may interfere with absorption of drug.

    Theophylline (Uniphyl, Uni-Dur)[4] Tannins in herb may interfere with absorption of drug.

Oats *Avena sativa*

    USES: Hypercholesterolemia (H-bran).

    PART USED: Spikelets.

    SAFETY: Take with adequate fluid. Effect on blood sugar is less than for most fiber-containing herbs and foods. AHPA Class: 1.[66]

    ADVERSE REACTIONS: Allergic reaction, contact dermatitis, distension, flatulence, increased frequency of bowel movements, increased stool bulk.

    INTERACTIONS:

    Seeds may decrease absorption of drugs.[710]

    Lovastatin (Mevacor)[710] Oat bran (50-100 mg/day) binds drug and decreases absorption.

    Morphine (MSIR, MS Contin, Oramorph, Roxanol)[709] In research using laboratory animals, a reconstituted tincture of oat antagonized the antinoceptive activity of morphine.

    Protease inhibitors[222] (see Appendix 22) Oat bran may assist in management of protease inhibitor-induced diarrhea.

Oleander *Nerium oleander*

PART USED: Leaf.

CONTRAINDICATIONS: Hypercalcemia (powdered extract).

SAFETY: Entire plant is toxic, and has caused fatal poisonings. Symptoms of poisoning: abdominal pain, cardiac abnormalities, cramping, diarrhea, N&V, pain in mouth.

ADVERSE REACTIONS: Abdominal pain, bradyarrhythmias, bradycardia, death, hyperkalemia, N&V, sedation, tachyarrhythmias.

INTERACTIONS:

Digoxin/Cardiac glycosides[34,711] Oleander contains the cardiac glycosides oleandrin and oleandrigenin. Theoretical additive effect.

Oleic Acid (OA)

INTERACTIONS:

Paclitaxel (Taxol)[337] OA and paclitaxel enhanced cytotoxic in T47D cells, MCF-7 cells, but not SK-Br3 cells. There was no effect in breast cancer cells preincubated with OA.

Oligofructose short-chain fructan

INTERACTIONS:

5-Fluorouracil[274] Research using mice showed synergistic effect of 5-fluorouracil and oligofructose (15% of diet) combination.

Cyclophosphamide (Cytoxan, Neosar)[274] Research using mice showed synergistic effect of cyclophosphamide and oligofructose (15% of diet) combination.

Oligofructose (cont'd.)

Cytarabine (Cytosar-U)[274] Research using mice showed additive effect of cytarabine and oligofructose (15% of diet) combination.

Doxorubicin (Adriamycin, Doxil, Rubex)[274] Research using mice showed additive effect of doxorubicin and oligofructose (15% of diet) combination.

Methotrexate (Rheumatrex)[274] Research using mice showed synergistic effect of methotrexate and oligofructose (15% of diet) combination.

Vincristine (Oncovin, Vincasar)[274] Research using mice showed additive effect of vincristine and oligofructose (15% of diet) combination.

Olive *Olea europaea*

USES: Essential arterial HTN (H-aqueous extract).

PART USED: Leaf.

CONTRAINDICATIONS: Hypoglycemia, hypotension.

ADVERSE REACTIONS: Gastric distress, hypoglycemia, hypotension.

INTERACTIONS:

Antihypertensives[242] (see Appendix 11) Olive leaf reduces hypertension. Concurrent use with antihypertensives should be monitored by health care professional.

Insulin/Oral hypoglycemic agents[70,105] (see Appendix 24) Oleuropeoside, a component of olive leaf, has hypoglycemic activity, as seen in research using laboratory animals. Herb may increase insulin secreted in response to glucose and increase peripheral uptake of glucose. Monitor patients with diabetes.

Onion *Allium cepa*

USES: Cardiovascular disease prevention (H).
PART USED: Bulb.
CONTRAINDICATIONS: Bleeding disorders, uncontrolled diabetes.
SAFETY: GRAS (oil, extract, oleoresin).
ADVERSE REACTIONS: Gastric distress.
INTERACTIONS:

Drugs metabolized by P450 isozymes CYP1A, CYP2B and CYP2E1[712] (see Appendix 38) In laboratory animals, onion powder induced CYP1A and CYP2B and inhibited CYP2E1. Serum levels of drugs metabolized by CYP1A and CYP2B may be decreased, and levels of drugs metabolized by CYP2E1 may be increased.

Anticoagulants and drugs that increase the risk of bleeding[212,240,328] (see Appendix 8) Onion (aqueous extract) may inhibit platelet aggregation. Thiosulfinates in fresh cut onion are probably responsible for antiplatelet activity, as seen in this research using human platelets. Propyl propane-TS, a component of onion, inhibited aggregation more potently than aspirin.

Insulin/Oral hypoglycemic agents[105,111,162,171,173] (see Appendix 24) In research animals, onion has a hypoglycemic effect, as well as a cholesterol lowering property. Monitor patients with diabetes.

Opium Poppy *Papaver somniferum*

PART USED: Seed.
CONTRAINDICATIONS: Pregnancy, lactation, children.
SAFETY: Contains alkaloids/narcotics. AHPA Class: 1.[66]

Opium Poppy (cont'd.)
  ADVERSE REACTIONS: Dependence, Guillain-Barré syndrome, occupational asthma, respiratory depression, sedation.
  INTERACTIONS:
    CNS depressants[713] (see Appendix 15) Herb contains morphine, which has sedative activity. Theoretical increased sedation.

Oregon Grape *Berberis aquifolium*
  USES: Psoriasis (H).
  PART USED: Root.
  CONTRAINDICATIONS: Safety in pregnancy and lactation not established. Bleeding disorders, gallbladder disease, hyperbilirubinemia, jaundice, kidney disease, liver disease.
  SAFETY: Contains berberine, which has a hypotensive effect.
  ADVERSE REACTIONS: Skin irritation. Increased bilirubin. Caution is urged with use of other herbs containing berberine (Amur cork tree, barberry, celandine, Chinese goldthread, goldenseal). Berberine may increase the risk of photosensitivity.
  INTERACTIONS:
    Berberine, a component of Oregon grape, may inhibit P450 enzymes.[122] (see Appendix 38)
    Acetaminophen/Paracetamol[122] Berberine, a component of herb, decreased the hepatotoxicity of acetaminophen.
    Alpha-adrenergic agonists[122,123] (see Appendix 36) Berberine (herb component), blocked muscle contraction by phenylephrine, norepinephrine and caffeine.

Oregon Grape (cont'd.)

Antiarrhythmics[130] (see Appendix 6) Berberine, a component of herb, has antiarrhythmic activity, which theoretically may be additive with antiarrhythmic drugs.

Antibiotics See Tetracycline and Pyrimethamine, below. Herb increased effectiveness of antibiotics.

Anticoagulants and drugs that increase the risk of bleeding[133] (see Appendix 8) Berberine, a component of herb, may inhibit platelet aggregation, which may increase bleeding.

Antihypertensives[130] (see Appendix 11) Berberine, a component of herb has a hypotensive effect, which theoretically may be additive with antihypertensive drugs.

Cyclophosphamide (Cytoxan, Neosar)[128,132] Berberine, a component of herb, decreased urotoxicity of drug in rats. In another study, berberine decreased retention of chemotherapeutic agents. Concurrent use is not suggested.

Digoxin/Cardiac glycosides[130] Berberine, a component of herb, may have an additive effect with cardiac glycosides.

General anesthetics[130] (see Appendix 20) Berberine, a component of herb, may potentiate hypotensive action of anesthetics.

MAOIs[134] (see Appendix 9) Berberine, a component of herb, competitively inhibited MAO-A in rat brain mitochondria. Avoid concurrent use.

Pentobarbital[122] Berberine, a component of herb, increased pentobarbital-induced sleep time.

Photosensitivity, drugs causing[127] (see Appendix 29) Preliminary research revealed a potential increase in photosensitivity with use of berberine (a component

Oregon Grape (cont'd.)

of herb), which theoretically may be additive with drugs that also increase photosensitivity. Avoid concurrent use.

Pyrimethamine (Daraprim, Fansidar)[126] Berberine, a component of herb, when combined with drug was more effective than combinations with other antibiotics in treating chloroquine-resistant malaria.

Tetracycline[125] (see Appendix 7) Simultaneous administration of tetracycline and herb (berberine) decreased efficacy of drug.

Papaya Extract/ Papain (proteolytic enzyme from papaya) *Carica papaya*
USES: PART USED: Leaf, fruit.
CONTRAINDICATIONS: Bleeding disorders (fruit/papain), pregnancy.
SAFETY: AHPA Class: 1.[66]
ADVERSE REACTIONS: Allergic reaction, gastritis, increased bleeding.
INTERACTIONS:

Anticoagulants and drugs that increase the risk of bleeding[177] (see Appendix 8) Papain inhibits platelet aggregation, which may further increase the risk of bleeding in patients also taking drugs that inhibit platelet aggregation.

Cyclophosphamide[715] Concurrent administration with papain caused severe damage to lung tissue in rats.

Diuretics[714] (see Appendix 11) In research using rats, herb had diuretic effect, which theoretically may be additive.

PART USED: Fruit/seed, root.

CONTRAINDICATIONS: CHF, pregnancy, kidney inflammation (herb and root), renal insufficiency, renal failure.

SAFETY: GRAS (spice, seasoning, flavoring, oil, extract, oleoresin). AHPA Class: 2b, 2d—not with inflammatory kidney disease.[66]

ADVERSE REACTIONS: Allergic reaction, anuria, bleeding of mucous membranes, cardiac arrhythmias, emaciation, fatty liver, GI bleeding, hemoglobinuria, kidney irritation, methemoglobinuria, photodermatitis, photosensitivity, vascular congestion, weight loss.

INTERACTIONS:

Warfarin[716,916] Herb contains 540 µg vitamin K per 100 g raw and 900 µg vitamin K per 100 g cooked parsley (provisional data). Vitamin K antagonizes the anticoagulant effect of warfarin. It is important to eat a consistent amount of vitamin K to prevent fluctuations in therapeutic effect of drug. Note that vitamin K content of plants varies. Herb also contains components that have an anticoagulant activity (rosmarinic acid) and antiplatelet activity (bergapten and imperatorin), which may offset coagulant activity to some extent.

Photosensitivity, drugs increasing[717] (see Appendix 29) Herb has caused photodermatitis in laboratory animals. Theoretical increased risk of photosensitivity with concurrent use.

Passion Flower *Passiflora incarnata*

USES: Generalized anxiety disorder (H), opiate withdrawal (H).

PART USED: Herb.

CONTRAINDICATIONS: Pregnancy.

SAFETY: Case report of 34 year old female with prolonged QTc and nonsustained ventricular tachycardia after consumption of therapeutic dose of passion flower. GRAS (flavoring). AHPA Class: 1.[66]

ADVERSE REACTIONS: Altered consciousness, CNS depression, drowsiness, GI distress, increased respiratory rate, may inhibit GI motility, reduced arterial blood pressure, ventricular tachycardia, vasculitis.

INTERACTIONS:

Anticoagulants-Warfarin (Coumadin), not heparin[719] (see Appendix 8) Herb contains variable amounts of vitamin K, which antagonizes the anticoagulant effect of warfarin.

Anxiolytics[721] (see Appendix 13) In research using mice, methanolic extract of herb exhibited anxiolytic properties. It is not known if this may be additive when combined with drugs having an anxiolytic effect.

CNS depressants[718] (see Appendix 15) Theoretical additive sedation.

Opiate withdrawal[720] Passionflower used as an adjunct to clonidine was superior to clonidine alone for mental symptoms of opiate withdrawal.

Pentobarbital (Nembutal)[718] Herb induced sleep with subtherapeutic dose of pentobarbital in mice.

Pau d'Arco Tabebuia spp.

USES: Antiinflammatory (A).

PART USED: Bark.

CONTRAINDICATIONS: Bleeding disorders, pregnancy.

SAFETY: There are two cases of hepatitis and death reported to the FDA. AHPA Class: 1.[66]

ADVERSE REACTIONS: Anemia, increased bleeding, N&V.

INTERACTIONS:

Anticoagulants/Warfarin (Coumadin), not heparin[722] (see Appendix 8) Herb contains lapachol, which is an antagonist of vitamin K and may increase risk of bleeding.

Pectin (powder from apple and citrus) Various

INTERACTIONS:

Herb may reduce intestinal absorption of other drugs.[723,724]

Acetaminophen/Paracetamol[724] The absorption of paracetamol has been delayed by pectin.

Lovastatin (Mevacor)[723] Herb may decrease absorption of drug.

Pennyroyal *Mentha pulegium*

PART USED: Herb.

CONTRAINDICATIONS: Children, epilepsy, HTN, kidney disease, lactation, liver disease, pregnancy.

SAFETY: Essential oil of leaf contains pulegone, which is metabolized into toxic

Pennyroyal (cont'd.)

metabolites by P450 isozymes, depleting the liver of glutathione. Pulegone has caused serious toxicity and death. One metabolite, menthofuran, exhibits hepatotoxicity. GRAS (flavoring). AHPA Class: 2b.[66]

ADVERSE REACTIONS: Abdominal pain, convulsions, death, dermatitis, disseminated intravascular coagulation, encephalopathy, hepatitis, increased blood pressure and pulse, N&V, paralysis. Large amounts may cause abortion, kidney damage, liver damage. Small amounts of oil may cause delirium, dizziness, hallucinations, seizures, shock, unconsciousness.

INTERACTIONS:

Hepatotoxic drugs[725] (see Appendix 21) Essential oil of herb has been associated with hepatotoxicity. Hepatotoxic drugs should be avoided.

Iron[269] Pennyroyal tea decreased absorption of non-heme iron by 73% in 77 human subjects, due to polyphenol content.

Peppermint *Mentha piperita*

USES: IBS (H-enteric oil capsules), cough (H-menthol), dyspepsia (H-oil), IBS (H-enteric oil), gastric ulcer (A), postoperative nausea (H-oil), nasal congestion (H), postoperative nausea (H), colonoscopy (H-oil), barium enema (H-oil), diverticular disease (H), tension headache (H), enhanced iron absorption (H-extract) , gallbladder and bile duct spasm (leaf).

PART USED: Oil (enteric coated), leaf.

CONTRAINDICATIONS: Bile duct obstruction (oil), external use on children (oil), gallbladder inflammation (oil), gallstones-cholecystitis (oil or leaf), liver disease (oil), achlorhydria (enteric coating my dissolve in stomach instead of small intestines), hiatal hernia, GERD. Safety of amounts exceeding those in food has not been established for pregnancy, lactation and children.

SAFETY: GRAS (spice, seasoning, flavoring, oil, extract, oleoresin). AHPA Class: 1.[66]

ADVERSE REACTIONS: Allergic response, dermatitis, mouth ulcers, GI distress, headache, flushing, heartburn.

INTERACTIONS:

Drugs metabolized by P450 CYP1A2 and CYP2E[313] (see Appendix 38) In liver microsomes or cytosol from rats given peppermint tea, CYP1A2 activity was 24% and CYP2E was 60% that of control animals. It is not known if inhibition also occurs in humans. Monitor patients taking peppermint and drugs that are substrates of these P450 enzymes, as serum levels may increase due to inhibition of metabolism.

Decreased gastric acid, drugs causing[911] (see Appendix 1) Drugs may cause dissolution of enteric coating prematurely.

Iron[269] Peppermint tea decreased absorption of non-heme iron by 84% in 77 human subjects, due to polyphenol content.

Periwinkle *Vinca minor*

USES: Mild to moderate dementia (H), stroke (H).

PART USED: Herb.

CONTRAINDICATIONS: Pregnancy. Hypotension or low blood pressure, constipation.

SAFETY: For use only under supervision of health care provider. AHPA Class: 2d—not with low BP and constipation.[66]

Periwinkle (cont'd.)

ADVERSE REACTIONS: Acute dyspnea, immune system suppression, N&V, leukocytopenia, lymphocytopenia, decreased levels of various globulins.

INTERACTIONS:

Digoxin (Lanoxin)[727] High dose chemotherapeutic agents have been found to decrease absorption of digoxin tablet (not capsule). It is possible that high doses of herb will also decrease absorption of digoxin, due to the alkaloids with chemotherapeutic action contained in herb.

Vincristine[726] Drug is an alkaloid derivative of herb. Effect would most likely be additive.

Vinblastine[726] Drug is an alkaloid derivative of herb. Effect would most likely be additive.

PG27, PG490, PG490-88 Natural and synthetic derivatives from *Tripterygium wilfordii*.

INTERACTIONS:

Cyclosporine (Neoral)[331] PG27, fraction purified from *Tripterygium wilfordii* extract, administered intraperitoneally in rats with heart or kidney transplant was associated with increased survival time. Herb fraction was synergistic with immunosuppressant drug. PG490 herbal extract (Triptolide) enhanced efficacy of cyclosporin. PG490-88, a semi-synthetic derivative of PG490, prolonged allograph survival.

Pheasant's Eye *Adonis vernalis*

PART USED: Above ground herb.

CONTRAINDICATIONS: Hypokalemia. Safety in pregnancy, lactation and children not established.

SAFETY: Contains cardiac glycosides.

ADVERSE REACTIONS: Overdose may cause arrhythmias. Diarrhea, GI distress, N&V.

INTERACTIONS:

Albuterol (Proventil, Ventolin)[910] Drug decreased serum digoxin, which is similar to the cardiac glycosides in pheasant's eye.

Amiodarone[911] Amiodarone reduces clearance and increases bioavailability of digoxin, a cardiac glycoside.

Aminoglycosides[912] (see Appendix 7) Aminoglycosides decrease absorption of digoxin in the GI tract. Digoxin is similar to the cardiac glycosides in pheasant's eye.

Amphotericin B (Amphocin, Fungizone)[912] Drug increases the risk of hypokalemia, which would increase the toxicity of pheasant's eye, based on interactions with digoxin, a cardiac glycoside drug.

Antacids[911] Magnesium and aluminum salts bind to digoxin in the GI tract, decreasing absorption. Digoxin is similar to cardiac glycosides in pheasant's eye.

Antiarrhythmics[912] (see Appendix 6) Possible synergistic or additive effect. Based on interactions with digoxin, a cardiac glycoside similar to those found in pheasant's eye.

Bleomycin (Blenoxane)[915] Use of drug with digoxin has decreased effectiveness of digoxin. Pheasant's eye contains cardiac glycosides similar to digoxin.

Pheasant's Eye (cont'd.)

Calcium[1] Concurrent use with herb increases risk of cardiac toxicity.

Calcium channel blockers[911] (see Appendix 11) Drug inhibits renal clearance of digoxin, which is similar to cardiac glycosides in pheasant's eye.

Carmustine (BiCNU)[912] Use of drug with digoxin has decreased effectiveness of digoxin. Pheasant's eye contains cardiac glycosides similar to digoxin.

Cholestyramine (Questran)[911] Drug decreases absorption of digoxin, a drug similar to the cardiac glycosides in pheasant's eye.

Colestipol (Colestid)[911] Drug decreases absorption of digoxin, a drug similar to the cardiac glycosides in pheasant's eye.

Cyclophosphamide (Cytoxan, Neosar)[912] Use of drug with digoxin has decreased effectiveness of digoxin. Pheasant's eye contains cardiac glycosides similar to digoxin.

Cyclosporine (Neoral)[912] Drug has been found to increase toxicity of digoxin, a drug similar to cardiac glycosides found in pheasant's eye.

Cytarabine (Cytosar-U)[914] Use of drug with digoxin has decreased effectiveness of digoxin. Pheasant's eye contains cardiac glycosides similar to digoxin.

Digoxin/Cardiac glycosides[728] Herb contains cardiac glycosides, which increase the effects and side effects of drug.

Diuretics[34] (see Appendix 11) Herb contains cardiac glycosides which may increase potassium loss, possibly additive with potassium-depleting diuretics.

Doxorubicin (Adriamycin)[913] Use of drug with digoxin has decreased effectiveness of digoxin. Pheasant's eye contains cardiac glycosides similar to digoxin.

Pheasant's Eye (cont'd.)

Erythromycin (E-mycin, ERYC, Ery-Tab)[911] Drug may increase serum cardiac glycosides (from herbs such as pheasant's eye/digitalis) by increasing bioavailability, possibly increasing risk of side effects.

Flecainide (Tambocor)[912] Drug increases clearance of digoxin, a cardiac glycoside similar to those found in pheasant's eye.

Glucocorticoids[1] Extended use increases effectiveness and side effects of drug.

Hydroxychloroquine (Plaquenil)[912] Drug has been found to decrease clearance of digoxin, a drug similar to cardiac glycosides in pheasant's eye.

Ibuprofen[912] Drug increases serum digoxin, which is similar to cardiac glycosides in pheasant's eye.

Indomethacin (Indocin)[912] Drug increases serum digoxin, which is similar to cardiac glycosides in pheasant's eye.

Itraconazole (Sporanox)[911] Drug may increase serum digoxin levels, thereby increasing toxicity of digoxin. Cardiac glycosides in pheasant's eye are similar to digoxin.

Laxatives[1] Herb increases the effects/side effects of drug.

Licorice[728] Licorice depletes potassium, which may increase toxicity of pheasant's eye (cardiac glycoside content).

Macrolide antibiotics and tetracycline[912] (see Appendix 7) Drug may increase serum cardiac glycosides (from herbs such as pheasant's eye/digitalis) by increasing bioavailability, possibly increasing the risk of side effects.

Nefazodone (Serzone)[448] Nefazodone increases serum digoxin, but clinical

Pheasant's Eye (cont'd.)

significance has not been established. Pheasant's eye contains cardiac glycosides similar to digoxin.

Penicillamine (Cuprimine)[911] Drug may decrease serum levels of digoxin, which is similar to the cardiac glycosides in pheasant's eye.

Phenytoin (Dilantin)[912] Drug has been found to decrease serum levels of digoxin, a cardiac glycoside similar to those in pheasant's eye.

Procarbazine (Matulane)[912] Use of drug with digoxin has decreased effectiveness of digoxin. Pheasant's eye contains cardiac glycosides similar to digoxin.

Propafenone (Rythmol)[911] Drug increases clearance of digoxin, a cardiac glycoside similar to those in pheasant's eye.

Quinidine (Quinaglute)[1] Herb increases the effects/side effects of drug.

Quinine[911] Drug may decrease clearance of digoxin, which may increase toxicity of digoxin. Herb contains digitoxin, another cardiac glycoside similar to digoxin.

Saluretics[1] Herb increases the effects/side effects of drug.

Stimulant laxatives Excessive use of laxatives increases the risk of hypokalemia, which may increase toxicity of drug.

Trazodone (Desyrel)[912] Drug may increase serum levels of digoxin, a cardiac glycoside similar to those in pheasant's eye.

Verapamil (Calan, Verelan)[911] Drug decreases clearance of digoxin, a cardiac glycoside similar to those in pheasant's eye.

Vincristine (Oncovin, Vincasar)[912] Use of drug with digoxin has decreased effectiveness of digoxin. Pheasant's eye contains cardiac glycosides similar to digoxin.

Phlogenzym® Includes: 90 mg bromelain, 48 mg trypsin, 100 mg rutin

INTERACTIONS:

Cyclosporine (Neoral) [265,728] Research on rats suggests Phlogenzym® may decrease the amount of cyclosporine needed to achieve therapeutic outcome in rheumatoid arthritis patients, which may decrease side effects of drug.

Phyllanthus *Phyllanthus niruri, Phyllanthus amarus*

USES: HTN (H), hepatitis (H).

PART USED: Leaf.

INTERACTIONS:

Insulin/Oral hypoglycemic agents [730] (see Appendix 24) Herb has a hypoglycemic effect. Monitor blood glucose in those on diabetes medication.

Pigeon Pea *Cajanus cajan*

INTERACTIONS:

Insulin/Oral hypoglycemic agents [78,105] (see Appendix 24) Unroasted nuts had hypoglycemic effect in mice. Roasted seeds, in contrast, had a hyperglycemic effect. Monitor patients with diabetes.

Plantain *Plantago lanceolata, Plantago major*

PART USED: Leaf.

SAFETY: AHPA Class: 1. [66]

ADVERSE REACTIONS: Anaphylaxis, chest congestion, constipation, flatulence, lip swelling, rash, sneezing, watering eyes.

Plantain (cont'd.)
  INTERACTIONS:
    Carbamazepine (Tegretol)[731] Herb may decrease plasma levels of drug.
    Lithium (Eskalith, Lithobid, Lithonate, Lithotabs)[731] Herb may decrease absorption and plasma concentration of drug.

Pleurisy Root *Asclepias tuberosa*
  PART USED: Root.
  CONTRAINDICATIONS: Pregnancy.
  SAFETY: Contains cardiac glycosides. Emetic. AHPA Class: 2b, 2d—possible N&V.[66]
  INTERACTIONS:
    Digoxin/Cardiac glycosides[54] Herb contains digoxin-like factors, whose effects may be additive when combined with drug.

Poplar *Populus spp.*
  PART USED: Bud.
  CONTRAINDICATIONS: Allergy to poplar buds, propolis, Peruvian balsam or salicylates.
  SAFETY: Contains salicylates, but not known to increase risk of bleeding. GRAS (buds as flavoring in alcoholic beverages).
  ADVERSE REACTIONS: Allergic reaction, skin allergy.

Prickly Pear *Opuntia spp.*

PART USED: Fruit, stem.

ADVERSE REACTIONS: Cactus granuloma, dermatitis, hypoglycemia, keratoconjunctivitis. Has been found to be nephrotoxic in rats.

INTERACTIONS:

Insulin/Oral hypoglycemic agents[173,333,732] (see Appendix 24) In research using rats, herb had a hypoglycemic action. Possible hypoglycemia or loss of blood glucose control. In case report of 57 year old male with type II diabetes given 200 ml of prickly pear sap tid before meals, mean fasting glucose went from 205 mg/dl to 105 mg/dl after 8th week of administration. Monitor patients on diabetes medications.

Psyllium *Plantago indica* (black seed), *Plantago ispaghula* (blonde seed and blonde seed husk), *Plantago ovata* (blonde seed husk), *Plantago psyllium* (black seed)

USES: Constipation (H), fecal incontinence (H), IBS (H), diarrhea (H-enterally fed), hemorrhoids (H), hypercholesterolemia (H), ulcerative colitis (H).

PART USED: Seed, seed husk.

CONTRAINDICATIONS: Esophageal stenosis, ileus (blonde), GI stenosis (blonde or black).

SAFETY: AHPA Class: 2d—take with 8oz. liquid, not with bowel obstruction.[66]

ADVERSE REACTIONS: Allergic reaction.

INTERACTIONS:

Delayed absorption of other drugs[1,66] (blonde seed and seed husk) Take drugs at least one hour before psyllium.

Psyllium (cont'd.)

Calcium[343] Relative calcium absorption was less than 90% when diet contained 10% psyllium or Metamucil® in study using rats. Other research has found no impact on calcium absorption.

Carbamazepine (Tegretol)[116] May decrease absorption (rate and amount).

Cholestyramine (Questran)[735,737] Concurrent intake of cholestyramine and psyllium increased cholesterol-lowering effect in hamsters. In human research, psyllium decreased GI side effects of drug.

Colestid (Colestipol)[736] In human research, psyllium and ½ dose of drug was effective in the treatment of high cholesterol and decreased side effects of drug.

Copper[116] Herb decreases absorption.

Coumarin derivatives[116] May decrease absorption.

Digoxin/Cardiac glycosides[116,734] One source warns of a decrease in absorption of drug. In research using elderly patients, psyllium had no effect on serum levels of digoxin.

Ethinyl estradiol[733] In research using rabbits, psyllium slightly increased amount of drug absorbed and decreased rate of absorption.

Insulin/Oral hypoglycemic agents[162,738,740,742,743] (see Appendix 24) Psyllium taken before a meal may decrease postprandial blood glucose, which may require an adjustment in diabetes medication. Monitor patient.

Lithium (Eskalith, Lithobid, Lithonate, Lithotabs)[104,116,6,741] Herb may decrease absorption and plasma concentration of drug.

Magnesium[116] Herb may decrease absorption.

Orlistat (Xenical)[738] In research, obese patients were given orlistat and psyllium hydrophilic mucilloid or placebo. It was found that 12 g of psyllium in water at bedtime, along with a moderate fat diet, was effective in decreasing GI events associated with orlistat use.

Protease inhibitors[222] (see Appendix 22) Psyllium may assist in management of protease inhibitor-induced diarrhea.

Vitamin B₁₂[116] Herb may decrease absorption.

Zinc[116] Herb may decrease absorption.

Quassia *Quassia amara*

PART USED: Bark, root, wood.

CONTRAINDICATIONS: Pregnancy.

SAFETY: GRAS (flavoring). AHPA Class: 2b.[66]

ADVERSE REACTIONS: Gastric irritation, vomiting.

Quercetin[346] Herbs containing quercetin: (Note: research used isolated quercetin, not specific herbs.) Evening Primrose leaf (*Oenothera biennis*) 207,000 ppm; Mayapple resin exudate/sap (*Podophyllum peltatum*) 50,000 ppm; Onion, Shallot bulb (*Allium cepa*) 48,100 ppm; Tea leaf (*Camellia sinensis*) 10,000 ppm; Himalayan Mayapple rhizome (*Podophyllum hexandrum*) 5,600-12,000 ppm; Neem flower (*Azadirachta indica*) 1,000 ppm; Girasol, Sunflower (*Helianthus annuus*) flower - 400 ppm, leaf - 210 ppm; Oats hay (*Avena sativa*) 310 ppm; Apple pericarp (*Malus domestica*) 263 ppm; American Cranberry, Cranberry, Large Cranberry fruit (*Vaccinium macrocarpon*) 250 ppm; Garlic bulb (*Allium sativum*) 200 ppm; Cabbage, Red Cabbage, White Cabbage leaf (*Brassica oleracea var. capitata*) 100 ppm; Cayenne, Chili, Hot Pepper, Red Chili, Spur Pepper, Tabasco (*Capsicum frutescens*) 63 ppm.

USES: Interstitial cystitis (H- Cysta-Q), category III chronic prostatitis syndromes (H).

INTERACTIONS:

Acetaminophen and other drugs metabolized by P450 CYP1A2[744] (see Appendix 38) In research using rat hepatic microsomes, quercetin inhibited oxidation of acetaminophen by 65%. In research using human hepatic microsomes, CYP3A4 oxidation of acetaminophen was inhibited. Serum levels of drugs metabolized by CYP1A2 and CYP3A4.

Cisplatin (Platinol)[314] In rats, quercetin was cytoprotective against cisplatin-induced renal damage.

Tamoxifen (Nolvadex)[308] Human non-small-cell lung cancer cells with type II binding sites were treated in vitro with tamoxifen. Quercetin increased the inhibition of cancer cell growth.

Raspberry *Rubus idaeus*

PART USED: Fruit, leaf.

CONTRAINDICATIONS: Pregnancy.

SAFETY: Contains tannins; avoid high dose for extended period. AHPA Class: 1.[66]

INTERACTIONS:

Alkaloids (see Appendix 4)[4] High tannin content of herb may cause alkaloids to become insoluble and precipitate.

Red Clover *Trifolium pratense*

PART USED: Flower, herb.

CONTRAINDICATIONS: Estrogen-sensitive cancers, pregnancy, lactation, children.

SAFETY: Herb contains coumestrol, which doesn't affect bleeding. GRAS (spice, seasoning, flavoring, oil, extract, oleoresin). AHPA Class: 2b.[66]

ADVERSE REACTIONS: Abnormal lactation, altered growth pattern in animals, dystonia, infertility, prolapsed uterus.

INTERACTIONS:

Drugs which are substrates of P450 CYP3A4 isozymes[227] (see Appendix 38) Preliminary in vitro research has shown that red clover may alter metabolism and/or effectiveness of drugs which are substrates of CYP3A4 isozymes. Further research is needed to determine if interaction will also occur in humans.

Estrogen replacement therapy[247] In research using ovariectomized mice, red clover was found to have weak estrogenic activity. It is not known what the effect is when combined with estrogen replacement therapy.

Oral contraceptives[247] In research using ovariectomized mice, red clover was found to have weak estrogenic activity. It is not known what the effect is when combined with oral contraceptives.

UV radiation[745] In research using mice, isoflavonoids contained in herb, applied topically, had a protective effect against inflammation and immune suppression induced by UV radiation.

Red Sandlewood *Pterocarpus santalinus*
  PART USED: Heart wood.
  SAFETY: GRAS (flavoring in alcoholic beverages). AHPA Class: 1.[66]
  ADVERSE REACTIONS: Allergic reaction, contact dermatitis.
  INTERACTIONS:
    Oral hypoglycemic agents[256] (see Appendix 24) Ethanolic bark extract decreased serum glucose the greatest at 7 hours. Use of herb with oral hypoglycemic agents should only be made under the supervision of a knowledgeable health care professional. Action of herb is believed to be regeneration of beta cells in pancreas, insulin-like activity or the conversion of proinsulin to insulin.

Red Yeast Rice fermented with *Monascus purpureus*
  USES: Hypercholesterolemia (H).
  CONTRAINDICATIONS: Safety in pregnancy, lactation and children not established.
  SAFETY: May contain citrinin, which is toxic to kidney. Monitor LFTs. Muscle pain should be reported to health care professional immediately. Herb contains low levels of monacolin K, also known as lovastatin, as well as other monacolins.
  ADVERSE REACTIONS: Anaphylaxis, headache, pneumonia, rash.
  INTERACTIONS:
    Drugs that inhibit P450 CYP3A4 (Grapefruit juice also inhibits CYP3A4)[746,751] (see Appendix 38) Lovastatin, a component of red yeast rice, is a substrate of CYP3A4, and serum levels may be increased by drugs that inhibit CYP3A4.
    Drugs that increase the risk of rhabdomyolysis[752] (see Appendix 31) May increase the risk of rhabdomyolysis. Avoid concurrent use. Interaction based

Red Yeast Rice (cont'd.)

on lovastatin content.

Hormone replacement therapy[747] Concurrent use of statin drug (herb contains lovastatin) with hormone replacement therapy may have a positive impact on lipid metabolism in postmenopausal women.

Lipid-lowering drugs, especially statins[751] (see Appendix 25) Herb contains low levels of monacolin K, also known as lovastatin, as well as other monacolins. Herb's effect would most likely be additive. Avoid concurrent use.

Niacin[749,750] The addition of niacin to simvastatin therapy (a statin drug similar to statin contained in red yeast rice) in patients with coronary artery disease was found to be beneficial, especially for raising HDLs. High doses of niacin may increase the risk of myopathy, and concurrent use should only be made under the supervision of a health care professional. Any muscle pain should be reported immediately.

Warfarin[748] Simvastatin (statin drug) may alter INR in patients also taking warfarin. Red yeast rice also contains lovastatin. Monitor INR.

Redheaded Cotton Bush *Asclepias curassavica*

SAFETY: Contains cardioactive substance (asclepin).

INTERACTIONS:

Digoxin/Cardiac glycosides[34,753] Herb contains asclepin, a cardenolide, which may increase the toxicity of drug.

Reishi *Ganoderma lucidum*

  USES: Prostate cancer (H-as part of PC-SPEC).

  PART USED: Fruiting body, mycelium.

  CONTRAINDICATIONS: Bleeding disorders, lactation, pregnancy.

  SAFETY: AHPA Class: 1.[66]

  ADVERSE REACTIONS: Bone pain, constipation, diarrhea, dizziness, GI distress, nosebleed, skin irritation.

  INTERACTIONS:

  Acyclovir (Zovirax)[760] Acidic protein bound polysaccharide isolated from reishi mushroom combined with acyclovir was found to have a synergistic effect against HSV-1 and HSV-2 in vero cells.

  Anticoagulants and drugs that increase the risk of bleeding[754,761] (see Appendix 8) Mushroom may inhibit platelet aggregation and has anticoagulant activity. In a study of 5 HIV-positive hemophiliacs, consumption of mushroom had no effect on platelet aggregation.

  Antihypertensives[244] (see Appendix 11) Water extract of mycelia may decrease blood pressure. Concurrent use with antihypertensives should be monitored by health care professional.

  Antibiotics[756] (see Appendix 7) Aqueous extract from carpophores of mushroom, had an additive or synergistic effect when combined with various antibiotics in in vitro study.

  Cefazolin[756] An aqueous extract from carpophores of *Ganoderma lucidum* was synergistic against *Bacillus subtilis* and *Klebseilla oxytoca*.

  Immunosuppressants[758] (see Appendix 23) Mushroom has been found to stimulate the immune system; It is not known if this activity may decrease the effectiveness of chemotherapy. More research is needed.

Insulin/Oral hypoglycemic agents[759] (see Appendix 24) Ganoderan B, a component of reishi mushroom, increased serum insulin levels in mice, which may decrease serum glucose. Patient with type 2 diabetes may need an adjustment in diabetes medications. Monitor blood glucose.

Interferon[757] Acidic protein bound polysaccharide of mushroom showed synergistic effect with interferon against herpes simplex virus types 1 and 2 in in vitro test.

Lipid-lowering drugs[755] (see Appendix 25) In in vitro research, ganoderic acid and its derivatives decreased cholesterol synthesis. Mushroom also contains chitosan, which has been found to lower cholesterol.

Rhinax Formula Water extract of: *Withania somnifera root, Asparagus racemosus root, Mucuna prurience root, Phyllanthus emblica fruit, Terminalia chebula fruit, Myristic fragrance seed, Glycyrrhiza glabra root.*

INTERACTIONS:

Alcohol[310] Rhinax formula reduced incidence and severity of alcohol-induced ulcers in rats by 47%.

Aspirin[310] Rhinax formula reduced incidence and severity of aspirin-induced ulcers in rats by 34%.

Rhubarb *Rheum officinale*

USES: Constipation (H), pregnancy-induced hypertension (H), diuretic (A), chronic renal failure (H), ulcers (H), pancreatitis (A), antiinflammatory (A), immunostimulant (A), antibacterial (H), antitrichomonal (A-emodin), cancer (A-emodin).

PART USED: Rhizomes, root.

CONTRAINDICATIONS: Abdominal pain of unknown origin, appendicitis, children under 12, Crohn's disease, GI inflammation, gastric or duodenal ulcers, ileus, intestinal obstruction, lactation, pregnancy, renal stones, ulcerative colitis.

SAFETY: Short-term use only (not more than 8-10 days). Contains oxalates and tannins. GRAS (flavoring in alcoholic beverages). Not high dose for extended period. AHPA Class: 2b, 2d—not with intestinal obstruction, abdominal pain of unknown origin, inflammatory disease of GI tract (appendicitis, irritable bowel, colitis, Crohn's disease, not in children <12 years old, not long-term or excessive amounts, caution with h/o kidney stones.[66]

ADVERSE REACTIONS: Albuminuria, cardiac irregularities, cramping, electrolyte imbalance, hypokalemia (can lead to heart dysfunction and muscular weakness). Chronic use may lead to pseudomelanosis coli, hematuria.

INTERACTIONS:

Herb may decrease intestinal absorption of other drugs.[116]

Antiarrhythmics[116] (see Appendix 6) Chronic use of herb may cause hypokalemia, which would increase toxicity of drug.

Cisplatin (Platinol)[917] In research using mice, concurrent use of rhubarb decreased toxicity without decreasing effectiveness of drug.

Corticosteroids[1,116] (see Appendix 18) Chronic use of herb may increase the

Rhubarb (cont'd.)

risk of hypokalemia when taken concurrently with corticosteroids.

Digoxin/Cardiac glycosides[116] Chronic use of herb may cause hypokalemia, which may increase toxicity of drug.

Diuretics[116] (see Appendix 11) Chronic use of herb concurrently with diuretics that increase the loss of potassium increases the risk of hypokalemia.

Laxatives[116] Concurrent use may increase risk of hypokalemia.

Quinidine (Quinaglute)[116] Herb potentiates drug.

Roman Chamomile *Chamaemelum nobile*

PART USED: Flower.

CONTRAINDICATIONS: Pregnancy. Allergy to *Asteraceae/Compositae* family.

SAFETY: AHPA Class: 2b.[66]

ADVERSE REACTIONS: Anaphylaxis, contact dermatitis, rhinitis.

INTERACTIONS:

Decreases effects of other drugs due to alteration of drug metabolizing enzymes[436] (see Appendix 38) Research on rat liver cells indicates (a 1,8-cineole (a component of Roman chamomile) may induce drug metabolizing enzymes such as CYP2B1. In one study, P450 enzymes were increased. This may decrease serum levels of drugs which are substrates of this isozyme.

CNS depressants[762] (see Appendix 15) Essential oil has been found to have a sedative effect. Theoretical additive effect.

Insulin/Oral hypoglycemic agents[87] (see Appendix 24) Chamaemeloside, a flavonoid from herb, has hypoglycemic activity. Monitor patients with diabetes.

Rosemary *Rosmarinus officinalis*

   PART USED: Leaf.

   CONTRAINDICATIONS: Pregnancy, female infertility.

   SAFETY: GRAS (spice, seasoning, flavoring, oil, extract, oleoresin). AHPA Class: 2b.[66]

   ADVERSE REACTIONS: Large amounts may cause abortion, contact dermatitis, gastric and GI irritation, kidney damage, seizures.

   INTERACTIONS:

   Drugs metabolized by P450 CYP1A, CYP2B, CYP2E and CYP3A isozymes[300,763] (see Appendix 38) Water extract of rosemary enhanced effectiveness of both phase I and phase 2 enzymes in rat liver. CYP1A1 activity was increased 4.5 x, CYP1A2 was increased 1.7 x, CYP2B1/2 was increased 7.9 x, CYP2E1 was increased 1.3 x and CYP3A was increased 1.3 x. Rosemary extract and purified rosmaric acid may alter the metabolism of numerous hepatic enzymes. The essential oil induced various isozymes, especially CYP2B.

   Drugs that are substrates of PGP[766] (see Appendix 38) Rosemary decreased the influx into cells of drugs that are substrates of PGP. Rosemary inhibited PGP activity by preventing the binding of PGP substrates. No actual interactions have been reported.

   Cyclophosphamide (Cytoxan, Neosar)[764] In research using rats, essential oil and ethanolic extract of rosemary decreased hepatotoxicity and the suppression of bone marrow cells induced by drug. Phenolic compounds in herb have antioxidant activity.

   Diuretics[765] (see Appendix 11) In research using rats, aqueous extract was

Rosemary (cont'd.)

found to have a diuretic effect. Theoretical additive effect.

Insulin/Oral hypoglycemic agents[71] (see Appendix 24) Volatile oil induced hyperglycemia in rabbits. Monitor patients being treated for diabetes.

Iron[268] In study of 27 women, rosemary tea decreased absorption of non-heme iron by 21%. Rosemary contains phenolic compounds which decrease absorption of iron.

Rubber Vine *Cryptostegia grandiflora*

SAFETY: Herb contains several cardiac glycosides.

INTERACTIONS:

Digoxin/Cardiac glycosides[34,767] Herb increases risk of drug toxicity.

Rue *Ruta graveolens*

PART USED: Herb.

CONTRAINDICATIONS: Bleeding disorders, kidney disease, children, lactation, pregnancy.

SAFETY: GRAS (as flavoring, 2-10 ppm). Hepatotoxic. Contains furanocoumarins, which increase photosensitization and are mutagenic. AHPA Class: 2b, 2d—not with compromised kidney function.[66]

ADVERSE REACTIONS: Abortion, allergic skin reactions, clammy skin, contact dermatitis (oil), dizziness, fainting, fatigue, GI irritation, hypotension, increased photosensitivity, irritation of stomach, kidney damage (oil), liver damage, low pulse, melancholy, muscle spasms, sleep disturbance, tongue swelling.

Rue (cont'd.)

INTERACTIONS:

Anticoagulants and drugs that increase the risk of bleeding[768] (see Appendix 8) Rue has been reported to contain coumarins that increase the risk of bleeding, but the coumarins in rue are furanocoumarins, which are not associated with bleeding.

Rupturewort *Herniaria glabra*

INTERACTIONS:

Antihypertensives[769] (see Appendix 11) In hypertensive rats, herb decreased blood pressure. Theoretically, this effect could be additive with hypertensive drugs.

Sacred Basil *Ocimum sanctum*

PART USED: Leaf.

CONTRAINDICATIONS: Children, lactation, pregnancy, thyroid disease.

SAFETY: Essential oil contains estragole, which has a mutagenic action after being metabolized. Not for extended use.

INTERACTIONS:

Anticoagulants and drugs that increase the risk of bleeding[773] (see Appendix 8) Fixed oil of herb increased clotting time and possibly may inhibit platelet aggregation, as seen in laboratory animals. Clinical significance unknown.

Bromocriptine[770] In mice, ethanolic extract of herb, when combined with drug, had a synergistic effect, which suggests that herb may have D2 agonist activity.

Doxorubicin (Adriamycin)[771] In in vitro research, ursolic acid from herb

228

showed a 13% protection of the liver cells and 17% protection of the heart cells.

Insulin/Oral hypoglycemic agents[53,105,192,772,775] (see Appendix 24) Herb lowered blood glucose in human subjects with type 2 diabetes, fasting by 17.6% and postprandial 7.3%. Patients taking diabetes medications should be monitored closely to prevent possible hypoglycemia.

Isoproterenol[774] In research using rats, herb was cardioprotective in isoproterenol-induced myocardial infarction.

Pentobarbital[770] In research using mice, ethanolic extract of herb increased lost reflex time induced by drug.

Pentobarbitone[773] In research using laboratory animals, fixed oil of herb increased pentobarbitone-induced sleep time. Clinical significance unknown.

Thyroid medications[776] In mice, leaf extract of herb decreased serum T_4. Monitor patients using herb leaf extract.

Safflower Carthamus tinctorius

PART USED: Flower.

CONTRAINDICATIONS: Bleeding disorders, gastric ulcers, pregnancy.

SAFETY: AHPA Class: 2b, 2d.[66]

ADVERSE REACTIONS: Allergic reactions, N&V.

INTERACTIONS:

Anticoagulants and drugs that increase the risk of bleeding[66] (see Appendix 8) Herb may increase risk of bleeding by delaying coagulation time.

Sage *Salvia officinalis*
   PART USED: Leaf.
   CONTRAINDICATIONS: Alcohol extract in pregnancy, lactation, children.
   SAFETY: Contains thujone. GRAS (spice, seasoning, flavoring, oil, extract, oleoresin).
   AHPA Class: 2b, 2d—no long-term use or excessive dosage.[66]
   ADVERSE REACTIONS: If ingested over a long period of time, alcohol extract or
   essential oil may cause convulsions. Cheilitis, N&V, stomatitis.
   INTERACTIONS:
      Alkaloids (see Appendix 4)[4] High tannin content of herb may cause alkaloids to
      become insoluble and precipitate.

Saiboku-To Formula contains: *Bupleuri radix, Pinelliae tuber, Hoelen, Scutellariae radix,
   Magnoliae cortex, Zizyphi fructus, Glycyrrhizae radix, Perillae herba, Zingiberis
   rhizoma.*
   ADVERSE REACTIONS: Pneumonia.
   INTERACTIONS:
      Diazepam (Valium)[285] In research conducted with male Sprague Dawley rats,
      saiboku-to was found to increase the anxiolytic effect of diazepam. Effect was not
      due to alterations in hepatic metabolism of drug. Authors suggest that herbal
      preparation may exert action through activation of GABA-A receptors and inhibition
      of histamine release.

      Prednisolone[23,176,211] Herb formula (containing *Panax ginseng, Ziziphus jujuba,
      Glycyrrhiza uralensis, Scutellaria baicalensis,* and *Bupleurum chinese*) affects
      pharmacokinetics of drug

Sairei-To TJ-114 (Contains glycyrrhizin)

USES: Muscle cramps from cirrhosis (H), pediatric IgA nephropathy (H), secretory otitis media (H-pediatric).

ADVERSE REACTIONS: GI distress.

INTERACTIONS:

Gentamicin (Garamycin)[777] In research using rats, sairei-to was found to be protective against nephrotoxicity of gentamicin.

Prednisolone[211] Herb had no effect on pharmacokinetics of drug.

Salt Bush Leaf *Atriplex halimus*

INTERACTIONS:

Insulin/Oral hypoglycemic agents[107,778] (see Appendix 24) Salt bush may potentiate insulin, as seen in in vitro research. Effect is most likely due to mineral content. More research is needed to determine if herb has a hypoglycemic effect in humans. Monitor blood glucose.

SAMe S-Adenosyl-L-methionine

USES: Depression (H), liver disease (A), cadmium chelation (H), nicotinic acid-induced hyperbilirubinemia in Gilbert's syndrome (H), osteoarthritis (H).

CONTRAINDICATIONS: Bipolar disorder. Safety in pregnancy, lactation and children not established.

ADVERSE REACTIONS: Diarrhea, GI distress, nausea, manic episode in bipolar disorder.

INTERACTIONS:

SAMe (cont'd.)

Acetaminophen/Paracetamol[784] In research using mice, SAMe administration was hepatoprotective against overdose of paracetamol, as seen by decreased mortality and liver necrosis. Further research is needed to determine if protective effect may be found in humans administered drugs with hepatotoxic effects.

Cyclosporine (Neoral)[781] In research using rats, SAMe decreased biliary bile abnormalities, liver secretions and protein secretions.

Imipramine and possibly other antidepressants[785] (see Appendix 9) In depressed patients administered IV SAMe, depressive symptoms were relieved sooner.

Interferon-alpha2b[782] Concurrent administration caused a decrease in the beneficial effects of each alone, which is in direct contrast to expected results (bile duct-ligated rats).

Levodopa (Lodosyn)[779,780] In research using mice, levodopa was found to increase methionine adenosyl transferase activity. In more recent research, SAMe improved depression in patients with Parkinson's disease.

Oral contraceptives[783] In a small preliminary study, SAMe decreased cholesterol supersaturation of gallbladder bile caused by oral contraceptives.

Sarsaparilla *Smilax febrifuga, Smilax regelii*
  PART USED: Root.
  SAFETY: GRAS (flavoring in alcoholic beverages). AHPA Class: 1.[66]
  ADVERSE REACTIONS: Diuresis, GI irritation, occupational asthma, skin irritation, temporary kidney impairment.

Sarsaparilla (cont'd.)

INTERACTIONS:

Bismuth[1] Herb may increase absorption of drug.

Digoxin/Cardiac glycosides[1] Herb may increase absorption of drug.

Hypnotics[1] Herb may increase excretion of simultaneously taken hypnotics.

Sassafras *Sassafras albidum*

PART USED: Leaf, root.

CONTRAINDICATIONS: Safety in pregnancy, lactation and children not established.

SAFETY: Contains safrole, which has been found to cause liver tumors. GRAS (leaves-flavoring safrole free). AHPA Class: 2d—not long term or excessive dose.[66]

ADVERSE REACTIONS: Abortion, cancer, dermatitis, diaphoresis, sedation, vomiting.

INTERACTIONS:

Drugs metabolized by P450 isozymes[786,787,788] (see Appendix 38) Eugenol, a component of herb, inhibits P450 enzymes, which may increase serum levels of drugs metabolized by these enzymes. Other research found no significant effect on P450 enzymes. Safrole, another component of herb, has also been found to induce these enzymes.

Saw Palmetto *Serenoa repens, Sabal serrulata*

USES: BPH (H).

PART USED: Fruit/berry.

CONTRAINDICATIONS: Bleeding disorders. Safety in pregnancy, lactation and children not established.

Saw Palmetto (cont'd.)

SAFETY: AHPA Class: 1.[66]

ADVERSE REACTIONS: GI distress, case report of excessive bleeding during surgery.

INTERACTIONS:

Drugs which are substrates of P450 CYP3A4 isozymes[227] (see Appendix 38) Preliminary in vitro research has shown that saw palmetto may alter metabolism and/or effectiveness of drugs that are substrates of CYP3A4 isozymes. Further research is needed to determine if interaction will also occur in humans.

Alkaloids (see Appendix 4)[4] High tannin content of herb may cause alkaloids to become insoluble and precipitate.

Anticoagulants and drugs that increase the risk of bleeding[789] (see Appendix 8) Case report of 54 year old male with intraoperative hemorrhage during surgery for left petroclival meningioma. Monitor patients taking the above drugs.

Doxazosin (Cardura)[41] Effect of concurrent use is unknown.

Estrogen replacement therapy[791] Herb has antiandrogenic effect. Effect of concurrent use is unknown.

Finasteride (Proscar)[790] It is unknown if herb (liposterolic extract) alters effectiveness of drug. Herb causes biochemical changes similar to those of drug.

Immunosuppressants/Immunostimulants[213] (see Appendix 23) Herb has immunostimulant activity, which may alter effects of drug.

Oral contraceptives[791] Herb has antiandrogenic effect. Effect of concurrent use is unknown.

Terazosin (Hytrin)[41] Effect of concurrent use is unknown.

Scopolia *Scopolia carniolica*

PART USED: Rhizome, root.
CONTRAINDICATIONS: GI stenosis, megacolon, narrow-angle glaucoma, prostate adenoma, tachycardia.
SAFETY: AHPA Class: 3.[66]
ADVERSE REACTIONS: Blurred vision, difficulty urinating, fever, glaucoma, hyperthermia, hypotension, red skin, reduced perspiration, tachycardia, xerostomia.
INTERACTIONS:
Amantadine[1] Increased anticholinergic activity of drug.
Quinidine (Quinaglute)[1] Increased anticholinergic activity of drug.
Tricyclic antidepressants[1] (see Appendix 9) Increased anticholinergic activity of drug.

Scotch Broom *Cytisus scoparius*

PART USED: Flowering tops, herb.
CONTRAINDICATIONS: CHF, HTN. Safety in pregnancy, lactation and children not established
SAFETY: Sparteine (alkaloid in herb) poisonings have been treated with prenalterol and isoprenaline. AHPA Class: 3.[66]
ADVERSE REACTIONS: Smoking herb may cause cardiac arrhythmias, headache, uterine stimulation.
INTERACTIONS:
Drugs that inhibit or induce P450 CYP2D6[793] (see Appendix 38) Sparteine, an alkaloid in herb, is metabolized by the CYP2D6 isozyme. Drugs that induce this

Scotch Broom (cont'd.)

isozyme will decrease serum levels of sparteine and drugs that inhibit this isozyme will increase serum level of sparteine, which could lead to circulatory collapse.

MAOIs[1] (see Appendix 9) Increased blood pressure or possible hypertensive crisis due to tyramine content of herb.

Sympathomimetics[792] (see Appendix 36) Theoretical increased risk of hypertension with concurrent use.

Scullcap *Scutellaria lateriflora*

PART USED: Herb.

CONTRAINDICATIONS: Safety in pregnancy, lactation and children not established.

SAFETY: Hepatotoxicity report may be a case of adulteration with germander. AHPA Class: 1.[66]

ADVERSE REACTIONS: Confusion, giddiness, pneumonitis, stupor, twitching.

INTERACTIONS:

CNS depressants[104] (see Appendix 15) Theoretical increase in sedation.

Sea Mango *Cerebra manghas*

INTERACTIONS:

Digoxin/Cardiac glycosides[34] Herb may increase drug toxicity.

Senega Snakeroot *Polygala senega*

PART USED: Root.

CONTRAINDICATIONS: Children, gastric ulcers, inflammatory bowel disease, lactation, pregnancy.

SAFETY: AHPA Class: 2b, 2d—not with gastritis or gastric ulcers. No long-term use.[66]

ADVERSE REACTIONS: Long-term use may lead to GI irritation.

INTERACTIONS:

Insulin/Oral hypoglycemic agents[794] (see Appendix 24) N-butanol extract of senega rhizomes had hypoglycemic action in mice. Insulin must be present for hypoglycemic action. Monitor patients with diabetes.

Senna *Cassia spp., Senna spp.*

USES: Constipation (H).

PART USED: Fruit, leaf, pod.

CONTRAINDICATIONS: Abdominal pain of unknown origin, pregnancy, lactation, children < 12, appendicitis, Crohn's disease, ulcerative colitis, ileus, intestinal inflammation or obstruction.

SAFETY: Short-term only, not more than 2 weeks or with abdominal pain of unknown origin. GRAS (flavoring). AHPA Class: 2b, 2c, 2d—not with intestinal obstruction, abdominal pain of unknown origin, inflammatory disease (appendicitis, colitis, Crohn's disease, IB), not with hemorrhoids, not < 12 years old, not longer than 8 days.[66]

ADVERSE REACTIONS: Albuminuria, cachexia, cramps, electrolyte imbalance, cardiac irregularities, hematuria, hypokalemia (can lead to heart dysfunction), laxative dependency and muscle weakness), pseudomelanosis coli, reversible finger clubbing.

Senna (cont'd.)
  INTERACTIONS:
    Herb may reduce intestinal absorption of other drugs.[4]
    Antiarrhythmics[175] (see Appendix 6) Herb may potentiate drug.
    Corticosteroids[175] (see Appendix 18) Herb use with drug may cause hypokalemia.
    Digoxin/Cardiac glycosides[175] Chronic herb use may increase effects of cardiac glycosides.
    Diuretics[175] (see Appendix 11) Herb may interfere with potassium-sparing effect of drug.
    Licorice[1] Licorice increases the loss of potassium, which may be additive when combined with senna.

Shankhapushpi Ayurvedic herbal formula (containing *Convolvulus pluricaulis* [chois], *Centella asiatica* [urban], *Nardostachys jatamansi* [DC], *Nepeta hinostana* [haimes], *Nepeta elliptica* [Royle], *Onosma bracteatum* [wall])
  INTERACTIONS:
    Phenytoin (Dilantin)[69] Multiple doses of herb decreased serum drug level.

Shark Cartilage
  USES: Analgesic (A), cancer adjunct (H-equivocal), psoriasis (H), weak antiinflammatory (A).
  CONTRAINDICATIONS: Liver disease. Safety in pregnancy, lactation and children not established.
  ADVERSE REACTIONS: Diarrhea, hepatitis, N&V.

INTERACTIONS:

Alcohol[316,319] Daidzein and daidzin, components of herb, decreased alcohol-induced sleep time in rats, which may be due to delayed gastric emptying. Daidzin caused blood alcohol to peak later and lower than in controls. Neither isoflavonoid altered alcohol dehydrogenase or aldehyde dehydrogenase activity. The isoflavonoids, daidzin, daidzein and puerarin decreased the alcohol intake in alcohol-preferring rats, indicating potential for use in the treatment of alcoholism. In hamster, *Radix puerariae* potentiated the bioavailability of daidzin, which suppressed alcohol intake in a dose dependent manner. Based on this interaction, it is possible that *Radix puerariae* may enhance the bioavailability of other drugs.

Shiitake Mushrooms *Lentinus edodes*

USES: Cancer (H—lentinan), HIV (H), hypercholesterolemia (H—fiber), impaired NK activity following cardiopulmonary bypass (H—lentinan preoperatively).

PART USED: Fruiting body, mycelium.

CONTRAINDICATIONS: Bleeding disorders.

SAFETY: AHPA Class: 1.[66]

ADVERSE REACTIONS: Lentinan—anaphylactoid reaction, back pain, leg pain, depression, rigor, fever, chills, granulocytopenia and elevated liver enzymes.

INTERACTIONS:

Anticoagulants and drugs that increase the risk of bleeding[796] (see Appendix 8) In vitro study of mushroom showed an inhibition of platelet aggregation.

Shiitake Mushrooms (cont'd.)

Chemotherapy[797] (see Appendix 16) May offset side effects of chemotherapy.

Didanosine (Videx)[795] Lentinan, a component of shiitake mushroom, may increase CD4 immune cell count when taken concurrently with didanosine.

Sho-saiko-To TJ-9 (contains glycyrrhizin) Contains: *Bupleurum falcatum, Pinella ternata, Scutellaria baicalensis, Zizphus vulgaris, Panax ginseng, Glycyrrhiza glabra, Zingiber officinale*

USES: Hepatitis (H).

ADVERSE REACTIONS: Pneumonitis, pulmonary edema, thrombocytopenic purpura.

INTERACTIONS:

Drugs metabolized by P450 CYP3A4 and CYP1A2[800] (see Appendix 38) Components of *Scutellaria baicalensis*, baicalein and wogonin, were found to alter P450 isozymes at high doses in rats. More research is need to determine if this alteration of P450 activity occurs in humans at therapeutic doses.

Insulin/Oral hypoglycemic agents[801] (see Appendix 24) In research using rats, herb formula lowered blood glucose. Monitor patients with diabetes.

Lamivudine (3TC)[799] In HIV patients, sho-saiko-to combined with 3TC enhanced anti-HIV-1 activity.

Interferon-alpha[798] Concurrent use of herbal remedy and drug may increase the risk of drug-induced pneumonitis.

Prednisolone[211] Herbal combination decreased serum concentration of drug.

Tolbutamide (Orinase)[303] Sho-saiko-To increased the intestinal absorption of tolbutamide, potentiating the hypoglycemic effect in rats. Plasma levels of tolbutamide were increased at one hour. This herbal combination may increase the risk of hypoglycemia when taken with OHA.

Siberian Ginseng *Eleutherococcus senticosus*

USES: Herpes (H)

PART USED: Root, root bark.

CONTRAINDICATIONS: Pregnancy, lactation, febrile state, HTN, MI.

SAFETY: Not for long term use. Not suggested for people less than 40 years of age. AHPA Class: 1.66

ADVERSE REACTIONS: Diarrhea, drowsiness, headache, hypoglycemia, HTN, skin eruptions. High doses can cause anxiety, insomnia and irritability.

INTERACTIONS:

N6-(delta 2-isopentenyl)-adenosine[805] Additive antiproliferative effect in L1210 leukemia cells.

CNS depressants[804] (see Appendix 15) Herb increased hexobarbital sleep time. Theoretical increased sedation with sedating drugs.

Cytarabine (Cytosar-U)[805] Additive antiproliferative effect in L1210 leukemia cells.

Digoxin (Lanoxin)[56,225] Silk vine (*Periploca sepium*) that was misidentified as Siberian ginseng was most likely cause of case report of interaction. No other reports of interaction between Siberian ginseng and digoxin noted.

Hexobarbital[804] Herb increased hexobarbital sleep time. Effect may be due to enzyme inhibition.

Insulin/Oral hypoglycemic agents[803] (see Appendix 24) In mice, intraperitoneal

Siberian Ginseng (cont'd.)

injection of herb had hypoglycemic action. It is not known if this effect is additive with diabetes medications. Monitor blood glucose.

Kanamycin (Kantrex)[802] Concurrent administration of herb with drug increased effectiveness of antibiotic treatment for dysentery and *Proteus* infection in children.

Monomycin[802] Concurrent administration of herb with drug increased effectiveness of antibiotic treatment for dysentery and *Proteus* infection in children.

Nifedipine and other drugs metabolized by P450 CYP3A4[278] (see Appendix 38) Research on 22 healthy human subjects showed a 29% increase in mean plasma levels of nifedipine with concurrent use of herb, suggesting inhibition of CYP3A4.

Si-Wu-Tang contains: Danggui (*Angelica sinensis*), Baishaoyao (*Paeonia lactifolia*), huanxiong (*Cnidium officinale*), Shoudenhaung (*Rehmannia glutinosa*), Si-Jun-Zi-Tang (SJZT)

INTERACTIONS:

Radiation therapy[284] In research using female mice, Si-Wu-Tang (administered prior to radiation therapy) was found to decrease the toxicity of radiation therapy. Ingredients responsible for effect are believed to be Danggui (*Angelica sinensis*) and Baishaoyao (*Paeonia lactifolia*).

Silk Cotton Tree *Bombax ceiba*

PART USED: Leaf.

INTERACTIONS:
Insulin/Oral hypoglycemic agents[19] (see Appendix 24) Shamimin, a glucoside of silk cotton, may decrease blood glucose, as seen in laboratory animals. Monitor blood glucose.

Slippery Elm *Ulmus fulva, Ulmus rubra* Part of Essaic Formula

PART USED: Bark.

SAFETY: AHPA Class: 1.[66]

ADVERSE REACTIONS: Allergic reaction, contact dermatitis, urticaria.

INTERACTIONS:
Herb may reduce intestinal absorption of other drugs due to hydrocolloidal fiber content (theoretical).[4]

Soybeans *Glycine max*

USES: Antibiotic-induced diarrhea (H—soy fiber added to infant formula), chronic renal disease (H-soy protein), hot flashes (H), hypercholesterolemia (H), osteoporosis (H).

PART USED: Bean.

CONTRAINDICATIONS: History of calcium oxalate kidney or urinary stones. Safety of use with patients that have estrogen-sensitive cancers not established.

ADVERSE REACTIONS: Diarrhea (soy phospholipid), GI distress (soy phospholipid), flatulence, increased risk of kidney stones. May decrease absorption of zinc, calcium and iron.

Soybeans (cont'd.)
INTERACTIONS:

Cisplatin (Platinol)[807] In one study using human medulloblastoma cells, genistein (isoflavone contained in soy) enhanced the antiproliferative and cytotoxic action of drug. More research is needed before genistein can be safely used in humans.

Estrogen replacement therapy/Oral contraceptives[809, 811]—potencies of estradiol 100, genistein 0.084, and daidzein 0.013 Soy contains genistein and daidzein. Isoflavones in soy may displace conjugated estrogens from receptors. In one study of premenopausal women on oral contraceptives, no changes in menstrual cycle or serum sex hormones was noted.

Oral hypoglycemic agents[292,806,813] (see Appendix 24) Touchi extract (from fermented soybean) decreased postprandial blood glucose in humans (with either borderline diabetes or non-insulin dependent diabetes) and in rats. Activity of Touchi is similar to oral hypoglycemic agents with alpha-glucosidase inhibitory action. Therapeutic use of Touchi should only be made under the supervision of a health care provider. The effect when combined with diabetes medications is unknown and may require an alteration of drug dosage.

MAOIs[810] (see Appendix 9) Soy products such as tofu and soy sauce may contain tyramine, which when combined with MAOIs may lead to hypertensive crisis.

Tamoxifen (Nolvadex)[297] In vitro research using human breast cell carcinoma showed a synergistic effect in concurrent use of purified genistein (isoflavone contained in soybean) and tamoxifen. Greater antiproliferative and cytotoxic effects were noted than with tamoxifen alone.

Thyroid replacement therapy[808,812] Take thyroid medications 2-3 hours prior to soy consumption. There is a case report of a 34 year old female on levothyroxine needing an increased dose after use of soy protein supplement immediately after ingestion of drug. Separation of soy product and thyroid medication resolved the need for additional drug. Children with congenital hypothyroidism may need changes in thyroid replacement therapy if fed soy formula. Iodine intake may alter effect.

Squill *Urginea maritima*

PART USED: Bulb

CONTRAINDICATIONS: Hypercalcemia, hyperkalemia, children, lactation, pregnancy.

SAFETY: Contains cardiac glycosides. Animals have been poisoned by herb.

ADVERSE REACTIONS: Atrioventricular block, CNS effects, convulsions, diarrhea, GI distress, irregular pulse, hyperkalemia, N&V, pseudolupus, seizures, ventricular arrhythmias and death.

INTERACTIONS:

Digoxin/Cardiac glycosides[1] Herb contains cardiac glycosides, which theoretically may increase toxicity of drug.

Glucocorticoids[1] Extended use of herb increases effectiveness and side effects of drug.

Laxatives[1] Increased effectiveness and side effects.

Quinidine (Quinaglute)[1] Increased effectiveness and side effects.

Saluretics[1] Increased effectiveness and side effects.

St. John's Wort *Hypericum perforatum*

USES: Anxiety (A), climacteric symptoms of menopause (H), mild to moderate depression (H), obsessive-compulsive disorder (H), seasonal affective disorder (H), smoking cessation (H).

PART USED: Herb, flowering tops.

CONTRAINDICATIONS: Pregnancy (research in animals showed no effect on fetal growth), lactation, bipolar disorders, male infertility, schizophrenia, thyroid disease.

SAFETY: Contains tannins; avoid high dose for extended period. MAOI activity of SJW is very weak and should not have clinical significance unless amounts exceeding those used therapeutically are ingested. SJW is a cadmium assimilator. GRAS (flavoring-hypericin free). AHPA Class: 2b—may potentiate MAOIs.[66]

ADVERSE REACTIONS: Photosensitizing potential in light-skinned individuals and in amounts exceeding recommended dosage. Abdominal pain, allergic reaction, alopecia, anorexia, anxiety, apathy, confusion, constipation, decreased sperm motility, diarrhea, dizziness, dry mouth, mania, fatigue, GI distress, headache, increased TSH, insomnia, itching, mania, pruritus, redness of skin, reduced intestinal motility, restlessness, sedation, tiredness, tremor. sexual dysfunction (improved by 20-50 mg sildenafil).

INTERACTIONS:

-Administration of SJW for 14 days, to 13 subjects, revealed an increased urinary 6-ß-hydroxycortisol/cortisol ratio, which suggests induction of CYP3A4.[846]

-In vitro research using human hepatocytes resulted in SJW activating pregnane X receptor, which regulates CYP3A4 expression. Hyperforin contained in SJW is responsible for PXR activation. Suggests induction of CYP3A4. [838]

246

-In vitro research using cultured human cells suggests a dose-dependent activation of steroid X receptor (SXR) by SJW, which can induce gene expression of cytochrome P450 enzymes. This in vivo research found that hyperforin, not hypericin, is responsible for this activation.[851]

-Studies covering less than 2 weeks have not been found to be reliable in predicting interactions.[207,827,828]

- In vitro research has not accurately predicted results in humans.[227,822,823,842]

Drugs metabolized by P450 CYP3A4 and transported by PGP[180,592] (see Appendix 38) SJW may induce CYP3A4 and PGP, which would decrease serum levels of drugs that are substrates of CYP3A4 and PGP.

Alcohol[246] SJW decreased alcohol intake in rats.

Alprazolam (Xanax)[207] Length of study was insufficient to alter metabolism of drug.

Amsacrine[844] In in vitro research, SJW was found to antagonize cleavage complex stabilization of etoposide. Patients on topo II-directed chemotherapy should use other means for the treatment of depression until further research is conducted to determine the safe use of SJW with this type of chemotherapy.

Amitriptyline (Elavil)[832] Hypericum extract and amitriptyline were administered concurrently for 14 days to 12 depressed patients, resulting in 22% decrease in AUC of amitriptyline and 41% decrease in AUC of nortriptyline (a metabolite).

Amphetamines[849] Survey of 862 psychiatrists in Australia and New Zealand reported 1 interaction between SJW and drug.

Caffeine[850] Clinical study of 12 healthy subjects resulted in no significant changes in serum concentrations of caffeine after a single dose or 2 weeks of SJW. Less than 2 week administration of SJW is insufficient amount of time to alter metabolism of caffeine.[827,828]

Carbamazepine (Tegretol)[821] In a clinical study of 8 healthy males, administration of SJW for 14 days did not alter serum level of carbamazepine. Results are in conflict with most research, which has suggested that SJW acts as an inducer of CYP3A4. Some possible explanations given by the authors include: 1) Carbamazepine is not induced by P-glycoprotein (SJW might not induce CYP3A4). 2) Carbamazepine may have increased elimination of SJW intermediate metabolite(s) responsible for induction of CYP3A4. 3) SJW may not be a strong enough inducer of CYP3A4 to induce isozymes already autoinduced by carbamazepine.

Cyclosporine (Neoral)[179,815,814,817,818,819, 833,836,839,845] Numerous case reports of decreased serum cyclosporine after initiation of SJW.

Dextromethorphan[850] Clinical study of 12 healthy subjects showed no significant changes in urinary dextromethorphan to dextrorphan after a single dose or 2 weeks of SJW. Suggests no induction of CYP2D6.

Digoxin (Lanoxin)[205,826,834,849] I n a study using 8 rats, a 3.8-fold increase in P-glycoprotein and 2.5-fold increase in hepatic CYP3A2 expression. In 8 healthy males given SJW for 14 days there was an 18% decrease in digoxin (single dose of 0.5 mg digoxin). There was a 1.4-fold increase in the expression of duodenal P-glycoproteim/MDR1, a 1.5-fold increase in activity of duodenal CYP3A4 and a 1.4-fold increase in activity of hepatic CYP3A4.[198] In research using 25 subjects, serum digoxin was reduced in 25 healthy subjects taking SJW concurrently. Ten-day **248**

St. John's Wort (cont'd.)

administration of SJW decreased AUC 25%. Statistically significant effect did not occur until the tenth day of SJW administration.

Etoposide (Vepesid)[844] In in vitro research, SJW was found to antagonize cleavage complex stabilization of etoposide. Patients on topo II-directed chemotherapy should use other means for the treatment of depression until further research is conducted to determine the safe use of SJW with this type of chemotherapy.

Fexofenadine (Allegra)[852] Clinical study of 10 subjects. SJW was administered for 12 days. Subjects were then given fexofenadine. AUC decreased more than 48%.

General anesthesia (see Appendix 20)[830] Case report of 23 year old female admitted for hysteroscopy under general anesthesia. Patient took SJW for 6 months prior to surgery and was not on any medications. The following drugs were administered: 150 µg fentanyl, 150 mg propofol, 3 mg d-tubocurarine and 120 mg succinylcholine. The patient was intubated and anesthesia maintained with nitrous oxide, oxygen and isoflurane. Patient became hypotensive (60/20 mm Hg and HR 60 bpm) for about 10 minutes and was administered saline, hydroxyethyl starch, ephedrine and phenylephrine, after which the patient became stabilized. Patient had been administered the same general anesthetics during a previous surgery without adverse reaction. It is theorized by the author that SJW may have caused an adrenergic desensitization/decreased responsiveness to vasopressors.

Indinavir (Crixivan)[180] Clinical study of 8 subjects. Administration of SJW for 14 days decreased serum indinavir (reduced the AUC by a mean of 57%). Results suggest induction of CYP3A4, but induction of PGP can not be ruled out. Other protease inhibitors and non-nucleoside reverse transcriptase inhibitors are metabolized similarly to indinavir.

Kava[849] Survey of 862 psychiatrists in Australia and New Zealand reported 1 interaction between SJW and drug.

L-Tryptophan[849] Survey of 862 psychiatrists in Australia and New Zealand reported 1 interaction between SJW and drug.

Lithium (Eskalith, Lithobid, Lithonate, Lithotabs)[849] Survey of 862 psychiatrists in Australia and New Zealand reported 1 interaction between SJW and drug.

MAOIs[840,849] (see Appendix 9) Survey of 862 psychiatrists in Australia and New Zealand reported 2 interactions between SJW and MAOIs. St. John's wort has very little MAOI activity, but concurrent use may theoretically increase the risk of serotonin syndrome.

Mianserin[849] Survey of 862 psychiatrists in Australia and New Zealand reported 1 interaction between SJW and drug.

Midazolam (Versed)[850,852] I n clinical study of 10 subjects, SJW was administered for 12 days. Subjects were then given midazolam. AUC decreased from 54(PO)/45(IV) to 24(PO)/34(IV). In clinical study of 12 healthy subjects, no significant changes in serum concentrations of midazolam were noted after a singe dose (oral or IV) of SJW. AUC for orally administered midazolam was decreased 50% and AUC of IV administered midazolam was decreased 21% after 2 weeks of concurrent SJW administration. These results suggest that CYP3A4 in intestinal wall is induced by SJW, thereby decreasing serum levels of orally administered drugs that are substrates of this isozyme.

Moclobemide[849] Survey of 862 psychiatrists in Australia and New Zealand reported 5 interactions between SJW and moclobemide.

Morphine (MS Contin)[829] In research using rats, SJW (171 mg/kg) for 7 days enhanced the analgesic effect of morphine. No significant effect was found with single or multiple doses of 85.5 mg/kg or single dose of 171 mg/kg.

Nevirapine (Viramune)[824] Case report of 5 males infected with HIV who consumed SJW, thereby decreasing plasma levels of nevirapine by 35%.

Nifedipine (Adalat, Procardia)[278] In research using 22 human subjects, SJW was administered for 18 days. Subjects were then given nifedipine. Concurrent SJW decreased serum nifedipine by 53% from baseline.

NNRTIs Drugs metabolized similarly to NNRTIs have been found to have decreased serum levels when combined with SJW, which induces both P450 CYP3A4 and PGP. See **Indinavir**, above.

Nortriptyline (Pamelor, Aventyl) see **Amitriptyline**, above.

Offenfluramine[816] Case report (telephone survey) of concurrent use of offenfluramine with 600 mg SJW. Nausea, headache, and increased anxiety reported by female subject.

Oral Contraceptives[181,854,929] Eight reports of intermenstrual bleeding with concurrent use of SJW and oral contraceptives reported to MPA (Swedish Medical Products Agency) since 1998. Three reports of intermenstrual bleeding with concurrent use of SJW and oral contraceptives. In research using 12 healthy females, 7 subjects had breakthrough bleeding with concurrent use of SJW and oral contraceptives. There was also an increased oral clearance of norethindrone. This

St. John's Wort (cont'd.)

research suggests induction of CYP3A on intestinal wall.

Phenprocoumon[837] Clinical study of 10 subjects. Concurrent administration of SJW resulted in a decrease in AUC of phenprocoumon by about 17%.

Photosensitivity, drugs increasing (see Appendix 29)[835,847] Three case reports of increased photosensitivity after administration of SJW.[820] Clinical study of 50 subjects. After 15 days there was a slight but significant increase in solar and UVA light sensitivity which could be compensated for by decreasing sun exposure by 21%. Note that dosage of SJW (3600 mg SJW extract/11.25 mg hypericin) is 4 times greater than those typically used. Results for pure hypericin may differ from the results of this study, as it is not known if other components of SJW may be protective against photosensitivity.[831] In one study, 6 out of 7 subjects who received 0.10 mg hypericin/kg/day had a phototoxic reaction. Photosensitivity has not been found in studies using standard therapeutic amounts. Concurrent use with drugs that increase the risk of photosensitivity should be avoided. Risk is theoretical.

Protease inhibitors (PIs) Drugs metabolized similarly to protease inhibitors have been found to have decreased serum levels when combined with SJW, which induces both P450 CYP3A4 and PGP. See **Indinavir**, above.

Reserpine (Enduronyl)[843] In research using rats, Psychotonin M (extract of *Hypericum perforatum*) prolonged sleep-time and at a specific dose antagonized reserpine.

Serotonin syndrome, drugs increasing the risk of[195,853] (see Appendix 32) There have been 5 case reports of serotonin syndrome and 1 case of serotonin excess with concurrent use of SJW and drug.

Sildenafil (Viagra)[271] Case report of improvement in sexual dysfunction, assumed from use of SJW with use of sildenafil.

Simvastatin (Zocor)[848] 16 Healthy males were given SJW 300 mg TID for 14 days. On day 14, subjects were given 10 mg simvastatin and 20 mg pravastatin. Peak concentration and AUC of simvastatin hydroxy acid was decreased. Plasma concentrations of pravastatin was not altered, which is consistent with an induction of CYP3A4 in liver and intestines.

Surgery, drugs used during[307] Review of herbs discusses the need to discontinue herb at least 5 days prior to surgery. Drugs used during surgery metabolized by CYP3A4 include alfentanil, midazolam, lidocaine, and calcium channel blockers.

Tramadol (Ultram)[816—telephone survey,849] Case report of interaction between tramadol and SJW.

SSRIs[849] Survey of 862 psychiatrists in Australia and New Zealand reported 33 interactions between SJW and SSRIs.

Theophylline (Elixophyllin, Slo-bid, Theo-Dur)[841] Case report of 42 year old female with decreased serum theophylline. Patient was on a complicated drug regimen and added SJW. Theophylline dose increased to 800 mg Theo-Dur bid from 300 mg/day (prior to administration of SJW) to maintain therapeutic effect. Significance of this report not established.

Tolbutamide (Orinase)[850] No significant changes in serum tolbutamide concentrations noted after a single dose or 2 weeks of SJW.

Trazodone (Desyrel)[825] Case report of serotonin syndrome with concurrent SJW and trazodone.

St. John's Wort (cont'd.)
Tricyclic antidepressants[849] (see Appendix 9) Survey of 862 psychiatrists in Australia and New Zealand reported 5 interactions between SJW and tricyclic antidepressants.

Venlafaxine (Effexor)[849] Survey of 862 psychiatrists in Australia and New Zealand reported 1 interaction between SJW and drug.

Warfarin (Coumadin)[181] Case report of 74 year old female with decreased serum warfarin with concurrent use of SJW. Seven case reports of increased INR with concurrent use of warfarin and SJW reported to MPA (Swedish Medical Products Agency) since 1998.[854]

Stephania *Stephania tetrandra*
PART USED: Root.

SAFETY: Misidentification and adulteration with Guang fang ji (*Aristolochia fangchi*), containing the nephrotoxic aristolochic acid, has occurred. Guang fang ji is considered interchangeable with stephania in some herbal formulas. AHPA Class: 1.[66]

INTERACTIONS:

Anticoagulants and drugs that increase the risk of bleeding[855] (see Appendix 8) Tetrandrine and fangchinoline, components of herb, inhibit platelet aggregation. Theoretical additive effect.

Calcium channel blockers[856] (see Appendix 11) Tetrandrine, a component of herb, blocks calcium channels, which theoretically may interfere with drug.

Strophanthus *Strophanthus hispidus, Strophanthus kombe*

PART USED: Seed.
SAFETY: Contains cardiac glycosides.
INTERACTIONS:
Anticoagulants and drugs that increase the risk of bleeding[857] (see Appendix 8) Herb may prolong clotting time. Theoretical increased risk of bleeding if combined with strophanthus.

Digoxin/Cardiac glycosides[104,858] Herb contains cardiac glycosides, which theoretically may be additive with drugs that contain cardiac glycosides.

Sweet Basil *Ocimum basilicum*

PART USED: Leaf.
CONTRAINDICATIONS: Children, pregnancy, lactation. Allergy to *Labiatae* family.
SAFETY: Not for long-term use. Contains estragole and safrole. GRAS (oil, extract, spice, flavoring, oleoresin). AHPA Class: 2b, 2c, 2d.[66]
INTERACTIONS:
Drugs metabolized by P450 isozymes[859] (see Appendix 38) Components of sweet basil, including 1,8-cineole and eugenol, induce P450 enzymes, which may decrease serum levels of drugs that are substrates of these enzymes.

Sweet Broom *Scoparia dulcis*

INTERACTIONS:
CNS depressants[860] (see Appendix 15) Scoparinol, a component of herb, increased pentobarbital-induced sleep time in laboratory animals. Theoretical additive effect.

Sweet Broom (cont'd.)

Diuretics[860] (see Appendix 11) In research using animals, herb had a diuretic effect, which theoretically may be additive with drug.

Insulin/Oral hypoglycemic agents[105,861] (see Appendix 24) Possible hypoglycemia or loss of blood glucose control.

Sweet Clover *Melilotus officinalis*
ADVERSE REACTIONS: Headaches.
INTERACTIONS:

Anticoagulants and drugs that increase the risk of bleeding[862,923] (see Appendix 8) Dicoumarol formed when sweet clover spoiled (molded) caused hemorrhagic disease in cattle. Free coumarin may be released during drying of the herb. Monitor labs of patient.

Tansy *Tanacetum vulgare*
PART USED: Herb.
CONTRAINDICATIONS: Pregnancy.
SAFETY: May contain thujone, which has neurotoxic activity. Lethal dose is 15-30 g of essential oil. 10 drops of oil may be lethal. Poisoning causes rapid pulse and convulsions. AHPA Class: 2b.[66]
ADVERSE REACTIONS: Abortion, cardiac arrhythmias, dermatitis, nausea. Large amounts may cause abdominal pain, abortion, clonic-tonic spasms, gastroenteritis, increased respiration, irregular heartbeat, kidney damage, liver damage, loss of consciousness, mydriasis, pupillary rigidity, red face, uterine bleeding, vomiting

PART USED: Herb.

SAFETY: Contains estragole. GRAS (spice, seasoning, flavoring, oil, extract and oleoresin). AHPA Class: 1.[66]

INTERACTIONS:
Benzodiazepines[339] (see Appendix 13) Benzodiazepines (delorazepam and temazepam) were found in cultured plant cells in the range of 100–200 ng/g.

Tea *Camellia sinensis*

USES: Cardiovascular disease (H-epidemiological), gingival inflammation (H), photoprotection (H-green).

PART USED: Leaf, stems.

CONTRAINDICATIONS: Gastric ulcer, children. Limit intake in pregnancy and lactation.

SAFETY: Contains caffeine 9–50 mg per cup of tea, which is a stimulant.[172] Contains tannins; avoid high dose for extended period. Catechin tannin linked to esophageal cancer. Tea may decrease zinc bioavailability. GRAS (oil, extract, oleoresin). AHPA Class: 2d—fermented black tea not long-term or excessive.[66]

INTERACTIONS:
Herb may reduce intestinal absorption of other drugs.[649]
Drugs metabolized by P450 CYP1A1, CYP1A2 and CYP2B1[647,648] (see Appendix 38) In research using rats, activity of the above isozymes was increased, which may decrease serum level of drugs that are substrates of these isozymes.

Tea (cont'd.)

Anticoagulants and drugs that increase the risk of bleeding[332,641,644,646-green tea] (see Appendix 8) Large amounts of green tea may increase the risk of bleeding if used concurrently with drugs which also increase the risk of bleeding. Catechin and epigallocatechin gallate are believed to be the components responsible for antithrombic activity. Black tea was given to 49 patients with coronary artery disease taking aspirin in a crossover design study. There were no changes in markers of platelet activation and function of whole blood aggregation. A major limitation of this study was that subjects were already taking aspirin, which is known to inhibit platelet aggregation, and it was not a blinded study.

Acetaminophen/Paracetamol[636] Caffeine in tea may increase pain relief.

Aspirin[638] Caffeine in tea increases effectiveness of ASA pain relief. Tea may also increase absorption and bioavailability of ASA in GI tract.

Atopic dermatitis drugs[253] 118 Subjects consumed oolong tea for six months. At 1 month 63% showed marked to moderate improvement, and at 6 months 54% remained improved.

Benzodiazepines[637] (see Appendix 13) Theoretical decrease in sedative and antianxiolytic effects.

Beta-adrenergic agonists[101] (see Appendix 36) Concurrent use may increase the risk of cardiac arrhythmias.

Cimetidine (Tagamet)[658] Drug may decrease clearance of caffeine, a component of tea. Theoretically this may increase serum caffeine and result in increased caffeine side effects. Results of research have been equivocal.

Cisplatin (Platinol)[193] In rats, green tea tannins reduced nephrotoxicity of drug **258**

Clozapine, and possibly other drugs metabolized by P450 CYP1A2[296,350] (see Appendix 38) Caffeine intakes greater than 400 mg may decrease clearance of clozapine (and possibly induce other drugs metabolized by CYP1A2). In randomized crossover research of 12 males, the AUC of clozapine was increased 19% and oral clearance of clozapine was decreased 14% with concurrent caffeine intake. Tea leaf contains 93,000 ppm caffeine, and shoots contain 47,900 ppm.

Disulfiram (Antabuse)[654] Drug may decrease metabolism of caffeine, a component of herb. The result may increase serum caffeine and caffeine side effects.

Doxorubicin (Adriamycin)[639,640] Theanine, a component of tea, increased drug concentration within cancer cells and increased antitumor activity.

Ephedra/Ephedrine[434] Concurrent use of high amounts of products containing caffeine and stimulants, such as ephedra or ephedrine, may have an additive stimulant effect.

Ergotamine (Ergomar)[653] Caffeine, a component of tea, increases serum level and efficacy of drug. The drug Wigraine contains both ergotamine and caffeine.

Estrogen[658] Ethinyl estradiol and estradiol cause an impaired CYP1A2 clearance of caffeine, a component of tea. This may increase serum caffeine and increase caffeine side effects

Fluvoxamine (Luvox)[658] Drug decreases metabolism of caffeine, a component of the tea. This may increase serum caffeine and increase caffeine side effects.

Furafylline[658] Drug inhibits CYP1A2, which decreases the metabolism of caffeine, a component of tea. This may increase serum levels of caffeine and increase

Tea (cont'd.)

caffeine side effects.

Grapefruit juice[531] Grapefruit juice inhibits CYP1A2, which decreases the metabolism of caffeine, a component of tea, thereby increasing caffeine side effects.

Ibuprofen[650] Concurrent use of both tea and drug may enhance pain relief.

Idrocilamide[658] Drug alters caffeine metabolism, increasing serum levels of caffeine and caffeine side effects.

Insulin/Oral hypoglycemic agents[84,651] (see Appendix 24) Caffeine, a component of tea, may increase insulin resistance. Monitor patients with diabetes.

Iron[268,269] Green tea decreased absorption of non-heme iron by 28% in 27 female subjects. In 77 human subjects, black tea decreased absorption of non-heme iron by 79-94%. Tea contains tannins, polyphenols and phenolic monomers, which form insoluble complexes with iron, preventing absorption.

Lithium (Eskalith, Lithobid, Lithonate, Lithotabs)[658] Caffeine, a component of tea, increases the renal excretion of lithium, which may decrease serum levels of drug. Discontinuation of herb use may then increase serum levels of drug.

MAOIs[109] (see Appendix 9) Excessive amounts of coffee may increase risk of hypertension.

Methotrexate (Rheumatrex)[224] Caffeine in tea may decrease effectiveness of drug.

Methoxsalen (8-MOP, Oxsoralen)[658] Drug inhibits metabolism of caffeine, a component of tea. Increased serum caffeine may increase side effects.

Metoprolol (Lopressor, Toprol)[101] Caffeine my increase blood pressure.

Methoxsalen (8-MOP, Oxsoralen)[658] Drug inhibits metabolism of caffeine, a component of tea. Increased serum caffeine may increase side effects.

Mexiletine (Mexitil)[656] Drug delays metabolism of caffeine, a component of tea. This may increase side effects of caffeine.

Oral contraceptives[658] Long-term use of oral contraceptives (ethinyl estradiol or estradiol) causes an impaired CYP1A2 clearance of caffeine, a component of tea. Concurrent use may increase serum caffeine and increase caffeine side effects.

Phenylpropanolamine[658] Drug may inhibit the metabolism of caffeine, increasing serum levels of caffeine and side effects. On 11/6/00, the FDA released an advisory to remove phenylpropanolamine from all products.[657]

Propranolol (Inderal)[101] Blood pressure may be increased by caffeine in tea.

Quinolones (ciprofloxacin, enoxacin, grepafloxacin, norfloxacin, pefloxacin, tosufloxacin)[658] Drugs may decrease clearance of caffeine, a component of herb. This may increase the side effects of caffeine due to increased serum caffeine.

Terbinafine (Lamisil)[658] Drug may inhibit the metabolism of caffeine, a component of tea. This may increase serum levels of caffeine and increase caffeine side effects. Research on this interaction has been equivocal.

Theophylline (Uniphyl, Uni-Dur)[658] Concurrent use of theophylline and caffeine may lead to an increase in serum levels of both.

Verapamil (Calan, Isoptin, Verelan)[658] Drug delays clearance of caffeine, a component of tea. This may increase caffeine side effects.

Tea Tree *Melaleuca alternifolia*
   USES: Acne (H), tinea pedis (H), toe nail onychomycosis (H).
   PART USED: Essential oil.
   SAFETY: External use only.
   ADVERSE REACTIONS: Allergic response, contact dermatitis, eczema.

Thorny Burnet *Sarcopoterium spinosum*
   PART USED: Bark, root.
   INTERACTIONS:
     Insulin/Oral hypoglycemic agents[863] (see Appendix 24) Herb may decrease blood glucose. Monitor patients with diabetes.

Tobacco *Nicotiana tabacum*
   PART USED: Leaf.
   CONTRAINDICATIONS: Asthma, cardiovascular disease, children, COPD, heart disease, infertility, lactation, lung disease, peptic ulcer, pregnancy, slow wound healing, stroke.
   SAFETY: Long-term use may cause cancer.
   ADVERSE REACTIONS: Central nervous system stimulation, chronic bronchitis, dependence, emphysema, increased cancer risk, low birth weight, premature labor.
   INTERACTIONS:
     Drugs metabolized by P450 CYP1A1 and CYP1A2[868] (see Appendix 38) Polycyclic amines in herb are believed to be responsible for induction of 1A1 and 1A2. Monitor patients taking drugs which are substrates of these isozymes as

Tobacco (cont'd.)

263

serum levels may be reduced.

Benzodiazepines[868] (see Appendix 13) Cigarette smoke decreases sedation of drug

Beta blockers[868] (see Appendix 11) Cigarette smoking decreases the effectiveness of drug.

Caffeine[868] Increased metabolism of caffeine.

Cimetidine (Tagamet)[867] Decreased serum level of drug.

Dextropropoxyphene[872] Cigarette smoke decreases efficacy of drug

Estrogen replacement therapy[868] Increased metabolism of drug.

Flecainide (Tambocor)[868] Increased metabolism of drug.

Furosemide (Lasix)[866] Decreased diuresis.

Glutethimide[866] Tobacco may decrease effectiveness of drug.

Haloperidol (Haldol)[868] Increased metabolism of drug.

Heparin[868] Cigarette smoking increases clearance of heparin.

Insulin[868] Tobacco causes slow absorption of insulin due to vasoconstriction.

Lidocaine (Xylocaine)[866] Cigarette smoke interferes with protein binding of drug.

Methamphetamine[870] Cigarette smoke lessened the decrease in dopamine caused by drug.

Olanzapine (Zyprexa)[869] Clearance of drug is increased by tobacco smoking.

Opioids[868] Cigarette smoke decreases analgesic effect of drug.

Oral contraceptives[868] Tobacco increases metabolism of estrogen.

Pentazocine (Talwin)[868] Increased metabolism of drug.

Tobacco (cont'd.)

Phenothiazines[865] (see Appendix 28) Cigarette smoking increases the metabolism of chlorpromazine, a phenothiazine.

Phenylbutazone[866] Increased metabolism of drug.

Propranolol (Inderal)[868] Increased metabolism of drug.

Propoxyphene (Darvon)[866] Tobacco may decrease effectiveness of drug.

Quinine[864] Increased elimination of drug.

Ropivacaine[871] Tobacco increased one of the metabolites of drug, most likely through induction of P450 CYP1A2.

Tacrine (Cognex)[868] Increased metabolism of drug.

Theophylline (Uniphyl, Uni-Dur)[868] Increased metabolism of drug.

Tricyclic antidepressants[868] (see Appendix 9) Increased metabolism of drug.

Tonka *Dipteryx odorata, Dipteryx oppositifolia*

PART USED: Seed.

SAFETY: Large amounts of fluid extract may cause cardiac paralysis. AHPA Class: 3.[66]

INTERACTIONS:

Anticoagulants and other drugs that increase the risk of bleeding.[916] (see Appendix 8) Seed contains coumarin (10,000-35,000 ppm). Use caution in concurrent use of drugs that increase the risk of bleeding.

Tree Peony *Paeonia suffruticosa*

PART USED: Bark.

SAFETY: AHPA Class: 2b.[66]

INTERACTIONS:

HIV therapies[338] (see Appendix 22) Suggests that antioxidant activity of herb may delay progress of HIV to AIDS. In rats, the herb inhibited erythrocyte hemolysis, decreased lipid peroxidation in brain and kidney, and decreased generation of superoxide peroxidation and hydroxyl radicals.

Tremella Mushroom *Tremella fuciformis*

INTERACTIONS:

Anticoagulants and drugs that increase the risk of bleeding[873] (see Appendix 8) In vitro study of mushroom showed an inhibition of platelet aggregation.

Trikatu Ayurvedic preparation containing: *Piper longum* (long pepper), *Piper nigrum* (Black pepper), *Zingiber officinalis* (ginger). See individual herbs.

INTERACTIONS:

Drugs metabolized by P450 enzymes[149,151,152] (see Appendix 38) In research using laboratory animals, CYP2E1 expression was suppressed and CYP2B and CYP1A expression was enhanced. Metabolism of drugs which are substrates of these isozymes may be altered. In research by Atal, piperine was found to be a nonspecific inhibitor of P450 enzymes. Use caution with concurrent use of drugs that are substrates of various P450 isozymes.

Trikatu (cont'd.)

Aspirin[629] In mice, water decoction of herb was protective against aspirin-induced ulcers.

Coenzyme Q10[157] Five mg of piperine, a component of long and black pepper, administered for 21 days increased serum levels of coenzyme Q10.

Hexobarbital[149,151] Piperine, a component of black and long pepper, increased hexobarbital-induced sleep time.

Indomethacin (Indocin)[153] In research using mice, piperine (a component of long and black pepper) was protective against drug-induced ulcers.

Isoniazid (Nydrazid)[312] In rabbits, serum levels of isoniazid were decreased by trikatu. Mean Cmax was reduced from 8.42 to 5.48, and mean AUC was reduced from 24.76 to 15.04. Effect was most likely due to delayed gastric emptying or alterations in intestinal motility.

Pentobarbitone[158] Piperine (contained in long and black pepper) prolonged drug sleep time, possibly through the inhibition of liver enzymes.

Phenytoin (Dilantin)[151] Piperine, a component of long and black pepper, may enhance bioavailability of drug.

Propranolol (Inderal)[154] Piperine, a component of long and black pepper, enhanced systemic availability of drug, which may result in a lower amount of drug needed to reach therapeutic levels.

Rifampicin[874] In rabbits, trikatu caused a decrease in the rate of bioavailability of drug.

Theophylline (Uniphyl, Uni-Dur)[114,154] Piperine enhanced availability of drug, which may result in a lower dose of drug needed to reach therapeutic levels. **266**

Trikatu (cont'd.)

Zoxazolamine[149] Piperine, a component of black and long pepper, increased drug-induced sleep time.

Tronadora Leaf *Tecoma stans*
INTERACTIONS:
Insulin/Oral hypoglycemic agents[88,162,173] (see Appendix 24) Possible hypoglycemia or loss of blood glucose control.

Turmeric *Curcuma longa*
USES: Cancer prevention (H), chronic anterior uveitis (H-curcumin), gastric ulcer (H).
PART USED: Rhizome.
CONTRAINDICATIONS: Bile duct obstruction, bleeding disorders, gallbladder disease, gastric hyperacidity, pregnancy, ulcers.
SAFETY: GRAS (spice, seasoning, flavoring). AHPA Class: 2b, 2d.[66]
ADVERSE REACTIONS: Allergic response, GI disturbance, contact dermatitis.
INTERACTIONS:
Drugs metabolized by P450 CYP1A1, CYP1A2 and CYP2B1[879,880,928] (see Appendix 38) In research using mice and rats, turmeric inhibited CYP1A2 and CYP2B1. This may increase serum level of drugs which are substrates of this isozyme. In vitro research has shown effect most likely due to curcumin, a component of turmeric.
Anticoagulants and drugs that increase the risk of bleeding[881,882] Turmeric inhibits platelet aggregation and alters the biosynthesis of eicosanoids. Concurrent

Turmeric (cont'd.)

use with these drugs may increase risk of bleeding.

Cyclosporine (Neoral)[875] Curcumin, a component of turmeric, blocked cyclosporine A-resistant CD28 costimulatory pathway of human T-cell proliferation. Curcumin may be a useful adjunct to chemotherapy.

Genistein[876] Concurrent use of genistein and curcumin caused a synergistic inhibition of breast cancer cell growth (exposed to estrogenic pesticides).

Indomethacin (Indocin)[877] Ethanol extract of herb may decrease risk of drug-induced GI ulcers.

Piperine[878] Piperine (in black and long pepper) enhances absorption and bioavailability of curcumin (component of herb).

Reserpine (Enduronyl)[877] Root extract may decrease risk of GI ulcers.

Uva Ursi *Arctostaphylos uva ursi*

USES: UTI prophylaxis (H).

PART USED: Leaf.

CONTRAINDICATIONS: Pregnancy, lactation, children. Not with renal or hepatic disease or GI irritation.

SAFETY: Contains tannins; not for long-term use. Contains GI irritants. AHPA Class: 2b, 2d—not with kidney disorders, GI irritation, acidic urine; prolonged use only under medical supervision.[66]

ADVERSE REACTIONS: Convulsions, cyanosis, death, GI distress, green urine, N&V, pigmentation of eye, ringing in ears.

INTERACTIONS:

Uva Ursi (cont'd.)

Beta-Lactams[883] (see Appendix 7) Coriiagin potentiated drugs against methicillin-resistant *Staphylococcus aureus*.

Drugs causing acidic urine[1,66] (Vitamin C/cranberry) Medications that acidify urine decrease the effectiveness of uva ursi.

Alkaloids (see Appendix 4)[4] High tannin content of herb may cause alkaloids to become insoluble and precipitate.

Dexamethasone ointment[886] Water extract of herb increased the inhibitory effect of dexamethasone ointment on the allergic and inflammatory response in laboratory animals.

Dexamethasone (Decadron)[884] Arbutin, isolated from the leaves of uva ursi, increased the action of dexamethasone in laboratory animals.

Indomethacin (Indocin)[885] Arbutin, isolated from the leaves of uva ursi, increased the action of indomethacin in laboratory animals.

Prednisolone[884] Arbutin, isolated from the leaves of uva ursi, increased the action of prednisolone in laboratory animals.

Vahl *Thonningia sanguinea*

INTERACTIONS:

Drugs metabolized by P450 CYP1A1/2, CYP2B1/2 and CYP3A4[320] (see Appendix 38) In rats, vahl extract inhibited CYP1A1/2 and CYP2B1/2. CYP3A4 was induced, as shown by an increased pentobarbital sleep time, but levels upon awakening were the same as in controls.

Valerian Root *Valeriana officinalis*
   USES: Insomnia & sleep disorders (H), anxiety(H).
   PART USED: Rhizome, root.
   CONTRAINDICATIONS: In a small percentage of individuals, valerian has a stimulating effect.
   SAFETY: GRAS (flavoring). AHPA Class: 1.[66]
   ADVERSE REACTIONS: Abdominal pain, cardiac disturbances, chest tightness, excitability, headache, insomnia, mydriasis, tremors, uneasiness. Possible withdrawal symptoms after long-term use. Stimulant effect in small minority. Toxicity: ataxia, hypothermia, increased muscle relaxation.
   INTERACTIONS:
   Drugs which are substrates of P450 CYP3A4 isozymes[227] (see Appendix 38)
   Preliminary in vitro research has shown that valerian may alter metabolism and/or effectiveness of drugs which are substrates of CYP3A4 isozymes. Further research is needed to determine if interaction will also occur in humans.
   Barbiturates[888] (see Appendix 12) Concurrent use increased sleep time in mice. Herb has sedative activity, theoretical additive sedation.
   Benzodiazepines[888] (see Appendix 13) Large doses of valepotriates, from herb, decreased withdrawal symptoms in rats. Herb has sedative activity; theoretical additive sedation.
   CNS depressants[888] (see Appendix 15) Herb has sedative action. Valerenic acid, contained in herb, inhibits the breakdown of GABA, and hydroxypinoresinol binds to benzodiazepine receptor. Herb also contains GABA, but bioavailability has been questioned. Urge caution in concurrent use of herb with drugs that also

Valerian Root (cont'd.)

increase sedation; theoretical increased sedation.

Diazepam (Valium)[889] Large doses of a mixture of valepotriates, from herb, decreased symptoms of withdrawal from drug in rats.

Flunitrazepam[887] At low doses valerian enhances binding of drug, but at high doses valerian inhibits binding of drug.

Surgery, drugs used during[307] The effect of sedatives may be enhanced. Duration of effect not known.

Thiopental[890] Concurrent use increased sleep time in mice.

Vervain Verbena officinalis

PART USED: Herb.

CONTRAINDICATIONS: Pregnancy.

SAFETY: GRAS (flavoring in alcoholic beverage). AHPA class: 2b.[66]

ADVERSE REACTIONS: Contact dermatitis.

INTERACTIONS:

Anticoagulants/Warfarin (Coumadin), not heparin[719] (see Appendix 8) Herb contains variable amounts of vitamin K, which antagonizes the anticoagulant effect of warfarin.

Iron[269] Vervain tea decreased absorption of non-heme iron by 59% in 77 human subjects due to polyphenol content.

Viñ-viño *Aristeguietia discolor*
  INTERACTIONS:
    Morphine (MSIR,MS Contin, Oramorph, Roxanol)[281] In vitro research (guinea pig ileum) suggests that flavonoid from herb may decrease symptoms of morphine withdrawal.

Wallflower *Cheiranthus cheiri*
  INTERACTIONS:
    Digoxin/Cardiac glycosides[11] Herb may increase risk of drug toxicity.

Watercress *Nasturtium officinale*
  PART USED: Leaf.
  CONTRAINDICATIONS: Children, gastric or duodenal ulcers, kidney inflammation, pregnancy.
  SAFETY: AHPA Class: 2b, 2d—not with gastric or duodenal ulcers, inflammatory kidney disease, not < 4 years old.[66]
  ADVERSE REACTIONS: Large amounts for extended periods may cause gastric irritation.
  INTERACTIONS:

    Drugs metabolized by P450 CYP1A1/2 and CYP2E1[892,893] (see Appendix 38) Watercress has been found to inhibit CYP2E1, which may increase serum levels of drugs that are substrates of CYP2E1.

    Acetaminophen/Paracetamol[891] Watercress caused a decrease in breakdown products of drug, possibly by inhibiting the oxidation metabolism of drug. **272**

Chlorzoxazone (Parafon Forte)[892] Research using 10 healthy subjects, found that watercress increased the AUC of drug by 56%. This research suggests that watercress is an inhibitor of cytochrome P450 CYP2E1.

Warfarin (Coumadin)[716] Watercress contains 250 µg of vitamin K per 100 g of watercress (provisional data). It is important to maintain a constant intake of vitamin K to maintain therapeutic effect of drug because vitamin K antagonizes the anticoagulant effect of warfarin.

White Button Mushroom *Agaricus bisporus*
INTERACTIONS:
Insulin/Oral hypoglycemic agents[401] (see Appendix 24) Possible hypoglycemia or loss of blood glucose control.

Wild Carrot *Daucus carota*
PART USED: Fruit/seed.
CONTRAINDICATIONS: Pregnancy.
SAFETY: GRAS (oil, extract, oleoresin). AHPA Class: 2b.[66]
ADVERSE REACTIONS: Photosensitivity.
INTERACTIONS:
Antihypertensives[894] (see Appendix 11) Herb has a hypotensive effect, as seen in laboratory animals. Excessive doses of herb may disturb hypertension control.
Hypotensive therapy[894] Herb has a hypotensive effect, as seen in laboratory animals. Excessive doses of herb may disturb blood pressure control.

Wild Cherry *Prunus serotina*
    PART USED: Bark.
    CONTRAINDICATIONS: Children, lactation, pregnancy.
    SAFETY: Contains cyanogenic glycosides. GRAS (oil, extract, oleoresin). AHPA
Class: 2d—not long-term or excessive dose.[66]
    ADVERSE REACTIONS:
    INTERACTIONS:
        Drugs which are substrates of P450 CYP3A4 isozymes[227] (see Appendix 38)
        Preliminary in vitro research has shown that wild cherry bark may alter metabolism
        and/or effectiveness of drugs which are substrates of CYP3A4 isozymes. Further
        research is needed to determine if interaction will also occur in humans.

Wild Yam *Dioscorea spp.*
USES: Hyperlipoproteinemia (H).
    PART USED: Rhizome, root.
    CONTRAINDICATIONS: Children, gallbladder and hepatic disease, lactation,
pregnancy.
    SAFETY: No progesterone is contained in wild yam, but some wild yam products have
synthetic progesterone added. AHPA class: 1.[66]
    ADVERSE REACTIONS: Diarrhea, GI distress, N&V.
    INTERACTIONS:
        Clofibrate (Atromid-S)[895] Diosgenin, a sapogenin from herb, combined with
        clofibrate caused a greater decrease in LDL than either substance alone in rats.

Wild Yam (cont'd.)

Hormone replacement therapy/Oral contraceptives[415] In vitro research using wild yam, showed an antiestrogenic effect. Effect on exogenous hormone treatments is unknown.

Indomethacin (Indocin)[896] Diosgenin, a sapogenin from wild yam, prevented drug-induced ulcers and also lowered serum level of drug in rats.

Willow *Salix spp.*

USES: Low back pain (H-Assalix), migraine (H), osteoarthritis, (H).

PART USED: Bark.

CONTRAINDICATIONS: In children with influenza or varicella to avoid the possibility of Reye's syndrome due to salicylate content. Bleeding disorders, gastric ulcers, pregnancy, salicylate sensitivity/aspirin allergy, thrombocyte abnormality.

SAFETY: Contains salicylates. Contains tannins; avoid high dose for extended period. In one study, willow was found to inhibit platelet aggregation to a much smaller degree than aspirin. On FDA's list of herbs and clinical relevance has not been established. Associated with illness or injury (Reye's syndrome).[178]

AHPA Class: 1.[66]

ADVERSE REACTIONS: Allergic reaction, GI distress.

INTERACTIONS:

Tannin content may result in a decreased absorption of other drugs.[4]

Salicylate-containing drugs[897] Salicin is metabolized to salicylic acid which theoretically may be additive when combined with drugs containing salicylic acid, such as aspirin.

Wintergreen *Gaultheria procumbens*
   PART USED: Leaf.
   CONTRAINDICATIONS: Salicylate/aspirin sensitivity. Children, pregnancy, lactation.
   SAFETY: Contains salicylates.   Lectine, a component of herb, is mutagenic. Large dose of oil is toxic and has caused death. AHPA Class: 1.[66]
   ADVERSE REACTIONS: Allergic response.
   INTERACTIONS:
   Anticoagulants and drugs that increase the risk of bleeding[898] (see Appendix 8) Wintergreen leaf oil contains methyl salicylate, which may inhibit platelet aggregation and increase the risk of bleeding.

Wintersweet *Carissa spectabilis*
   INTERACTIONS:
   Digoxin/Cardiac glycosides[34] Herb increases risk of drug toxicity.

Witch Hazel *Hamamelis virginiana*
   PART USED: Bark, leaf.
   SAFETY: Contains tannins, avoid high dose for extended period. Not recommended for internal use. AHPA Class: 1.[66]
   ADVERSE REACTIONS: Constipation, GI irritation, hepatic damage, impaction, N&V.
   INTERACTIONS:
   Herb may reduce intestinal absorption of other drugs due to tannin content.[4]

Wormwood *Artemisia absinthium*

PART USED: Herb.

CONTRAINDICATIONS: Pregnancy, ulcers.

SAFETY: Contains thujone, which may cause convulsions. On FDA's list of herbs associated with illness or injury (numbness of extremities, delirium, paralysis and loss of intellect).[178] GRAS (flavoring, thujone free). AHPA Class: 2b, 2c, 2d—not long-term or excessive dose.[66]

ADVERSE REACTIONS: Agitation, cramping, headache, renal failure, restlessness, rhabdomyolysis, seizures, tremors, vertigo, vomiting.

INTERACTIONS:

Acetaminophen/Paracetamol[899] Plant extract decreased hepatotoxicity of acetaminophen in mice. Protective effect of wormwood may be mediated via alterations in microsomal drug metabolizing enzymes

Alkaloids (see Appendix 4)[4] High tannin content of herb may cause alkaloids to become insoluble and precipitate.

Pentobarbital (Nembutal)[899] Plant extract increased pentobarbital sleep time in mice.

Yacon *Smallantus sonchifolius*

INTERACTIONS:

Oral hypoglycemic agents[255] Water extract of herb had hypoglycemic effect. Maximal effect was found with greater than 30 days of administration. Action of herb is believed to increase release of insulin from pancreas or decrease breakdown of existing insulin.

Yarrow *Achillea millefolium*
    PART USED: Flower, herb.
    CONTRAINDICATIONS: Pregnancy and lactation. Allergy to *Asteraceae* family.
    SAFETY: GRAS (flavoring in alcoholic beverages-thujone free). AHPA Class: 2b.[66]
    ADVERSE REACTIONS: Contact dermatitis, photosensitivity.

Yellow Dock *Rumex crispus*
    PART USED: Root.
    CONTRAINDICATIONS: Safety in pregnancy, lactation and children not established.
Hypocalcemia, kidney stones.
    SAFETY: Contains oxalates and tannins; avoid high dose for extended period. AHPA
Class: 2d—not with h/o kidney stones.[66]
    ADVERSE REACTIONS: GI distress. Overdose may cause ataxia, diarrhea, hepatic
necrosis, hypocalcemia, kidney stones, metabolic acidosis, nausea, polyuria,
salivation, tremors and death.

Yellow Oleander *Thevetia peruviana*
    SAFETY: Fatal poisonings have occurred.
    ADVERSE REACTIONS: Cardiac dysrrhythmias, dizziness, palpitations, vomiting.
    INTERACTIONS:
        Digoxin/Cardiac glycosides[34] Herb contains cardiac glycosides.

INTERACTIONS:

Drugs metabolized by P450 CYP3A4 enzymes[282] (see Appendix 38) In research using human liver microsomes, Yi Mu Cao weakly inhibited CYP3A4 enzymes.

Yin Yang Huo *Herba eppimedii*

INTERACTIONS:

Drugs metabolized by P450 CYP3A4 enzymes[282] (see Appendix 38) In research using human liver microsomes, Yin Yang Huo strongly inhibited CYP3A4 enzymes.

Yohimbe *Pausinystalia yohimbe*

USES: Erectile dysfunction (H).

PART USED: Bark.

CONTRAINDICATIONS: Pregnancy, lactation, children, angina, anxiety, cardiovascular disease, diabetes, psychiatric disorders, HTN, hepatic disease, renal disease, schizophrenia.

SAFETY: High amounts may lower BP and affect GI and nervous systems. Use only under supervision of a health care professional. AHPA Class: 2d—not with kidney and liver disease, inflammation of prostate, not excessive or long-term.[66]

ADVERSE REACTIONS: Anorexia, anxiety, diarrhea, dizziness, flushing, GI distress, hallucinations, headache, hypothermia, HTN, insomnia, mydriasis, N&V, nervousness, palpitations, paresthesias, perspiration, piloerection, restlessness, rhinorrhea, salivation, sleep disturbance, tachycardia, tremor. High doses can cause abdominal pain, CNS stimulation, hypotension, kidney failure, lupus-like syndrome, paralysis,

Yohimbe (cont'd.)

psychosis and muscle weakness.

INTERACTIONS:

Alpha 2-Adrenergic-blocking agents (Phenoxybenzamine, Phentolamine, Bretylium, Atropine)[93,900-high doses] Moderate to high doses of drug increase toxicity of herb. Additive alpha-2a blocking.

Antihypertensives[900] (see Appendix 11) 15-20 Mg of yohimbe increases systolic blood pressure.

Beta blockers[93] (see Appendix 11) Drug may be protective against yohimbe toxicity.

Clonidine[900,906] Herb antagonizes effect of drug.

CNS stimulants[93] (amphetamines, cocaine) Drug increases toxicity risk.

Diazepam (Valium)[900,906] Herb antagonizes effect of drug.

Insulin/Oral hypoglycemic agents[907] (see Appendix 24) Yohimbine, a component of yohimbe, had a hypoglycemic effect and increased insulin release in type 2 diabetes and non-diabetic patients. The effect was additive when combined with glibenclamide (glyburide).

Levodopa[93,902] Yohimbe decreased dyskinetic side effect of drug in animal model of Parkinson's disease. Drug inhibited some of herb's effects.

Neuroleptics with a-adrenergic blocking activity[93] (chlorpromazine) Drug increases yohimbe toxicity.

MAOIs[93] (see Appendix 9) Drug increases toxicity of herb.

Morphine[904] In research using mice, pretreatment with yohimbe blocked the antinociceptive effect of drug.

Phenothiazines[93] (see Appendix 28)   Drug increases toxicity of herb (psychic and autonomic effects).

Reserpine (Enduronyl)[93]   Drug reduces anxiety and hypertension from herb use.

SSRIs[901] (see Appendix 9)   Herb has been found to improve sexual side effects of drug.

Sympathomimetics[93] (see Appendix 36)   Drug increases risk of herb's adverse effects and toxicity.

Tricyclic antidepressants[93] (see Appendix 9)   Yohimbe may increase sensitivity to drug, and concurrent use may increase the risk of hypertension and side effects of herb.

Venlafaxine (Effexor)[903]   Yohimbe decreases antinociceptive effect of drug.

Xylazine[905]   A combination of yohimbine, a component of yohimbe, and 4-aminopyridine decreased the drug-induced sedation of xylazine in goats.

Yoko *Paullinia yoko*

INTERACTIONS:

Clozapine, and possibly other drugs metabolized by P450 CYP1A2[296,350] (see Appendix 38)   Caffeine intakes greater than 400 mg may decrease clearance of clozapine (and possibly induce other drugs metabolized by CYP1A2.   In randomized crossover research of 12 males, the AUC of clozapine was increased by 19% and oral clearance of clozapine was decreased 14% with concurrent caffeine intake.   Yoko bark contains 27,300 ppm of caffeine.

Zygophyllum gaetulum
INTERACTIONS:

Insulin/Oral hypoglycemic agents[329,908] (see Appendix 24) In rats given herb .7g/kg, hypoglycemic effect was seen in normal and hypoglycemic rats. Mechanism of action is believed to be in part due to increased peripheral metabolism of glucose.

A - research using animals
ADHD - attention deficit hyperactive disorder
AHPA - American Herbal Products Association
AUC - area under the concentration-time curve
BP - blood pressure
BPH - benign prostatic hypertrophy
CHF - congestive heart failure
CNS - central nervous system
ER - estrogen receptor
ER+ - estrogen receptor positive
GERD - gastroesophageal reflux disease
GFR - glomerular filtration rate
GMPs – good manufacturing practices
GRAS - generally accepted as safe by U.S. Food and Drug Administration
H - human research
HAMA - Hamilton Anxiety Scale
HIV - human immunodeficiency virus
h/o - history of
HS - evening
HTN - hypertension
IBS - irritable bowel syndrome
IM - intramuscular

INR - international normalized rates (blood test)
LDCY - low doses of cyclophosphamide
LDH - lactate dehydrogenase (blood test that measures tissue damage)
LFT - liver function test
MI - myocardial infarction
MOP - type of chemotherapy
NK - natural killer cells
NO - nitric oxide
N&V - nausea and vomiting
OGTT - oral glucose tolerance test
OHA - oral hypoglycemic agent
PGP - P glycoprotein
RA - rheumatoid arthritis
RBC - red blood cells
SGOT or AST - serum glutamic-oxaloacetic transaminase (blood test)
SGPT or ALT - serum glutamate pyruvate transaminase (blood test)
SJW - St. John's wort
URTI - upper respiratory tract infection
WBC - white blood test

Appendix 1 Acid-inhibiting drugs

Histamine H2-receptor antagonists: Cimetidine (Tagamet), famotidine (Pepcid), nizatidine (Axid), ranitidine (Zantac).

Proton pump inhibitors: Esomeprazole (Nexium), lansoprazole (Prevacid), omeprazole (Prilosec), pantoprazole (Protonix), Rabeprazole (Aciphex).

Antimuscarinic agents: Pirenzepine.

Appendix 2 Adrenergics See Catecholamines under Sympathomimetics.

Appendix 3 Adrenergic agonists see Sympathomimetics.

Appendix 4 Alkaloids

Apomorphine, atropine (Sal-Tropine), cocaine, homatropine, hyoscyamine, morphine (MSIR, MS Contin, Oramorph, Roxanol), physostigmine (Antilirium), scopolamine (Scop, Scopace).

Appendix 5 Drugs with anticholinergic activity

Phenothiazines: (see Appendix 28).

Tricyclic antidepressants see Tricyclic Antidepressants (Appendix 9).

Others: Amantadine, anisotropine (Valpin), antihistamines, atropine, belladonna, clidinium (Quarzan), cyclopentolate (Cyclogyl), dicyclomine (Bentyl), flavoxate (Urispas), glycopyrrolate (Robinul), hexocyclium, homatropine (Isopto, Homatropine), isopropamide (Darbid),

Appendix 5 Drugs with anticholinergic activity (cont'd.)

l-Hyoscyamine (Anaspaz, Cystospaz, Lavsinex), ipratropium (Atrovent), mecamylamine (Inversine), mepenzolate (Cantil), methantheline (Banthine), methscopolamine (Pamine), oxybutynin (Ditropan), pralidoxime (Protopam), Procainamide (Procanbid, Pronestyl), propantheline (Pro-Banthine), quinidine (Quinaglute), scopolamine, tolterodine (Detrol), tridihexethyl (Pathilon), tropicamide (Mydriacyl Ophthalmic).

Appendix 6 Antiarrhythmics

Group I:

Sodium channel blockers: Disopyramide (Norpace), flecainide (Tambocor), lidocaine (Xylocaine), mexiletine (Mexitil), moricizine (Ethmozine), procainamide (Pronestyl), propafenone (Rythmol), quinidine (Quinidex), tocainide (Tonocard).

Group II

Beta blockers: Acebutolol (Sectral), esmolol (Brevibloc), propranolol (Inderal).

Group III

Amiodarone (Cordarone), bretylium (Bretylol), dofetilide (Tikosyn), ibutilide (Corvert), sotalol (Betapace)

Group IV

Calcium channel blockers: Bepridil (Vascor), diltiazem (Cardizem), verapamil (Calan, Isoptin).

Misc.: Adenosine (Adenocard), digoxin (Lanoxin).

Aminoglycosides: Amikacin (Amikin), gentamicin (Garamycin), kanamycin (Kantrex), neomycin (Mycifradin), netilmicin (Netromycin), paromomycin (Humatin), spectinomycin (Trobicin), streptomycin, tobramycin (Nebcin).

Beta-Lactam: Amoxicillin (Amoxil), amoxicillin/potassium clavulanate (Augmentin), ampicillin (Omnipen, Polycillin), ampicillin/subactam sodium (Unasyn), bacampicillin (Spectrobid), carbenicillin (Geocillin), cloxacillin (Tegopen), dicloxacillin (Dynapen), methicillin (Staphcillin), mezlocillin (Mezlin), monobactams, nafcillin (Unipen, Nafcil, Nallpen), oxacillin (Bactocill, Prostaphlin), penicillin (various), piperacillin (Pipracil), ticarcillin (Ticar).

Cephalosporins: Aztreonam (Azactam), cefaclor (Ceclor), cefadroxil (Duricef), cefamandole (Mandol), cefazolin (Ancef, Kefzol), cefdinir (Omnicef), cefepime (Maxipime), cefixime (Suprax), cefmetazole (Zefazone), cefonicid (Monocid), cefoperazone (Cefobid), cefotaxime (Claforan), cefotetan (Cefotan), cefoxitin (Mefoxin), cefpodoxime (Vantin), cefprozil (Cefzil), ceftazidime (Fortaz, Tazidime), ceftibuten (Cedax), ceftizoxime (Cefizox), ceftriaxone (Rocephin), cephalexin (Keflex), cephalothin (Keflin), cephapirin (Cefadyl), cephradine (Anspor, Velosef), loracarbef (Lorabid), moxalactam, proxetil.

Macrolides: Azithromycin (Zithromax), clarithromycin (Biaxin), erythromycin (Erythrocin, Ilotycin).

Quinolones & fluoroquinolones: cinoxacin (Cinobac), ciprofloxacin (Cipro), enoxacin (Penetrex), gatifloxacin (Tequin), levofloxacin (Levaquin), lomefloxacin (Maxaquin), moxifloxacin (Avelox), nalidixic acid (NegGram), norfloxacin (Noroxin), ofloxacin (Floxin), sparfloxacin (Zagam), trovafloxacin (Trovan).

Sulfonamides: Mafenide (Sulfamylon), Sulphasalazine (Azulfidine), sulfamethizole, sulfamethoxazole, sulfisoxazole (Gantrisin).

Appendix 7   Antibiotics (cont'd.)

Tetracyclines: Demeclocycline (Declomycin), doxycycline (Vibramycin), methacycline (Rondomycin), minocycline (Minocin), oxytetracycline (Terramycin), tetracycline (Achromycin).

Others and antimycobacterials: Aztreonam (Azactam), capreomycin (Capastat), chloramphenicol (Chloromycetin), clindamycin (Cleocin), clofazimine (Lamprene), cycloserine (Myambutol, Seromycin), dapsone, ethambutol (Myambutol), ethionamide (Trecator-SC), fosfomycin (Monurol), imipenem/cilastatin (Primaxin), isoniazid (Nydrazid), linezolid (Zyvox), meropenem (Merrem), novobiocin (Albamycin), pyrazinamide, quinupristin and dalfopristin (Synercid), rifabutin (Mycobutin), rifampin (Rifadin), rifapentine (Priftin), streptomycin, trimethoprim (Proloprim, Trimpex), trimethoprim/sulfamethoxazole (Bactrim, Septra, CoTrim), vancomycin (Vancocin, Vancoled).

Appendix 8   Anticoagulants and drugs that increase the risk of bleeding

Anticoagulants; Heparin, low molecular weight heparins, warfarin (Coumadin).
Antiplatelets: Abciximab (ReoPro), aspirin, cilostazol (Pletal), clopidogrel (plavix), dipyridamole (Persantine), eptifibatide (Integrilin), sulfinpyrazone (Anturane), ticlopidine (Ticlid), tirofiban (Aggrastat).
NSAIDs: Celecoxib (Celebrex), diclofenac (Cataflam), etodolac (Lodine), fenoprofen (Nalfon), flurbiprofen (Ansaid), ibuprofen, indomethacin (Indocin), ketoprofen (Orudis), ketorolac (Toradol), meclofenamate (Meclomen), mefenamic acid (Ponstel), meloxicam (Mobic), nabumetone (relafen), naproxen (naprosyn), oxaprozin (Daypro), piroxicam (Feldene), rofecoxib (Vioxx), sulindac (Clinoril), tolmetin (Tolectin).
Thrombolytics: Alteplase recombinant (Activase), anistreplase/APSAC (Eminase),

Appendix 8 Anticoagulants (cont'd.)

reteplase (Retavase), streptokinase (Streptase), urokinase (Abbokinase).

Herbs: Agrimony, andrographis, angelica, anise, arnica (not including homeopathic preparations), astragalus, asafoetida, astragalus, baikal skullcap, barberry, bilberry, black currant, black seed, bogbean, boldo, borage, bromelain, cayenne, celery, chamomile, cinchona bark, cloves, cocoa, coleus, cumin, dan shen, dandelion, devil's claw, dong quai, evening primrose oil, fenugreek, feverfew, fish oil supplements, flaxseed, fucus, gamma-linolenic acid, garlic, ginger, ginkgo, ginseng (Panax or Asian), goat's rue, goldenseal, grapeseed, green tea, guarana, hawthorn, horse chestnut, indian snakeroot, ivy, Japanese honeysuckle, kava, kelp, licorice, lovage, lycium, meadowsweet, motherwort, onion, Oregon grape, Papain, pau d'arco, reishi mushroom, rue, sacred basil, safflower, saw palmetto, shiitake mushroom, stephania, strophanthus, sweet clover, tonka bean, tremella mushroom, turmeric, wintergreen, vitamin E.

Appendix 9 Antidepressants

Monoamine oxidase inhibitors: Phenelzine (Nardil), isocarboxazid (Marplan), tranylcypromine (Parnate).

SSRIs: Citalopram (Celexa), fluoxetine (Prozac), fluvoxamine (Luvox), paroxetine (Paxil), sertraline (Zoloft).

Tricyclics: Amitriptyline (Elavil), clomipramine (Anafranil), desipramine (Norpramin, Pertofrane), doxepin (Adapin, Sinequan), imipramine (Tofranil), nortriptyline (Aventyl, Pamelor), protriptyline (Aventyl, Pamelor), trimipramine (Surmontil).

Others: Amoxapine (Asendin), bupropion (Wellbutrin), maprotiline (Ludiomil), mirtazapine (Remeron), nefazodone (Serzone), trazodone (Desyrel), venlafaxine (Effexor).

Appendix 10   Anticonvulsants

Carbamazepine (Tegretol), clonazepam (Klonopin), clorazepate dipotassium (Tranxene), ethosuximide (Zarontin), ethotoin (Peganone), felbamate (Felbatol), fosphenytoin (Cerebyx), gabapentin (Neurontin), lamotrigine (Lamotrigine), levetiracetam (Keppra), mephenytoin (Mesantoin), mephobarbital (Mebaral), methsuximide (Celontin Kapseals), oxcarbazepine (Trileptal), paramethadione (Paradione), phenacemide (Phenurone), phenobarbital (Nembutal), phensuximide (Milontin, Kapseals), phenytoin (Dilantin), primidone (Mysoline), tiagabine (Gabitril), topiramate (Topamax), valproic acid (Depakene, Depakote).

Appendix 11   Antihypertensives

ACE-inhibitors: Benazepril (Lotensin), captopril (Capoten), enalapril (Vasotec), fosinopril (Monopril), lisinopril (Prinivil, Zestril), moexipril (Univasc), quinapril (Accupril), ramipril (Altace), trandolapril (Mavik).

Alpha blockers: Doxazosin (Cardura), prazosin (Minipress), terazosin (Hytrin).

Angiotensin II receptor blockers: Candesartan (Atacand), eprosartan, irbesartan (Avapro), losartan (Cozaar), telmisartan (Micardis), valsartan (Diovan).

Beta blockers: Acebutolol (Sectral), atenolol (Tenormin), bisoprolol (Zebeta), carteolol (Cartrol), carvedilol (Coreg), labetalol (Normodyne, Trandate), metoprolol ER (Toprol XL), metoprolol (Lopressor), nadolol (Corgard), penbutolol (Levatol), pindolol (Visken), propranolol ER (Betachron ER, Inderal LA), propranolol (Inderal), timolol (Blocadren).

Calcium channel blockers: Amlodipine (Norvasc), diltiazem (Cardizem), diltiazem ER (Cardizem CD, Cardizem SR, Cartia XT, Dilacor XR, (Tiazac), felodipine (Plendil), isradipine (DynaCirc), nicardipine (Cardene), nifedipine ER (Adalat CC, Procardia XL), nisoldipine (Sular), verapamil (Calan, Isoptin), verapamil extended-release (Calan SR, Covera-HS,

Appendix 11 Antihypertensives (cont'd.)

Isoptin SR, Verapamil ER, Verelan, Verelan PM).

Diuretics: Amiloride and hydrochlorothiazide (Moduretic), bumetanide (Bumex), chlorthalidone (Hygroton), furosemide (Lasix), hydrochlorothiazide (Esidrix, Ezide, HydroDIURIL, Microzide, Oretic), indapamide (Lozol), metolazone (Mykrox, Zaroxolyn), spironolactone (Aldactone), torsemide (Demadex), triamterene (Dyrenium).

Appendix 12 Barbiturates

Amobarbital (Amytal), phenobarbital, pentobarbital (Nembutal), secobarbital, thiopental (Pentothal).

Appendix 13 Benzodiazepines

Alprazolam (Xanax), chlordiazepoxide (Librium), clonazepam (Klonopin), clorazepate dipotassium (Gen-Xene, Tranxene-T, Tranxene-SD), diazepam (Valium), estazolam (ProSom), flurazepam (Dalmane), halazepam (Paxipam), lorazepam (Ativan), oxazepam (Serax), quazepam (Doral), temazepam (Restoril), triazolam (Halcion).

Appendix 14 Cardiovascular drugs also see Antihypertensives and

Antiarrhythmics.

Cardiac glycosides: Digoxin (Lanoxin), digitoxin (Crystodigin).

Phosphodiesterase inhibitors: Amrinone (Inocor).

Vasodilating drugs: Alprostadil, amyl nitrate, dipyridamole (Persantine), isosorbide dinitrate (Isordil, Sorbitrate), isosorbide mononitrate (ISMO, Monoket), nitric oxide (Natrecor), papaverine, tolazoline (Priscoline).

Appendix 14   Cardiovascular drugs (cont'd.)

Cardioactive herbs: Balloon cotton, Bishop's weed, black hellebore, blue flag, cereus, dog bane, figwort, foxglove, frangipani, king's crown, lily of the valley, motherwort, oleander, Oregon grape, pheasant's eye, pleurisy root, redheaded cotton bush, rubber vine, sea mango, squill, strophanthus, wintersweet, yellow oleander.

Appendix 15   CNS depressants

Alcohol

Anesthetics (see Appendix 20).

Anticonvulsants (see Appendix 10).

Antiemetics

Antihistamines

Antipsychotics (see Appendix 19).

Antivertigo drugs

Barbiturates (see Appendix 12).

Benzodiazepines: (see Appendix 13).

Hypnotics: Meprobamate, zaleplon (Sonata), zolpidem (Ambien), also see barbiturates.

Opioids: Alfentanil (Alfenta), buprenorphine (Buprenex), butorphanol (Stadol), codeine, dezocine (Dalgan), fentanyl (Sublimaze), hydrocodone (various), hydromorphone (Dilaudid), levomethadyl (Orlaam), levorphanol (Levo-Dromoran), meperidine (Demerol), methadone (Dolophine), morphine, nalbuphine (Nubain), oxycodone, oxymorphone (Numorphan), pentazocine (Talwin), propoxyphene (Darvon/darvocet), remifentanil (Ultiva), sufentanil (Sufenta), tramadol (Ultram).

Tricyclic antidepressants (see Appendix 9).

Misc.: Ethchlorvynol (Placidyl), meprobamate (Miltown), paraldehyde (Paral).

Herbs: Ashwagandha, balloon flower, barberry, calamus, calendula, california poppy, catnip, cayenne, chamomile, goldenseal, gotu kola (large amounts), hawthorn, henbane, hops, indian snakeroot, Jamaica dogwood Bark, kava, king's crown, lavender, lemon Balm, motherwort, nettles, oleander, opium flower, passion flower, sassafras, scullcap, Siberian ginseng, St. John's wort, sweet broom, valerian, yerba mansa.

Appendix 16   Chemotherapy

Alkylating agents: Busulfan (Myleran), carboplatin (Paraplatin), carmustine (BiCNU), chlorambucil (Leukeran), cisplatin (Platinol), cyclophosphamide (Cytoxan, Neosar), ifosfamide (Ifex), lomustine (CeeNU), mechlorethamine (Mustargen), melphalan (Alkeran), procarbazine (Matulane), streptozocin (Zanosar), thiotepa (Thioplex).

Antibiotics: Bleomycin(Blenoxane), dactinomycin (actinomycin) (daunomycin) (daunomycin), Doxorubicin (Adriamycin, Rubex), idarubicin, mitoxantrone (Novantrone), mitomycin C, pentostatin (Nipent), plicamycin (mithracin).

Antimetabolites: 5-Fluoruricil (Adrucil), cytarabine (Cytosar), floxuridine (FUDR), mercaptopurine (Purinethol), methotrexate (Rheumatrex), thioguanine.

Hormones: Anastrozole (Arimidex), bicalutamide (Casodex), diethylstilbestrol (Stilphostrol), estramustine (emcyt), flutamide (eulexin), goserelin (Zoladex), irinotecan (Camptosar), letrozole (Femara), leuprolide (Lupron), medroxyprogesterone, megestrol (Megace), nilutamide (Nilandron), polyestradiol, prednisone (Deltasone, Medrol), tamoxifen (Nolvadex), testolactone (Teslac), topotecan (Hycamtin).

Mitotic inhibitors: Etoposide (Etopophos, VePesid), teniposide (Vumon), vinblastine (Velban),

Appendix 16   Chemotherapy (cont'd.)

vincristine (Oncovin, Vincasar), vindesine, vinorelbine (Navelbine).

Misc: Aldesleukin (Proleukin), altretamine (Hexalen), asparaginase (Elspar), BCG (Tice), cladribine (leustatin), dacarbazine (DTIC-Dome), gemcitabine (Gemzar), hydroxyurea (Droxia, Hydrea), interferon, interleukin, levamisole (Ergamisol), mitotane (Lysodren), paclitaxel (Taxol), pegaspargase (Oncaspar), tretinoin (Avita, Renova, Retin-A).

Appendix 17   Cholinergic drugs

Acetylcholine, bethanechol (Urecholine), donepezil (Aricept), echothiophate (Phospholine Iodide), edrophonium (Enlon, Reversol, Tensilon), neostigmine (Prostigmin), physostigmine (Antilirium), pyridostigmine (Mestinon, Regonol), succinylcholine (Anectine, Quelicin), tacrine (Cognex).

Appendix 18   Corticosteroids

Betamethasone (Celestone), cortisone (Cortone, Cortisone), dexamethasone (Decadron), fludrocortisone (Florinef), hydrocortisone (Cortef, Hydrocortone), methylprednisolone (Medrol, Depo-Medrol), prednisone (Deltasone), triamcinolone (Aristocort, Kenacort).

Appendix 19   Drugs with dopamine-receptor antagonist activity

Antipsychotics: Chlorpromazine (Thorazine), haloperidol (Haldol), loxapine (Loxitane), pimozide (Orap), prochlorperazine (Compazine).

Atypical antipsychotics: Clozapine (Clozaril), olanzapine (Zyprexa), quetiapine (Seroquel), risperidone (Risperdal), sertindole (Serlect), ziprasidone (Geodon).

Others: metoclopramide (reglan).

Desflurane (Suprane), enflurane (Ethrane), halothane (Fluothane), isoflurane (Forane), nitrous oxide, Sevoflurane (Ultane).

Appendix 21   Drugs that may cause hepatotoxicity

Acarbose (Precose), acetaminophen, amiodarone (Cordarone), atorvastatin (Lipitor), azathioprine (Imuran), carbamazepine (Tegretol), cerivastatin (Baycol), diclofenac (Voltaren), erythromycin (Erythrocin, others), estrogens, felbamate (Felbatol), fenofibrate (Tricor), fluconazole (Diflucan), fluvastatin (Lescol), gemfibrozil (Lopid), isoniazid (INH), itraconazole (Sporanox), ketoconazole (Nizoral), leflunomide (Arava), lovastatin (Mevacor), methotrexate (Rheumatrex), nevirapine (Viramune), niacin, nitrofurantoin (Macrodantin), phenytoin (Dilantin), pioglitazone (Actos), pravastatin (Pravachol), pyrazinamide, rifampin (Rifadin), ritonavir (Norvir), rosiglitazone (Avandia), simvastatin (Zocor), tacrine (Cognex), tamoxifen, terbinafine (Lamisil), valproic acid, and zileuton (Zyflo).

Appendix 22   HIV medications

Protease inhibitors: Amprenavir (Agenerase), indinavir (Crixivan), lopinavir + ritonavir (Kaletra), nelfinavir (Viracept), ritonavir (Norvir), saquinavir (Invirase, Fortovase).

Nucleoside reverse transcriptase inhibitors (NNRTIs): Abacavir (Ziagen), didanosine (Videx), emtricitabine (Coviracil), lamivudine (Epivir), stavudine (Zerit), zalcitabine (Hivid), zidovudine (Retrovir), zidovudine + lamivudine (Combivir).

Non-nucleoside reverse transcriptase inhibitors (NNRTIs): delavirdine (Rescriptor), Efavirenz (Sustiva), emivirine (Coactinon), nevirapine (Viramune).

Appendix 23   Immunosuppressant drugs

Azathioprine (Imuran), basiliximab (Stimulect), cyclosporine (Sandimmune, Neoral), daclizumab (Zenapax), interferon, muromonab-CD3 (OKT3, Orthoclone OKT3), mycophenolate (CellCept), sirolimus (Rapamune), tacrolimus (FK506, Prograf), also see Corticosteroids .(Appendix 18)

Appendix 24   Insulin/Oral hypoglycemic agents

Alpha-glucosidase inhibitors: Acarbose (Precose), miglitol (Glyset).
Biguanides: Metformin (Glucophage, Glucophage XR).
Meglitinides: Nateglinide (Starlix), Repaglinide (Prandin).
Sulfonylurea/Biguanide combination: Glyburide and metformin (Glucovance).
Sulfonylureas: Acetohexamide (Dymelor), chlorpropamide (Diabinese), glimepiride (Amaryl), glipizide (Glucotrol), glyburide (Diabeta, Glynase, Micronase), tolazamide (Tolinase), tolbutamide (Orinase).
Thiazolidinediones: Pioglitazone (Actos), rosiglitazone (Avandia).
Insulins: Insulin Aspart, Insulin Lente, Insulin lispro, NPH, regular, ultralente and various others.

Bile acid resins: Cholestyramine (Cholybar, LoCholest, LoCholest Light, Prevalite, Questran, Questran Light), colesevelam (WelChol), colestipol (Colestid).

Fibric acid derivatives: Clofibrate (Atromid-S), fenofibrate (Tricor), gemfibrozil (Lopid).

HMG-CoA reductase inhibitors: Atorvastatin (Lipitor), fluvastatin (Lescol, Lescol XL), lovastatin (Mevacor), pravastatin (Pravachol), simvastatin (Zocor).

Other: Niacin (Niaspan).

Appendix 26   Drugs that may cause nephrotoxicity

Aminoglycosides: Amikacin (Amikin), gentamicin (Garamycin, Gentak, others), tobramycin (Nebcin, others).

NSAIDs: Ibuprofen (Advil, Motrin, Nuprin, others), indomethacin (Indocin), naproxen (Aleve, Anaprox, Naprelan, Naprosyn), piroxicam (Feldene).

Others: Cyclosporine (Neoral, Sandimmune).

Appendix 27   NSAIDs see list of NSAIDs under **Anticoagulants and drugs that increase the risk of bleeding.**

Appendix 28   Phenothiazines

Chlorpromazine (Thorazine), fluphenazine (Permitil, Prolixin), mesoridazine besylate (Serentil), perphenazine (Trilafon), prochlorperazine (Compazine), promazine hydrochloride (Sparine), promethazine hydrochloride (Phenergan), thioridazine hydrochloride (Mellaril), trifluoperazine hydrochloride (Stelazine), triflupromazine hydrochloride (Vesprin).

Appendix 29   Drugs that may cause photosensitivity

Chlorpromazine (Thorazine), doxycycline (Vibramycin), felbamate (Felbatol), griseofulvin (Fulvicin, Grisactin), interferon, isotretinoin (Accutane), piroxicam (Feldene), porfimer (Photofrin), tetracyclines (see list under antibiotics), tretinoin (Renova, Retin-A).

Appendix 30   Highly protein bound drugs (clinical significance not established)

Chlordiazepoxide (Librium), chlorpropamide (Diabinese), cyclosporine (Neoral, Sandimmune), diazepam (Valium), dicloxacillin (Dynapen), digitoxin, fluoxetine (Prozac), furosemide (Lasix), midazolam (Versed), nifedipine (Adalat, Procardia), nortriptyline (Aventyl, Pamelor), prazosin (Minipress), propranolol (Inderal), tolbutamide (Orinase), valproic acid (Depakene, Depakote), warfarin (Coumadin).

Appendix 31   Drugs that may cause rhabdomyolysis

Azole anitfungals (itraconazole, ketoconazole, fluconazole), cyclosporine (Neoral, Sandimmune), HMG-CoA Reductase inhibitors (see Appendix 25), macrolide antibiotics (see Appendix 7), protease inhibitors (see Appendix 22).

Appendix 32   Drugs that may cause serotonin syndrome

Antidepressants (see Appendix 9), Triptans (see Appendix 37), 5-Hydroxy-Tryptophan, L-tryptophan, procarbazine (Matulane), sibutramine (Meridia), tramadol (Ultram).

Appendix 33   Serotonin agonist

Buspirone (BuSpar), gepirone, ipsapirone, quipazine, trazodone at high doses (Desyrel). Also see Triptans (Appendix 37).

Appendix 34 Serotonin antagonist

Alosetron (Lotronex), cyproheptadine (Periactin), fenfluramine, granisetron (Kytril), homochlorcyclizine, ketanserin, mescaline, methysergide (Sansert), mianserin, mirtazapine (Remeron), nefazodone (Serzone), ondansetron (Zofran), oxetorone, perlapine, pizotyline, trazodone at low doses (Desyrel).

Appendix 35 Drugs that may lower seizure threshold

Buproprion (Zyban). Antidepressants (see Appendix 9), antihistamines (sedating), antimalarials, antipsychotics, corticosteroids, MAOIs (see Appendix 9), quinolones (see Appendix 7), theophylline (Theo-Dur), systemic steroids (see Appendix 18), tramadol (Ultram). Aliphatic phenothiazines--chlorpromazine (Thorazine), prochlorperazine (Compazine), thioridazine (Mellaril).

Appendix 36 Sympathomimetics

Beta2-selective adrenergic agonists include: Albuterol (Proventil, Ventolin), bitolterol (Tornalate), formoterol (Foradil), metaproterenol (Alupent, Metaprel), pirbuterol (Maxair), salmeterol (Serevent), terbutaline (Brethine, Bricanyl).

Catecholamines: Dobutamine (Dobutrex), dopamine (Intropin), epinephrine (Adrenalin), fenoldopam, ibopamine, isoproterenol (Isuprel), norepinephrine (Levophed).

Others: Amphetamine, cocaine, ephedrine, isoetharine, levalbuterol (Xopenex), methamphetamine, methoxamine (Vasoxyl), methylphenidate (Ritalin), midodrine (ProAmatine), oxymetazoline (Afrin), pemoline (Cylert), phenmetrazine, phenylephrine, phenylpropanolamine, tyramine, xylometazoline (Otrivin).

Appendix 37 Triptans

Naratriptan (Amerge), rizatriptan (Maxalt), sumatriptan (Imitrex), zolmitriptan (Zomig).

Appendix 38 P450 and PGP substrates

CYP1A2; Acetaminophen (Tylenol), aminophylline (Truphylline), amitriptyline (Elavil), caffeine, clomipramine (Anafranil), clopidogrel (Plavix), clozapine (Clozaril), cyclobenzaprine (Flexeril), estradiol, flutamide (Eulexin), fluvoxamine (Luvox), haloperidol (Haldol), imipramine (Tofranil), ipriflavone, mexiletine (Mexitil), naproxen (Naprosyn), olanzapine (Zyprexa), ondansetron (Zofran), phenacetin, propranolol (Inderal), riluzole (Rilutek), ropivacaine (Naropin), ropinirole (Requip), tacrine (Cognex), theophylline (Theo-Dur), verapamil (Calan, Covera-HS, Isoptin, Verelan), R-warfarin (Coumadin), zileuton (Zyflo), zolmitriptan (Zomig).

CYP2C9: Celecoxib (Celebrex), diclofenac (Cataflam), fluvastatin (Lescol), glipizide (Glucotrol), ibuprofen, irbesartan (Avapro), losartan (Cozaar), naproxen (Naprosyn), phenytoin (Dilantin), piroxicam (Feldene), sulfamethoxazole (Gantanol), tamoxifen (Nolvadex), tolbutamide (Orinase), torsemide (Demadex), S-warfarin (Coumadin).

CYP2D6: Amitriptyline (Elavil), bufuralol, clomipramine (Anafranil), clozapine (Clozaril), codeine, debrisoquine, desipramine (Norpramin), dextromethorphan, encainide, flecainide (Tambocor), fluoxetine (Prozac), haloperidol (Haldol), imipramine (Tofranil), methoxyamphetamine, S-metoprolol (Lopressor, Toprol XL), mexiletine (Mexitil), minaprine, nortriptyline (Aventyl, Pamelor), ondansetron (Zofran), paroxetine (Paxil), perhexiline, perphenazine (Trilafon), propafenone (Rythmol), propranolol (Inderal), risperidone (Risperdal), sparteine, tamoxifen (Nolvadex), thioridazine (Mellaril), timolol (Blocadren), tramadol (Ultram), venlafaxine (Effexor).

CYP2E1: Acetaminophen, chlorzoxazone (Parafon), enflurane, ethanol, isoflurane, theophylline (Theo-Dur).

CYP3A4: Alfentanil (Alfenta), alprazolam (Xanax), amiodarone (Cordarone), amlodipine (Norvasc), amoxapine (Elavil, Pamelor), amprenavir (Agenerase), atorvastatin (Lipitor), bepridil (Vascor), carbamazepine (Tegretol), clarithromycin (Biaxin), clomipramine (Anafranil), clonazepam (Klonopin), corticosteroids (see Appendix 8), cortisone (Cortone), cyclophosphamide (Cytoxan), cyclosporine (Neoral, Sandimmune), delavirdine (Rescriptor), desipramine (Norpramin), dexamethasone (Decadron), diazepam (Valium), diltiazem (Cardizem), disopyramide (Norpace), doxorubicin (Adriamycin), efavirenz (Sustiva), erythromycin (Ilotycin), estradiol, etopophos/etoposide (Vepesid), felodipine (Plendil), fentanyl (Actiq, Duragesic), finasteride (Proscar), flutamide (Eulexin), granisetron (Kytril), haloperidol (Haldol), ifosfamide (Ifex), imipramine (Tofranil), indinavir (Crixivan), isradipine (DynaCir), ketoconazole (Nizoral), lidocaine (Xylocaine), loratadine (Claritin), losartan (Cozaar), lovastatin (Mevacor), methadone (Methadose), miconazole (Monistat), midazolam (Versed), nefazodone (Serzone), nelfinavir (Viracept), nevirapine (Viramune), nicardipine (Cardene), nifedipine (Adalat, Procardia), nimodipine (Nimotop), nisoldipine (Sular), nortriptyline (Aventyl, Pamelor), ondansetron (Zofran), oral contraceptives, paclitaxel (Taxol), paracetamol , pimozide (Orap), propafenone (Rythmol), protease inhibitors, quinine, quinidine (Quinidex), repaglinide (Prandin), retinoic acid, rifabutin (Mycobutin), ritonavir (Norvir), saquinavir (Fortovase, Invirase), sildenafil (Viagra), simvastatin (Zocor), sufentanil (Sufenta), tacrolimus (Prograf), tamoxifen (Nolvadex), teniposide (Vumon), terfenadine, testosterone, venlafaxine (Effexor), verapamil (Calan, Isoptin), vinblastine (Velban), vincristine (Oncovin, Vincasar), zolpidem (Ambien), zonisamide (Zonegran).

Appendix 38   P450 and PGP substrates (cont'd.)

PGP:

Amiodarone (Cordarone), amprenavir (Agenerase), atorvastatin (Lipitor), cyclosporine (Neoral, Sandimmune), dexamethasone (Decadron), digoxin (Lanoxin), diltiazem (Cardizem), doxorubicin (Adriamycin), erythromycin (Ilotycin), etopophos/etoposide (Vepesid), fexofenadine (Allegra), indinavir (Crixivan), Ivermectin, lidocaine (Xylocaine), loperamide (Imodium), lovastatin (Mevacor), morphine (MS Contin), nicardipine (Cardene), nifedipine (Adalat, Procardia), protease inhibitors, quinidine (Quinidex), ritonavir (Norvir), saquinavir (Fortovase, Invirase), tamoxifen (Nolvadex), teniposide (Vumon), terfenadine, verapamil (Calan, Isoptin), vinblastine (Velban), vincristine (Oncovin, Vincasar).

Numbers 1, 4, 66, 113, 116, 117, 118, 172 and 175, below, are general references, used throught this book.

1. Blumenthal M, Gruenwald J, Hall T, Riggins W, Busse W, Goldbert A, eds. *The Complete German Commission E Monographs: Therapeutic Guide to Herbal Medicines*. Austin, TX: American Botanical Council, 1998.

2. Sporer KA. The serotonin syndrome. Implicated drugs, pathophysiology and management. Drug Saf 1995 Aug;13(2):94-104.

3. Joly P, Lampert A, Thomine E, Lauret P. Development of pseudobullous morphea and scleroderma-like illness during therapy with L-5-hydroxytryptophan and carbidopa. J Am Acad Dermatol 1991 Aug;25(2 Pt 1):332-3.

4. Claus E, Tyler V, Brady L. Pharmacognosy. 6thed. Philadelphia:Lea & Febiger, 1970.

5. Mills J, Melville GN, Bennett C, West M, Castro A. Effect of hypoglycin A on insulin release. Biochem Pharmacol 1987 Feb 15;36(4):495-7.

6. Ubillas RP, Mendez CD, Jolad SD, et al. Antihyperglycemic acetylenic glucosides from *Bidens pilosa*. Planta Med 2000 Feb;66(1):82-3.

7. Yeih DF, Chiang FT, Huang SK. Successful treatment of aconitine induced life threatening ventricular tachyarrhythmia with amiodarone. Heart 2000 Oct;84(4):E8.

8. Hsu MF, Young JH, Wang JP, Teng CM. Effect of hsien-ho-t'sao (*Agrimonia pilosa*) on experimental thrombosis in mice. Am J Chin Med 1987;15(1-2):43-51.

9. House JK, George LW, Oslund KL, et al. Primary photosensitization related to ingestion of alfalfa silage by cattle. J Am Vet Med Assoc 1996 Nov 1;209(9):1604-7.

10. Haroon Y, Hauschka PV. Application of high-performance liquid chromatography to assay phylloquinone (vitamin K1) in rat liver. J Lipid Res 1983 Apr;24(4):481-4.

11. Mashour N, Lin G, Frishman W. Herbal medicine for the treatment of cardiovascular disease. Arch Intern Med. 1998;158:2225-2234.

12. Gray AM, Flatt PR. Pancreatic and extra-pancreatic effects of the traditional anti-diabetic plant, *Medicago sativa*

(lucerne). Br J Nutr 1997 Aug;78(2):325-34

13. Story JA, LePage SL, Petro MS, et al. Interactions of alfalfa plant and sprout saponins with cholesterol in vitro and in cholesterol-fed rats. Am J Clin Nutr. 1984;39:917–929.

14. Milk Thistle. The Review of Natural Products. Jan 1997;1-6.

15. Jacob DA, Temple JL, Patisaul HB, et al. Coumestrol antagonizes neuroendocrine actions of estrogen via the estrogen receptor alpha. Exp Biol Med (Maywood) 2001 Apr;226(4):301-6.

16. Bouraoui A, Brazier J, Zouaghi H, Rousseau M. Theophylline pharmacokinetics and metabolism in rabbits following single and repeated administration of capsicum fruit. Eur J Drug Metab Pharmacokinet. 1995;20:173-8.

17. Yamori Y, Nara Y, Tsubouchi T, Sogawa Y, Ikeda K, Horie R. Dietary prevention of stroke and its mechanisms in stroke-prone spontaneously hypertensive rats—preventive effect of dietary fibre and palmitoleic acid. J Hypertens Suppl 1986 Oct;4(3):S449-52.

18. Mandel KG, Daggy BP, Brodie DA, Jacoby HI. Review article: alginate-raft formulations in the treatment of heartburn and acid reflux. Aliment Pharmacol Ther 2000 Jun;14(6):669-90.

19. Saleem R, Ahmad M, Hussain S, Qazi A, Ahmad S, Qzai M, Ali M, Faizi S, Akhtar S, Husnain S. Hypotensive, hypoglycemic and toxicological studies on the flavonol c-glycoside shaminin from *Bombax ceiba*. Planta Med. 1999;65:331-4..

20. Davis RH, DiDonato JJ, Johnson RW, Stewart CB. Aloe vera, hydrocortisone, and sterol influence on wound tensile strength and anti-inflammation. J Am Podiatr Med Assoc 1994 Dec;84(12):614-21.

21. Gutierrez-Cabano CA. Thioctic acid protection against ethanol-induced gastric mucosal lesions involves sulfhydryl and prostaglandin participation. Acta Gastroenterol Latinoam 1997;27(1):31-7.

22. Almeida J, Grimsley E. Coma from the health food store: interaction between kava and alprazolam. Annals Intern Med. 1996;125:940-941.

23. Ernst E. Harmless herbs? A review of recent literature. Am J Med. 1998;104:170-178.

24. Dovinova I, Novotny L, Rauko P, Kvasnicka P. Combined effect of lipoic acid and doxorubicin in murine leukemia. Neoplasma 1999;46(4):237-41.

25. Rosenblatt M, Mindel J. Spontaneous hyphema associated with ingestion of *Ginkgo biloba* extract. N Engl J Med. 1997;336:1108.

26. *Ginkgo biloba* for dementia. Med Lett Drugs Ther. 1998;40:63-64.

27. Jones B, Runikis A. Interactions of ginseng with phenelzine. J Clin Psychopharmacol. 1987;7:201-202.

28. Rowin J, Lewis S. Spontaneous bilateral subdural hematomas associated with chronic *Ginkgo biloba* ingestion. Neurology. 1996;46:1775-1776.

29. Jacob S, Ruus P, Hermann R, et al. Oral administration of RAC-alpha-lipoic acid modulates insulin sensitivity in patients with type-2 diabetes mellitus: a placebo-controlled pilot trial. Free Radic Biol Med 1999 Aug;27(3-4):309-14.

30. Gleiter CH, Schreeb KH, Freudenthaler S, et al. Lack of interaction between thioctic acid, glibenclamide and acarbose. Br J Clin Pharmacol 1999 Dec;48(6):819-25.

31. Visen PK, Shukla B, Patnaik GK, Dhawan BN. Andrographolide protects rat hepatocytes against paracetamol-induced damage. J Ethnopharmacol 1993 Oct;40(2):131-6.

32. Amroyan E, Gabrielian E, Panossian A, Wikman G, Wagner H. Inhibitory effect of andrographolide from *Andrographis paniculata* on PAF-induced platelet aggregation. Phytomedicine 1999 Mar;6(1):27-31.

33. Puri A, Saxena R, Saxena RP, et al. Immunostimulant agents from *Andrographis paniculata*. J Nat Prod 1993 Jul;56(7):995-9.

34. Radford D, Gillies A, Hinds J, Duffy P. Naturally occurring cardiac glycosides. Med J Aust. 1986;144:540-544.

35. Zhang CY, Tan BK. Mechanisms of cardiovascular activity of *Andrographis paniculata* in the anaesthetized rat. J Ethnopharmacol 1997 Apr;56(2):97-101.

36. Zhan g XF, Tan BK. Anti-diabetic property of ethanolic extract of *Andrographis paniculata* in streptozotocin-diabetic rats. Acta Pharmacol Sin 2000 Dec;21(12):1157-64.

37. Ko FN, Wu TS, Liou MJ, Huang TF, Teng CM. Inhibition of platelet thromboxane formation and phosphoinositides breakdown by osthole from *Angelica pubescens*. Thromb Haemost 1989 Nov 24;62(3):996-9.

38. Eliason B. Transient hyperthyroidism in a patient taking dietary supplements containing kelp. J Am Board Fam Pract. 1998;11:478-80.

39. Hann SK, Park YK, Im S, Byun SW. Angelica-induced phytophotodermatitis. Photodermatol Photoimmunol Photomed 1991 Apr;8(2):84-5.

40. Okada Y, Miyauchi N, Suzuki K, et al. Search for naturally occurring substances to prevent the complications of diabetes. II. Inhibitory effect of coumarin and flavonoid derivatives on bovine lens aldose reductase and rabbit platelet aggregation. Chem Pharm Bull (Tokyo) 1995 Aug;43(8):1385-7.

41. Dhar SK. Anti-fertility activity and hormonal profile of trans-anethole in rats. Indian J Physiol Pharmacol 1995 Jan;39(1):63-7.

42. Pourgholami MH, Majzoob S, Javadi M, et al. The fruit essential oil of *Pimpinella anisum* exerts anticonvulsant effects in mice. J Ethnopharmacol 1999 Aug;66(2):211-5.

43. el-Shobaki FA, Saleh ZA, Saleh N. The effect of some beverage extracts on intestinal iron absorption. Z Ernahrungswiss 1990 Dec;29(4):264-9.

44. Morrison EY, Thompson H, Pascoe K, West M, Fletcher C. Extraction of an hyperglycaemic principle from the annatto (*Bixa orellana*), a medicinal plant in the West Indies. Trop Geogr Med 1991 Jan-Apr;43(1-2):184-8.

45. Schroder H, Losche W, Strobach H, et al. Helenalin and 11 alpha,13-dihydrohelenalin, two constituents from *Arnica montana* L., inhibit human platelet function via thiol-dependent pathways. Thromb Res 1990 Mar 15;57(6):839-45.

46. Englisch W, Beckers C, Unkauf M, Ruepp M, Zinserling V. Efficacy of artichoke dry extract in patients with hyper-lipoproteinemia. Arzneimittelforschung 2000 Mar;50(3):260-5.

47. Ziauddin M, Phansalkar N, Patki P, Diwanay S, Patwardhan B. Studies on the immunomodulatory effects of Ashwagandha. J Ethnopharmacol 1996 Feb;50(2):69-76.

48. Prasad S, Malhotra CL. Studies on *Withania ashwagandha* Kaul. VI. The effect of the alkaloidal fractions (acetone, alcohol and water soluble) on the central nervous system. Indian J Physiol Pharmacol 1968 Oct;12(4):175-81.

49. Uusitupa M, Sodervik H, Silvasti M, Karttunen P. Effects of a gel-forming dietary fiber, guar gum, on the absorption of glibenclamide and metabolic control and serum lipids in patients with non-insulin-dependent (type 2) diabetes. Int J Clin Pharmacol Ther Toxicol. 1990;28:153-7.

50. Andallu B, Radhika B. Hypoglycemic, diuretic and hypocholesterolemic effect of winter cherry (*Withania somnifera*, Dunal) root. Indian J Exp Biol 2000 Jun;38(6):607-9.

51. Sotaniemi E, Haapakoski E, Rautio A. Ginseng therapy in non-insulin-dependent diabetic patients. Diabetes Care. 1995;18:1373-5.

52. Malhotra CL, Mehta VL, Das PK, Dhalla NS. Studies on Withania-ashwagandha, Kaul. V. The effect of total alkaloids (ashwagandholine) on the central nervous system. Indian J Physiol Pharmacol 1965 Jul;9(3):127-36.

53. Kar A, Choudhary B, Bandyopadhyay N. Preliminary studies on the inorganic constituents of some indigenous hypo-glycaemic herbs on oral glucose tolerance test. J Ethnopharmacol. 1999;64:179-84.

54. Longerich L, Johnson E, Gault M. Digoxin-like factor in herbal teas. Clin Invest Med. 1993;16:210-8.

55. Alarcon-Aguilara F, Roman-Ramos R, Perez-Gutierrez S, Aguilar-Contreras A, Contreras-Weber C, Flores-Saenz J. Study of the anti-hyperglycemic effect of plants as antidiabetics. J Ethnopharmacol. 1998;61:101-10.

56. McRae S. Elevated serum digoxin levels in a patient taking digoxin and Siberian ginseng. Can Med Assoc J. 1996;155:293-5.

57. Gray A, Flatt P. Antihyperglycemic actions of *Eucalyptus globulus* (eucalyptus) are associated with pancreatic and extra-pancreatic effects in mice. J Nutr. 1998;128:2319-23.

58. Chan K, Lo A, Yeung H, Woo K. The effects of danshen (*Salvia miltiorrhiza*) on warfarin: pharmacodynamics and pharmacokinetics of warfarin enantiomers in rats. J Pharm Pharmacol. 1995;47:402-6.

59. Gupta YK, Sharma SS, Rai K, Katiyar CK. Reversal of paclitaxel induced neutropenia by *Withania somnifera* in mice. Indian J Physiol Pharmacol 2001 Apr;45(2):253-7.

60. Zuo, Li; Dong, Xichang; Sun, Xiaojian. The curative effects of *Astragalus membranaceus* Bungo A-6 in combination with acyclovir on the mice infected with HSV-1. Virologica Sinica. 1995;10(2):177-9.

61. Zhang WJ, Wojta J, Binder BR. Regulation of the fibrinolytic potential of cultured human umbilical vein endothelial cells: astragaloside IV downregulates plasminogen activator inhibitor-1 and upregulates tissue-type plasminogen activator expression. J Vasc Res 1997 Jul-Aug;34(4):273-80.

62. Yu C, Chan J, Sanderson J. Chinese herbs and warfarin potentiation by 'danshen'. J Intern Med. 1997;241:337-9.

63. Roman-Ramos R, Lara-Lemus A, Alarcon-Aguilar F, Flores-Saenz J. Hypoglycemic activity of some antidiabetic plants. Arch Med Res. 1992;23:105-9.

64. Chu DT, Wong WL, Mavligit GM. Immunotherapy with Chinese medicinal herbs. II. Reversal of cyclophosphamide-induced immune suppression by administration of fractionated *Astragalus membranaceus* in vivo. J Clin Lab Immunol 1988 Mar;25(3):125-9.

65. Qian ZW, Mao SJ, Cai XC, et al. Viral etiology of chronic cervicitis and its therapeutic response to a recombinant interferon. Chin Med J (Engl) 1990 Aug;103(8):647-51.

66. McGuffin M. *American Herbal Products Association's Botanical Safety Handbook.* Boca Raton, FL: CRC Press, 1997.

67. Wang Y, Qian XJ, Hadley HR, Lau BH. Phytochemicals potentiate interleukin-2 generated lymphokine-activated killer cell cytotoxicity against murine renal carcinoma. Mol Biother 1992 Sep;4(3):143-6.

68. McKenna DJ, Towers GH, Abbott F. Monoamine oxidase inhibitors in South American hallucinogenic plants: tryptamine and beta-carboline constituents of ayahuasca. J Ethnopharmacol 1984 Apr;10(2):195-223.

69. Dandekar U, Chandra R, Dalvi S, Joshi M, Gokhale P, Sharma A, Shah P, Kshirsagar N. Analysis of a clinically important interaction between phenytoin and shankhapushpi, an ayurvedic preparation. J Ethnopharmacol. 1992;35:285-8.

70. Gonzalez M, Zarzuelo A, Gamez M, Utrilla M, Jimenez J, Osuna I. Hypoglycemic activity of olive leaf. Planta Med. 1992;58:513-5.

71. Al-Hader A, Hasan Z, Aqel M. Hyperglycemic and insulin release inhibitory effects of *Rosmarinus officinalis*. J Ethnopharmacol. 1994;43:217-21.

72. Shaw D, Leon C, Kolev S, Murray V. Traditional remedies and food supplements. A 5-year toxicological study (1991-1995). Drug Saf. 1997;17:342-56.

73. Perharic L, Shaw D, Colbridge M, House I, Leon C, Murray V. Toxicological problems resulting from exposure to traditional remedies and food supplements. Drug Saf. 1994;11:284-94.

74. Guo LQ, Taniguchi M, Chen QY, Baba K, Yamazoe Y. Inhibitory potential of herbal medicines on human cytochrome P450-mediated oxidation: properties of umbelliferous or citrus crude drugs and their relative prescriptions. Jpn J Pharmacol 2001 Apr;85(4):399-408.

75. Roman-Ramos R, Flores-Saenz J, Alarcon-Aguilar F. Anti-hyperglycemic effect of some edible plants. J Ethnopharmacol. 1995;48:25-32.

76. Welihinda J, Karunanayake E, Sheriff M, Jayasinghe K. Effect of *Momordica charantia* on the glucose tolerance in maturity onset diabetes. J Ethnopharmacol. 1986;17:277-82.

77. Al-Khazraji S, Al-Shamaony L, Twaij H. Hypoglycaemic effect of *Artemisia herba alba*. I. Effect of different parts and influence of the solvent on hypoglycaemic activity. J Ethnopharmacol. 1993;40:163-6.

78. Amalraj T, Ignacimuthu S. Hypoglycemic activity of *Cajanus cajan* (seeds) in mice. Indian J Exp Biol. 1998;36:1032-3.

79. Lo A, Chan K, Yeung J, Woo K. Danggui (*Angelica Sinensis*) affects the pharmacodynamics but not the pharmokinetics of warfarin in rabbits. Eur J Drug Metab Pharmacokinet. 1995;20:55-60.

80. Huupponen R, Seppala P, Iisalo E. Effect of guar gum, a fibre preparation, on digoxin and penicillin absorption in man. Eur J Clin Pharmacol. 1984;26:279-81.

81. Gray A, Flatt P. Insulin-releasing and insulin-like activity of the traditional anti-diabetic plant *Coriandrum sativum* (coriander). Br J Nutr. 1999;81:203-9.

82. Gray A, Flatt P. Actions of the traditional anti-diabetic plant, *Agrimony eupatoria* (agrimony): effects on hyperglycaemia, cellular glucose metabolism and insulin secretion. Br J Nutr. 1998;80:109-14.

83. Leatherdale B, Panesar R, Singh G, Atkins T, Bailey C, Bignell A. Improvement in glucose tolerance due to *Momordica charantia* (Karela). Br Med J. 1981;282:1823-4.

84. Pizzioli A, Tikhonoff V, Palearì C, Russo E, Mazza A, Ginocchio G, Onesto C, Pavan L, Casiglia E, Pessina A. Effects of caffeine on glucose tolerance: a placebo-controlled study. Eur J Clin Nutr. 1998;52:846-9.

85. Kim BR, Kim DH, Park R, et al. Effect of an extract of the root of *Scutellaria baicalensis* and its flavonoids on aflatoxin B1 oxidizing cytochrome P450 enzymes. Planta Med 2001 Jul;67(5):396-9.

86. Gin H, Orgerie G, Aubertin J. The influence of guar gum on absorption of metformin from the gut in healthy volunteers. Hormone Metabolism. 1989;21:81-83.

87. Konig G, Wright A, Keller W, Judd R, Bates S, Day C. Hypoglycaemic activity of an HMG-containing flavonoid gluco-side. chamaemeloside. from *Chamaemelum nobile*. Planta Med. 1998;64:612-4.

88. Perez R, Ocegueda A, Munoz J, Avila J, Morrow W. A study of the hypoglycemic effect of some Mexican plants. J Ethnopharmacol. 1984;12:253-62.

89. Nishioka T, Kawabata J, Aoyama Y. Baicalein, an alpha-glucosidase inhibitor from *Scutellaria baicalensis*. J Nat Prod 1998 Nov;61(11):1413-5.

90. Razina TG, Udintsev SN, Prishchep TP, Iaremenko KV. [Enhancement of the selectivity of the action of the cytostatics cyclophosphane and 5-fluorouracil by using an extract of the Baikal skullcap in an experiment.] Vopr Onkol 1987;33(2):80-4.

91. DeSmet P, Keller K, Hansel R, Chandler R, eds. *Adverse Effects of Herbal Drugs.* Vol. 1. NY:Springer-Verlag, 1992.

92. DeSmet P, Keller K, Hansel R, Chandler R, eds. *Adverse Effects of Herbal Drugs.* Vol. 2. NY:Springer-Verlag, 1993.

93. DeSmet P, Keller K, Hansel R, Chandler R, eds. *Adverse Effects of Herbal Drugs.* Vol. 3. NY:Springer-Verlag, 1997.

94. Chen S, Hwang J, Deng PS. Inhibition of NAD(P)H:quinone acceptor oxidoreductase by flavones: a structure-activity study. Arch Biochem Biophys 1993 Apr;302(1):72-7.

95. Karunanayake E, Welihinda J, Sirimanne S, Sinnadorai G. Oral hypoglycaemic activity of some medicinal plants of Sri Lanka. J Ethnopharmacol. 1984;11:223-31.

96. Preuss H, Jarrell S, Scheckenbach R, Lieberman S, Anderson R. Comparative effects of chromium, vanadium and *Gymnema sylvestre* on sugar-induced blood pressure elevations in SHR. J Am Coll Nutr. 1998;17:116-23.

97. Hui KM, Wang XH, Xue H. Interaction of flavones from the roots of *Scutellaria baicalensis* with the benzodiazepine site. Planta Med 2000 Feb;66(1):91-3.

98. Taussig S, Batkin S. Bromelain, the enzyme complex of pineapple (*Ananas comosus*) and its clinical application. An update. J Ethnopharmacol. 1988;22:191-203.

99. D'arcy P. Adverse reactions and interactions with herbal medicines. Part 1. Adverse reactions. Adverse Drug React Toxicol Rev. 1991;10:189-208.

100. Chiu FC, Watson TR. Conformational factors in cardiac glycoside activity. J Med Chem 1985 Apr;28(4):509-15.

101. Sawyer DR, Conner CS, Rumack BH. Managing acute toxicity from nonprescription stimulants. Clin Pharm 1982 Nov-Dec;1(6):529-33.

102. Lee KJ, You HJ, Park SJ, et al. Hepatoprotective effects of *Platycodon grandiflorum* on acetaminophen-induced liver damage in mice. Cancer Lett 2001 Dec 10;174(1):73-81

103. Baker GB, Wong JT, Coutts RT, Pasutto FM. Simultaneous extraction and quantitation of several bioactive amines in cheese and chocolate. J Chromatogr 1987 Apr 17;392:317-31.

104. D'Arcy P. Adverse reactions and interactions with herbal medicines. Part 2. Drug interactions. Adverse Drug React Toxicol Rev. 1993;12:147-62.

105. Atta-Ur-Rahman, Khurshid Z. Medicinal plants with hypoglycemic activity. J Ethnopharmacol. *1989*;26:1-55.

106. Goel RK, Gupta S, Shankar R, Sanyal AK. Anti-ulcerogenic effect of banana powder (*Musa sapientum* var. *paradisiaca*) and its effect on mucosal resistance. J Ethnopharmacol 1986 Oct;18(1):33-44.

107. Day C. Traditional plant treatments for diabetes mellitus: pharmaceutical foods. Br J Nutr. 1998;80:5-6..

108. Pari L, Umamaheswari J. Antihyperglycaemic activity of *Musa sapientum* flowers: effect on lipid peroxidation in alloxan diabetic rats. Phytother Res 2000 Mar;14(2):136-8

109. Dawson JK, Earnshaw SM, Graham CS. Dangerous monoamine oxidase inhibitor interactions are still occurring in the 1990s. J Accid Emerg Med 1995 Mar;12(1):49-51.

110. Skogh M. Correspondence. Extracts of *Ginkgo biloba* and bleeding or haemorrhage. Lancet. 1998;352:1145-6.

111. Babu P, Srinivasan K. Influence of dietary capsaicin and onion on the metabolic abnormalities associated with streptozotocin induced diabetes mellitus. Mol Cell Biochem. 1997;175:49-57.

112. DeVries J. *Food Safety and Toxicity*. NewYork:Open University of the Netherlands. 1997.

113. Longwood Herbal Taskforce. In-depth Monograph (echinacea). http://www.mcp.edu/herbal/echinacea/echinacea.pdf

114. De Smet P. Health risks of herbal remedies. Drug Saf. 1995;13:81-93.

115. Emery EA, Ahmad S, Koethe JD, et al. Banana flakes control diarrhea in enterally fed patients. Nutr Clin Pract 1997 Apr;12(2):72-5.

116. World Health Organization. *WHO Monographs on Selected Medicinal Plants. Vol 1*. Geneva: World Health

117. Newall C, Anderson L, Phillipson J. *Herbal Medicines A Guide for Health-Care Professionals*. London: Pharmaceutical Press, 1996.

118. Grainger Bisset N, ed. *Herbal Drugs and Phytopharmaceuticals*. London: CRC Press and Stuttgart: Medpharm, 1994.

119. Geetha BS, Mathew BC, Augusti KT. Hypoglycemic effects of leucodelphinidin derivative isolated from *Ficus bengalensis* (Linn). Indian J Physiol Pharmacol 1994 Jul;38(3):220-2.

120. Augusti KT. Hypoglycaemic action of bengalenoside, a glucoside isolated from *Ficus bengalensis* Linn, in normal and alloxan diabetic rabbits. Indian J Physiol Pharmacol 1975 Oct-Dec;19(4):218-20.

121. Janbaz KH, Gilani AH. Studies on preventive and curative effects of berberine on chemical-induced hepatotoxicity in rodents. Fitoterapia 2000 Feb;71(1):25-33.

122. Olmez E, Ilhan M. Evaluation of the alpha-adrenoceptor antagonistic action of berberine in isolated organs. Arzneimittelforschung 1992 Sep;42(9):1095-7.

123. Ko WH, Yao XQ, Lau CW, et al. Vasorelaxant and antiproliferative effects of berberine. Eur J Pharmacol 2000 Jul 7;399(2-3):187-96.

124. Lin HL, Liu TY, Lui WY, Chi CW. Up-regulation of multidrug resistance transporter expression by berberine in human and murine hepatoma cells. Cancer 1999 May 1;85(9):1937-42.

125. Khin-Maung-U, Myo-Khin, Nyunt-Nyunt-Wai, Tin-U. Clinical trial of high-dose berberine and tetracycline in cholera. J Diarrhoeal Dis Res 1987 Sep;5(3):184-7.

126. Sheng WD, Jiddawi MS, Hong XQ, Abdulla SM. Treatment of chloroquine-resistant malaria using pyrimethamine in combination with berberine, tetracycline or cotrimoxazole. East Afr Med J 1997 May;74(5):283-4.

127. Inbaraj JJ, Kukielczak BM, Bilski P, Sandvik SL, Chignell CF. Photochemistry and phototoxicity of alkaloids from Goldenseal (Hydrastis canadensis L.) 1. Berberine. Chem Res Toxicol 2001 Nov;14(11):1529-34.

128. Xu X, Malave A. Protective effect of berberine on cyclophosphamide-induced haemorrhagic cystitis in rats. Pharmacol Toxicol 2001 May;88(5):232-7.

129. Shanbhag SM, Kulkarni HJ, Gaitonde BB. Pharmacological actions of berberine on the central nervous system. Jpn J Pharmacol 1970 Dec;20(4):482-7.

130. Lau CW, Yao XQ, Chen ZY, Ko WH, Huang Y. Cardiovascular actions of berberine. Cardiovasc Drug Rev 2001 Autumn;19(3):234-44.

131. Chan E. Displacement of bilirubin from albumin by berberine. Biol Neonate 1993;63(4):201-8.

132. Lin HL, Liu TY, Wu CW, Chi CW. Berberine modulates expression of mdr1 gene product and the responses of digestive tract cancer cells to Paclitaxel. Br J Cancer 1999 Oct;81(3):416-22.

133. Xuan B, Wang W, Li DX. Inhibitory effect of tetrahydroberberine on platelet aggregation and thrombosis. Zhongguo Yao Li Xue Bao 1994 Mar;15(2):133-5.

134. Kong LD, Cheng CH, Tan RX. Monoamine oxidase inhibitors from rhizoma of *Coptis chinensis*. Planta Med 2001 Feb;67(1):74-6.

135. Abdel-Haq H, Cometa MF, Palmery M, Leone MG, Silvestrini B, Saso L. Relaxant effects of *Hydrastis canadensis* L. and its major alkaloids on guinea pig isolated trachea. Pharmacol Toxicol 2000 Nov;87(5):218-22.

136. Singh A, Handa SS. Hepatoprotective activity of *Apium graveolens* and *Hygrophila auriculata* against paracetamol and thioacetamide intoxication in rats. J Ethnopharmacol 1995 Dec 15;49(3):119-26.

137. Shukla K, Narain JP, Puri P, et al. Glycaemic response to maize, bajra and barley. Indian J Physiol Pharmacol 1991 Oct;35(4):249-54.

138. Hapke HJ, Strathmann W. [Pharmacological effects of hordenine.] Dtsch Tierarztl Wochenschr 1995 Jun;102(6):228-32. Abstract.

139. Afifi FU, Khalil E, Tamimi SO, Disi A. Evaluation of the gastroprotective effect of *Laurus nobilis* seeds on ethanol induced gastric ulcer in rats. J Ethnopharmacol 1997 Sep;58(1):9-14.

140. Shader RI, Greenblatt DJ. Uses and toxicity of belladonna alkaloids and synthetic anticholinergics. Semin Psychiatry 1971 Nov;3(4):449-76.

141. Deahl M. Betel nut-induced extrapyramidal syndrome: an unusual drug interaction. Mov Disord 1989;4(4):330-2

142. Panda S, Kar A. Dual role of betel leaf extract on thyroid function in male mice. Pharmacol Res 1998 Dec;38(6):493-6.

143. Seeram NP, Momin RA, Nair MG, Bourquin LD. Cyclooxygenase inhibitory and antioxidant cyanidin glycosides in cherries and berries. Phytomedicine 2001 Sep;8(5):362-9.

144. Cignarella A, Nastasi M, Cavalli E, Puglisi L. Novel lipid-lowering properties of *Vaccinium myrtillus* L. leaves, a traditional antidiabetic treatment, in several models of rat dyslipidaemia: a comparison with ciprofibrate. Thromb Res 1996 Dec 1;84(5):311-22.

145. Ahmad N, Hassan MR, Halder H, Bennoor KS. Effect of *Momordica charantia* (Karolla) extracts on fasting and **312**

postprandial serum glucose levels in NIDDM patients. Bangladesh Med Res Counc Bull 1999 Apr;25(1):11-3.

146. Penzak SR, Jann MW, Cold JA, et al. Seville (sour) orange juice: synephrine content and cardiovascular effects in normotensive adults. J Clin Pharmacol 2001 Oct;41(10):1059-63.

147. Malhotra S, Bailey DG, Paine MF, Watkins PB. Seville orange juice-felodipine interaction: comparison with dilute grapefruit juice and involvement of furocoumarins. Clin Pharmacol Ther 2001 Jan;69(1):14-23.

148. Kockmann V, Spielmann D, Traitler H, Lagarde M. Inhibitory effect of stearidonic acid (18:4 n-3) on platelet aggregation and arachidonate oxygenation. Lipids 1989 Dec;24(12):1004-7.

149. Atal C, Dubey R, Singh J. Biochemical basis of enhanced drug bioavailability by piperine: evidence that piperine is a potent inhibitor of drug metabolism. J Pharmacol Exp Ther. 1985;232:258-62.

150. Hedman A, Meijer DK. Stereoselective inhibition by the diastereomers quinidine and quinine of uptake of cardiac glycosides into isolated rat hepatocytes. J Pharm Sci 1998 Apr;87(4):457-61.

151. Atal CK, Dubey RK, Singh J. Biochemical basis of enhanced drug bioavailability by piperine: evidence that piperine is a potent inhibitor of drug metabolism. J Pharmacol Exp Ther 1985 Jan;232(1):258-62.

152. Kang MH, Won SM, Park SS, et al. Piperine effects on the expression of P4502E1, P4502B and P4501A in rat. Xenobiotica 1994 Dec;24(12):1195-204.

153. Bai YF, Xu H. Protective action of piperine against experimental gastric ulcer. Acta Pharmacol Sin 2000 Apr;21(4):357-9.

154. Bano G, Raina RK, Zutshi U, Raina V, et al. Effect of piperine on bioavailability and pharmacokinetics of propranolol and theophylline in healthy volunteers. Eur J Clin Pharmacol 1991;41(6):615-7.

155. Bano G, Amla V, Raina RK, Zutshi U, Chopra CL. The effect of piperine on pharmacokinetics of phenytoin in healthy volunteers. Planta Med 1987 Dec;53(6):568-9.

156. Page R, Lawrence J. Potentiation of warfarin by dong quai. Pharmacotherapy. 1999;19:870-6.

157. Badmaev V V, Majeed M, Prakash L. Piperine derived from black pepper increases the plasma levels of coenzyme q10 following oral supplementation. J Nutr Biochem. 2000 Feb 1;11(2):109-113.

158. Mujumdar AM, Dhuley JN, Deshmukh VK, et al. Effect of piperine on pentobarbitone induced hypnosis in rats. Indian J Exp Biol 1990 May;28(5):486-7.

159. El-Dakhakhny M, Barakat M, Aly SM. Effects of Nigella sativa oil on gastric secretion and ethanol induced ulcer in rats. J Ethnopharmacol 2000 Sep;72(1-2):299-304.

160. Nair SC, Salomi MJ, Panikkar B, Panikkar KR. Modulatory effects of *Crocus sativus* and *Nigella sativa* extracts on cisplatin-induced toxicity in mice. J Ethnopharmacol 1991 Jan;31(1):75-83.

161. el Tahir KE, Ashour MM, al-Harbi MM. The cardiovascular actions of the volatile oil of the black seed (*Nigella sativa*) in rats: elucidation of the mechanism of action. Gen Pharmacol 1993 Sep;24(5):1123-31.

162. Ivorra M, Paya M, Villar A. A review of natural products and plants as potential antidiabetic drugs. J Ethnopharmocol. 1989;27:243-75.

163. Lasswell W, Weber S, Wilkins J. In vitro interactions of neuroleptics and tricyclic antidepressants with coffee, tea, and gallotannic acid. J Pharm Sci. 1984;73:1056-8.

164. Enomoto S, Asano R, Iwahori Y, et al. Hematological studies on black cumin oil from the seeds of *Nigella sativa* L. Biol Pharm Bull 2001 Mar;24(3):307-10.

165. Alonso R, Cadavid I, Calleja JM. A preliminary study of hypoglycemic activity of *Rubus fruticosus*. Planta Med 1980;Suppl:102-6.

166. Rao R, Hoffman R, Desiderio R, et al. Nicotinic toxicity from tincture of blue cohosh (*Caulophyllum thalictroides*) used as an abortifacient. Journal of Toxicology Clinical Toxicology. 1998;36(5): 455. Meeting Info.: Annual Meeting of the North American Congress of Clinical Toxicology Orlando, Florida, USA September 9-15, 1998.

167. Clinical trial of fenugreek for cholesterol and blood sugar levels of non-insulin-dependent diabetics. Herbalgram. 1997;41:18.

168. American Herbal Pharmocopoeia and Therapeutic Compendium. St. John's wort *hypericum perforatum* monograph. Herbalgram. 1997;40:27.

169. Kayahara H, Miao Z, Fujiwara G. Synthesis and biological activities of ferulic acid derivatives. Anticancer Res 1999 Sep-Oct;19(5A):3763-8.

170. Shukia B, Khanna NK, Godhwani JL. Effect of Brahmi Rasayan on the central nervous system. J Ethnopharmacol 1987 Sep-Oct;21(1):65-74..

171. Vats V, Grover JK, Rathi SS. Evaluation of anti-hyperglycemic and hypoglycemic effect of *Trigonella foenum-graecum* Linn, *Ocimum sanctum* Linn and *Pterocarpus marsupium* Linn in normal and alloxanized diabetic rats. J Ethnopharmacol 2002 Feb;79(1):95-100.

172. Pronsky Z. *Food Medication Interactions*. 12th ed. Birchrunville, Pa: Food-Medication Interactions, 2002.

173. Bailey C, Day C. Traditional plant medicines as treatments for diabetes. Diabetes Care. 1989;12:553-64.

174. United States Food and Drug Administration. CFR21- parts 182, 184 and 186.

175. Blumenthal M, Goldberg A, Brinckmann J, eds. *Herbal Medicine: Expanded Commission E Monographs.* Newton, MA: Integrative Medicine Communications, 2000.
http://www.access.gpo.gov/nara/cfr/waisidx_01/21cfrv3_01.html

176. Rovenska E, Svik K, Stancikova M, Rovensky J. Inhibitory effect of enzyme therapy and combination therapy with cyclosporin A on collagen-induced arthritis. Clin Exp Rheumatol 2001 May-Jun;19(3):303-9.

177. Metzig C, Grabowska A, Eckert K, Rehse K, Maurer HR. Bromelain proteases reduce human platelet aggregation in vitro, adhesion to bovine endothelial cells and thrombus formation in rat vessels in vivo. In Vivo 1999 Jan-Feb;13(1):7-12.

178. Food and Drug Administration. Supplements associated with illnesses and injuries. FDA Consumer. Sept - Oct 1998.

179. Ruschitzka F, Meier P, Turina M, Luscher T, Noll G. Acute heart transplant rejection due to Saint John's wort. Lancet. 2000;355:548-9.

180. Piscitelli S, Burstein A, Chaitt D, Alfaro R, Falloon J. Indinavir concentrations and St. John's wort. Lancet. 2000;355:547-548.

181. Ernst E. Second thoughts about safety of St. John's wort. Lancet. 1999;354:2014-6.

182. Aufmkolk M, Ingbar JC, Kubota K, Amir SM, Ingbar SH. Extracts and auto-oxidized constituents of certain plants inhibit the receptor-binding and the biological activity of Graves' immunoglobulins. Endocrinology 1985 May;116(5):1687-93.

183. Aufmkolk M, Kohrle J, Gumbinger H, Winterhoff H, Hesch RD. Antihormonal effects of plant extracts: iodothyronine deiodinase of rat liver is inhibited by extracts and secondary metabolites of plants. Horm Metab Res 1984 Apr;16(4):188-92.

184. Lin SC, Chung TC, Chung CC, et al. Hepatoprotective effects of *Arctium lappa* on carbon tetrachloride- and acetamino-phen-induced liver damage. Am J Chin Med 2000;28(2):163-73.

185. Miller VM, Rud KS, Gloviczki P. Pharmacological assessment of adrenergic receptors in human varicose veins. Int Angiol 2000 Jun;19(2):176-83.

186. Corina P, Dimitris S, Emanuil T, Nora R. [Treatment with acyclovir combined with a new Romanian product from plants]. Oftalmologia 1999;46(1):55-7. Abstract.

187. Iatsyno AI, Belova LF, Lipkina GS, et al. [Pharmacology of calenduloside B, a new triterpene glycoside from the roots

of Calendula officinalis]. Farmakol Toksikol 1978 Sep-Oct;41(5):556-60.

188. Yoshikawa M, Murakami T, Kishi A, et al. Medicinal flowers. III. Marigold. (1): hypoglycemic, gastric emptying inhibitory, and gastroprotective principles and new oleanane-type triterpene oligoglycosides, calendasaponins A, B, C, and D, from Egyptian *Calendula officinalis*. Chem Pharm Bull (Tokyo) 2001 Jul;49(7):863-70.

189. Brahmi. The Review of Natural Products. Jan 2000;1-2.

190. Rolland A, Fleurentin J, Lanhers MC, Misslin R, Mortier F. Neurophysiological effects of an extract of *Eschscholzia californica* Cham. (Papaveraceae). Phytother Res 2001 Aug;15(5):377-81.

191. Rolland A, Fleurentin J, Lanhers MC, et al. Behavioural effects of the American traditional plant *Eschscholzia californica*: sedative and anxiolytic properties. Planta Med 1991 Jun;57(3):212-6.

192. Chattopadhyay R. A comparative evaluation of some blood sugar lowering agents of plant origin. J Ethnopharmocol. 1999;67:367-72.

193. Yokozawa T, Nakagawa T, Lee K, Cho E, Terasawa K, Takeuchi S. Effects of green tea tannin on cisplatin-induced nephropathy in LLC_PK$_1$ cells and rats. J Pharm Pharmacol. 1999;51:1325-31.

194. Panda S, Kar A. *Withania somnifera* and *Bauhinia purpurea* in the regulation of circulating thyroid hormone concentrations in female mice. J Ethnopharmocol. 1999;67:233-9.

195. Lantz M, Buchalter E, Giambanco V. St. John's wort and antidepressant drug interactions in the elderly. J Geriatr Psychiatry Neurol. 1999;12:7-10.

196. Lee F, Ko J, Park J, Lee J. Effects of *Panax Ginseng* on blood alcohol clearance in man. Clin Exp Pharmacol Physiol. 1987;14:543-6.

197. Rolland A, Fleurentin J, Lanhers MC, et al. Behavioural effects of the American traditional plant *Eschscholzia californica*: sedative and anxiolytic properties. Planta Med 1991 Jun;57(3):212-6.

198. Johne A, Brockmoller J, Bauer S, Maurer A, Langheinrich M, Roots I. Pharmacokinetic interaction of digoxin with an herbal extract from St. John's wort (*Hypericum perforatum*). Clin Pharmacol Ther. 1999;66:338-45.

199. Kamtchouing P, Sokeng SD, Moundipa PF, et al. Protective role of *Anacardium occidentale* extract against streptozotocin-induced diabetes in rats. J Ethnopharmacol 1998 Sep;62(2):95-9.

200. Ammon HV, Thomas PJ, Phillips SF. Effects of oleic and ricinoleic acids on net jejunal water and electrolyte movement. Perfusion studies in man. J Clin Invest 1974 Feb;53(2):374-9.

201. Harney JW, Barofsky IM, Leary JD. Behavioral and toxicological studies of cyclopentanoid monoterpenes from *Nepeta cataria.* Lloydia 1978 Jul-Aug;41(4):367-74.

202. Sandoval-Chacon M, Thompson JH, Zhang XJ, et al. Antiinflammatory actions of cat's claw: the role of NF-kappaB. Aliment Pharmacol Ther 1998 Dec;12(12):1279-89.

203. Riva L, Coradini D, Di Fronzo G, et al. The antiproliferative effects of *Uncaria tomentosa* extracts and fractions on the growth of breast cancer cell line. Anticancer Res 2001 Jul-Aug;21(4A):2457-61.

204. Sheng Y, Pero RW, Wagner H. Treatment of chemotherapy-induced leukopenia in a rat model with aqueous extract from *Uncaria tomentosa.* Phytomedicine 2000 Apr;7(2):137-43

205. Lam Y. St. John's wort may decrease efficacy of digoxin. Psychopharmacology Update 1999;10:2-3.

206. Endo K, Oshima Y, Kikuchi H, Koshihara Y, Hikino H. Hypotensive principles of *Uncaria* hooks. Planta Med 1983 Nov;49(3):188-90.

207. Markowitz J, DeVane C, Boulton D, Carson S, Nahas Z, Risch S. Effect of St. John's wort (*Hypericum perforatum*) on cytochrome P-450 2D6 and 3A4 activity in healthy volunteers. Life Sci. 2000;21:PL133-9.

208. Aisaka K, Hattori Y, Kihara T, et al. Hypotensive action of 3 alpha-dihydrocadambine, an indole alkaloid glycoside of *Uncaria* hooks. Planta Med 1985 Oct;(5):424-7.

209. Cheng JT, Liu IM, Yen ST, et al. Stimulatory effect of D-ephedrine on beta3-adrenoceptors in adipose tissue of rats. Auton Neurosci 2001 Apr 12;88(1-2):1-5.

210. Fowler J, Wang G, Volkow N, et al. Evidence that *Ginkgo biloba* extract does not inhibit MAO A and B in living human brain. Life Sci. 2000;66:PL141-6.

211. Homma M, Oka K, Ikeshima K, Takahashi N, Niitsuma T, Fukuda T, Itoh H. Different effects of traditional Chinese medicines containing similar herbal constituents on prednisolone pharmacokinetics. J Pharm pharmacol. 1995;47:687-92.

212. Heck AM, DeWitt BA, Lukes AL. Potential interactions between alternative therapies and warfarin. Am J Health Syst Pharm. 2000 Jul 1;57(13):1221-7.

213. Lamm S, Sheng Y, Pero RW. Persistent response to pneumococcal vaccine in individuals supplemented with a novel water soluble extract of *Uncaria tomentosa*, C-Med-100. Phytomedicine 2001 Jul;8(4):267-74.

214. Tolan I, Ragoobirsingh D, Morrison EY. The effect of capsaicin on blood glucose, plasma insulin levels and insulin binding in dog models. Phytother Res 2001 Aug;15(5):391-4.

215. Park JS, Choi MA, Kim BS, et al. Capsaicin protects against ethanol-induced oxidative injury in the gastric mucosa of

rats. Life Sci 2000 Nov 10;67(25):3087-93.

216. Duda RB, Zhong Y, Navas V, Li MZ, Toy BR, Alavarez JG. American ginseng and breast cancer therapeutic agents synergistically inhibit MCF-7 breast cancer cell growth. J Surg Oncol. 1999 Dec;72(4):230-9.

217. Lombaert GA, Siemens KH, Pellaers P, Mankotia M, Ng W. Furanocoumarins in celery and parsnips: method and multiyear Canadian survey. J AOAC Int 2001 Jul-Aug;84(4):1135-43.

218. Gral N, Beani JC, Bonnot D, et al. [Plasma levels of psoralens after celery ingestion]. Ann Dermatol Venereol 1993;120(9):599-603. Abstract.

219. Singh A, Handa SS. Hepatoprotective activity of *Apium graveolens* and *Hygrophila auriculata* against paracetamol and thioacetamide intoxication in rats. J Ethnopharmacol 1995 Dec 15;49(3):119-26.

220. Noldner M, Chatterjee S. Inhibition of haloperidol-induced catalepsy in rats by root extracts from *Piper methysticum* F. Phytomedicine. 1999;6(4):285-286.

221. Teng CM, Ko FN, Wang JP, et al. Antihaemostatic and antithrombotic effect of some antiplatelet agents isolated from Chinese herbs. J Pharm Pharmacol 1991 Sep;43(9):667-9.

222. Sherman D, Fish D. Management of protease inhibitor-associated diarrhea. Clin Infect Dis. 2000 Jun;30(6):908-14. Review.

223. Kenny F, Pinder S, Ellis I, Gee J, Nicholson R, Bryce R, Robertson J. Gamma linolenic acid with tamoxifen as primary therapy in breast cancer. Int J Cancer 2000 Mar 1;85(5):643-8.

224. Montesinos M, Yap J, Desai A, Posadas I, McCrary C, Cronstein B. Reversal of the antiinflammatory effects of methotrexate by the nonselective adenosine receptor antagonists theophylline and caffeine: evidence that the antiinflammatory effects of methotrexate are mediated via multiple adenosine receptors in rat adjuvant arthritis. Arthritis Rheum 2000 Mar;43(3):656-63.

225. Awang D. Siberian ginseng toxicity may be case of mistaken identity. CMAJ 1996 Nov 1;155(9):1237.

226. Blumenthal M. Interactions between herbs and conventional drugs: introductory considerations. Selected herb-drug interactions. Herbalgram. 2000 49:52-63.

227. Budzinski J, Foster B, Vandenhoek S. An in vitro evaluation of human cytochrome P450 3A4 inhibition by selected commercial herbal extracts and tinctures. Phytomedicine. 2000;7(4):273-82.

228. Badary O, Abdel-Naim A, Abdel-Wahab M, Hamada F. The influence of thymoquinone on doxorubicin-induced hyperlipidemic nephropathy in rats. Toxicology. 2000;143:219-26.

318

229. Babu U, Mitchell G, Wiesenfeld P, Jenkins M, Gowda H. Nutritional and hematological impact of dietary flaxseed and defatted flaxseed meal in rats. Int J Food Sci Nutr. 2000;51: 109-17.

230. Schechter J. Treatment of disequilibrium and nausea in the SRI discontinuation syndrome. J Clin Psychiatry. 1998;59:531-2.

231. Galluzzi S, Zanetti O, Binetti G, Trabucchi M, Frisoni G. Coma in a patient with Alzheimer's disease taking low dose trazodone and gingko biloba. J Neurol Neurosurg Psychiatry. 2000;68:679-80.

232. Beckmann-Knopp S, Rietbrock S, Weyhenmeyer R, et al. Inhibitory effects of silibinin on cytochrome P-450 enzymes in microsomes. Pharmacol Toxicol. 2000;86:250-6.

233. Zhu M, Wong P, Li R. Effects of Taraxacum mongolicum on the bioavailability and disposition of ciprofloxacin in rats. J Pharm Sci. 1999;88:632-4.

234. Guivernau M, Meza N, Barja P, Roman O. Clinical and experimental study on the long-term effect of dietary gamma-linolenic acid on plasma lipids, platelet aggregation, thromboxane formation, and prostacyclin production. Prostaglandins leukot Essent Fatty Acids. 1994;51:311-6.

235. Datta P, Dasgupta A. Interactions between drugs and Asian medicine: displacement of digitoxin form protein binding site by bufalin, the constituent of Chinese medicines Chan Su and Lu-Shen-Wan. Ther Drug Monit. 2000;22:155-9.

236. Bolkent S, Yanardag R, Tabakçglu-Oguz A, et al. Effect of chard (Beta Vulgaris L. var. Cicla) extract on pancreatic B cells in streptozotocin-diabetic rats: a morphological and biochemical study. J Ethnopharmacol. 2000;73:251-259.

237. Ishihara K, Kushida H, Yuzurihara M, et al. Interaction of drugs and Chinese herbs: pharmacokinetic changes of tolbutamide and diazepam caused by extract of Angelica dahurica. Pharm Pharmacol. 2000;52:1023-9.

238. Fidler P, Loprinzi C, O'Fallon J, et al. Prospective evaluation of a chamomile mouthwash for prevention of 5-FU-induced oral mucositis. Cancer. 1996;77:522-5.

239. Carl W, Emrich L. Management of oral mucositis during local radiation and systemic chemotherapy: a study of 98 patients. J prosthet Dent. 1991;66:361-9.

240. Moon C, Jung Y, Kim M, et al. Mechanism for antiplatelet effect of onion: AA release inhibition, thromboxane A2 synthase inhibition and TXA2/PGH2 receptor blockade. Prostaglandins Leukot Essent Fatty Acids. 2000 May;62:277-83.

241. Dalvi S, Nayak V, Pohujani S, et al. Effect of gugulipid on bioavailability of diltizem and propranolol. J Assoc Physicians India. 1994;42:454-5.

242. Cherif S, Rahal N, Haouala M, et al. A clinical trial of a titrated of Olea extract in the treatment of essential arterial

hypertension. J Pharm Belg. 1996;51:69-71.

243. Tripathi Y, Malhotra O, Tripathi S. Thyroid stimulating action of Z-guggulsterone obtained from *Commiphora Mukul*. Planta Med. 1984;1:78-80.

244. Lee S, Rhee H. Cardiovascular effects of mycelium extract of *Ganoderma lucidum*: inhibition of sympathetic outflow as a mechanism of its hypotensive action. Chem Pharm Bull (Tokyo). 1990;38:1359-64.

245. Davis L, Kuttan G. Effect of *Withania somnifera* on cyclophosphamide-induced urotoxicity. Cancer Lett 2000 Jan 1;148(1):9-17.

246. Carai MA, Agabio R, Bombardelli E, et al. Potential use of medicinal plants in the treatment of alcoholism. Fitoterapia 2000 Aug;71 Suppl 1:S38-S42.

247. Burdette j, liu J, lantvit D. *Trifolium pratense* (Red Clover) exhibits estrogenic effects in vivo in ovariectomized Sprage-Dawley rats. J Nutr 2002;132:27-30.

248. Vuksan V, Sievenpiper JL, Wong J, et al. American ginseng (Panax quinquefolius L.) attenuates postprandial glycemia in a time-dependent but not dose-dependent manner in healthy individuals. Am J Clin Nutr 2001 Apr;73(4):753-8.

249. Vuksan V, Stavro MP, Sievenpiper JL, Beljan-Zdravkovic U, Leiter LA, Josse RG, Xu Z. Similar postprandial glycemic reductions with escalation of dose and administration time of American ginseng in type 2 diabetes. Diabetes Care 2000 Sep;23(9):1221-6.

250. Barwell CJ, Basma AN, Lafi MA, Leake LD. Deamination of hordenine by monoamine oxidase and its action on vasa deferentia of the rat. J Pharm Pharmacol 1989 Jun;41(6):421-3.

251. Beckmann-Knopp S, Rietbrock S, Weyhenmeyer R, Bocker RH, Beckurts KT, Lang W, Hunz M, Fuhr U. Inhibitory effects of silibinin on cytochrome P-450 enzymes in human liver microsomes. Pharmacol Toxicol. 2000 Jun;86(6):250-6.

252. Norred CL, Finlayson CA. Hemorrhage after the preoperative use of complementary and alternative medicines. AANA J. 2000 Jun;68(3):217-20.

253. Uehara M, Sugiura H, Sakurai K. A trial of oolong tea in the management of recalcitrant atopic dermatitis. Arch Dermatol. 2001;137:42-43.

254. Steuer-Vogt MK, Bonkowsky V, Ambrosch P, et al. The effect of an adjuvant mistletoe treatment programme in resected head and neck cancer patients. a randomised controlled clinical trial. Eur J Cancer. 2001 Jan;37(1):23-31.

255. Aybar MJ, Sanchez Riera AN, Grau A, et al. Hypoglycemic effect of the water extract of *Smallantus sonchifolius* (yacon) leaves in normal and diabetic rats. J Ethnopharmacol. 2001;74:125-132.

256. Kameswara Rao B, Giri R, Kesavulu MM, et al. Effect of oral administration of bark extracts of *Pterocarpus santalinus* L. on blood glucose level in experimental animals. J Ethnopharmacol. 2001;74:69-74. **321**

257. Sitasawad SL, Shewade Y, Bhonde R, et al. Role of bittergourd fruit juice in stz-induced diabetic state in vivo and in vitro. J Ethnopharmacol. 2000;73:71-9.

258. Alarcon-Aguilar FJ, Jimenez-Estrada M, Reyes-Chilpa R, et al. Hypoglycemic effect of extracts and fractions from *Psacalium decompositum* in healthy and alloxan-diabetic mice. J Ethnopharmacol. 2000;72:21-7.

259. Patel NM, Nozaki S, Shortle NH. Paclitaxel sensitivity of breast cancer cells with constitutively active NF-KB is enhanced by KBa super-repressor and parthenolide. Oncogene. 2000;19:4159-69.

260. Piscitelli SC, Burstein AH, Welden N, Gallicano KD, Falloon J. The Effect of Garlic Supplements on the Pharmacokinetics of Saquinavir. Clin Infect Dis 2002 Jan 15;34(2):234-238.

261. Guerra MC, Speroni E, Broccoli M, et al. Comparison between Chinese medical herb *Pueraria lobata* crude extract and its main isoflavone puerarin antioxidant properties and effects on rat liver CYP-catalysed drug metabolism. Life Sci. 2000 Nov 3;67(24):2997-3006.

262. De-Oliveira AC, Ribeiro-Pinto LF, Otto SS, et al. Induction of liver monooxygenases by β-myrcene. Toxicology. 1997 Dec 26;124(2):135-40.

263. Zhu M, Chan KW, Ng LS, et al. Possible influences of ginseng on the pharmacokinetics and pharmacodynamics of warfarin in rats. J Pharm Pharmacol. 1999 Feb;51(2):175-80.

264. Kudolo GB. The effect of 3-month ingestion of *Ginkgo biloba* extract on pancreatic beta-cell function in response to glucose loading in normal glucose tolerant individuals. J Clin Pharmacol. 2000 Jun;40(6):647-54.

265. Rovenska E, Svik K, Stancikova M, et al. Enzyme and combination therapy with cyclosporin A in the rat developing adjuvant arthritis. Int J Tissue React. 1999;21(4):105-11.

266. Henderson MC, Miranda CL, Stevens JF, et al. In vitro inhibition of human P450 enzymes by prenylated flavonoids from hops, *Humulus lupulus*. Xenobiotica. 2000 Mar;30(3):235-51.

267. Shon JH, Park JY, Kim KA, et al. Effect of licorice (*Radix Glycyrrhizae*) on the pharmacokinetics (PK) and pharmaco-dynamics (PD) of midazolam in healthy subjects. 2001 Annual Meeting of the American Society for Clinical Pharmacology and Therapeutics. Orlando, Florida, USA. March 6-10, 2001. Clin Pharmacol Ther 2001 Feb;69(2):P78 [abstract PIII-58].

268. Samman S, Sandstrom B, Toft MB, et al. Green tea or rosemary extract added to foods reduces nonheme-iron absorption. Am J Clin Nutr. 2001 Mar;73(3):607-12.

269. Hurrell RF, Reddy M, Cook JD. Inhibition of non-haem iron absorption in man by polyphenolic-containing beverages. Br J Nutr. 1999 Apr;81(4):289-95.

270. Wang EJ, Li Y, Lin M, et al. Protective effects of garlic and related organosulfur compounds on acetaminophen-induced hepatotoxicity in mice. Toxicol Appl Pharmacol. 1996 Jan;136(1):146-54.

271. Assalian P. Sildenafil for St. John's Wort-induced sexual dysfunction. J Sex Marital Ther. 2000 Oct-Dec;26(4):357-8.

272. Zhang XY, Zhou DF, Su JM, et al. The effect of extract of ginkgo biloba added to haloperidol on superoxide dismutase in inpatients with chronic schizophrenia. J Clin Psychopharmacol. 2001 Feb;21(1):85-8.

273. Fessenden JM, Wittenborn W, Clarke L. Gingko biloba: a case report of herbalmedicine and bleeding postoperatively from a laparoscopic cholecystectomy. Am Surg. 2001 Jan;67(1):33-5.

274. Taper HS, Roberfroid MB. Nontoxic potentiation of cancer chemotherapy by dietary oligofructose or inulin. Nutr Cancer. 2000;38(1):1-5.

275. Moses, G. Thyroxine interacts with celery seed tablets? Australian Prescriber. 2001;24(1):6-7.

276. Davis L, Kuttan G. Effect of Withania somnifera on cytokine production in normal and cyclophosphamide treated mice. Immunopharmacol Immunotoxicol. 1999 Nov;21(4):695-703.

277. Cheng JT, Yang RS. Hypoglycemic effect of guava juice in mice and human subjects. Am J Chin Med. 1983;11(1-4):74-6.

278. Smith M, Lin K, Zheng Y, et al. An open trial of nifedipine-herb interactions: nifedipine with St. John's wort, ginseng or ginkgo biloba. 2001 Annual Meeting of the American Society for Clinical Pharmacology and Therapeutics. Orlando, Florida, USA. March 6-10, 2001. Clin Pharmacol Ther. 2001 Feb;69(2):Abstract PIII-89.

279. Olajide OA, Awe SO, Makinde JM, et al. Evaluation of the anti-diabetic property of Morinda lucida leaves in streptozotocin-diabetic rats. J Pharm Pharmacol. 1999 Nov;51(11):1321-4.

280. Panda S, Kar A. How safe is neem extract with respect to thyroid function in male mice? Pharmacol Res. 2000 Apr;41(4):419-22.

281. Capasso A, Saturnino P, Simone FD, et al. Flavonol glycosides from Aristeguietia discolor reduce morphine withdrawal in vitro. Phytother Res. 2000 Nov;14(7):538-40.

282. Yoon YR, Kim MJ, Shin MS, et al. Screening of in vitro inhibitory effects of 15 herbal medicines on CYP3A4-catalyzed midazolam hydroxylation. 2001 Annual Meeting of the American Society for Clinical Pharmacology and Therapeutics. Orlando, Florida, USA. March 6-10, 2001. Clin Pharmacol Ther. 2001 Feb;69(2):Abstract PIII-97.

283. Park HJ, Kim DH, Choi JW, et al. A potent anti-diabetic agent from Kalopanax pictus. Arch Pharm Res. 1998 Feb;21(1):24-9.

284. Lee SE, Oh H, Yang JA, et al. Radioprotective effects of two traditional Chinese medicine prescriptions: si-wu-tang and si-jun-zi-tang. Am J Chin Med. 1999;27(3-4):387-96.

285. Yuzurihara M, Ikarashi Y, Ishihara K, et al. Effects of subacutely administered saiboku-to, an oriental herbal medicine, on pharmacodynamics and pharmacokinetics of diazepam in rodents. Eur J Drug Metab Pharmacokinet. 2000 Apr-Jun;25(2):127-36.

286. Ramelet AA, Buchheim G, Lorenz P, et al. Homeopathic Arnica in postoperative haematomas: a double-blind study. Dermatology. 2000;201(4):347-8.

287. Okyar A, Can A, Akev N, et al. Effect of Aloe vera leaves on blood glucose level in type I and type II diabetic rat models. Phytother Res. 2001 Mar;15(2):157-61.

288. Lewis DA, Shaw GP. A natural flavonoid and synthetic analogues protect the gastric mucosa from aspirin-induced erosions. J Nutr Biochem. 2001 Feb;12(2):95-100.

289. Kubinova R, Machala M, Minksova K, et al. Chemoprotective activity of boldine: modulation of drug-metabolizing enzymes. Pharmazie. 2001 Mar;56(3):242-3.

290. Lambert JP, Cormier A. Potential interaction between warfarin and boldo-fenugreek. Pharmacotherapy. 2001 Apr;21(4):509-12.

291. Amason JT, Assinewe V, Leiter LA, et al. Chinese ginseng (Panax ginseng C.A. Meyer) within a low dose range does not affect postprandial glycemia in subjects with normal glucose tolerance. FASEB Experimental Biology Meeting. Orlando, Florida, March 31-April 4, 2001. Brd. No. B423.

292. Fujita H, Yamagami T, Ohshima K. Fermented soybean-derived water-soluble Touchi extract inhibits alpha-glucosidase and is antiglycemic in rats and humans after single oral treatments. J Nutr. 2001 Apr:131(4):1211-3.

293. Arya SC. Controlling angiotensin-converting-enzyme-inhibitor induced cough by fennel fruit. Indian Journal of Pharmacology. 1999;31(2):1999.

294. Shetty R, Kumar KV, Naidu MU, et al. Effect of Ginkgo biloba extract on ethanol-induced gastric mucosal lesions in rats. Indian Journal of Pharmacology. 2000;32(5):313-7.

295. Ray SD, Kumar MA, Bagchi D. A novel proanthocyanidin IH636 grape seedextract increases in vivo Bcl-XL expression and prevents acetaminophen-induced programmed and unprogrammed cell death in mouse liver. Arch Biochem

Biophys. 1999 Sep 1;369(1):42-58.

296. Hagg S, Spigset O, Mjorndal T, Dahlqvist R. Effect of caffeine on clozapine pharmacokinetics in healthy volunteers. Br J Clin Pharmacol. 2000 Jan;49(1):59-63.

297. Shen F, Xue X, Weber G. Tamoxifen and genistein synergistically down-regulate signal transduction and proliferation in estrogen receptor-negative human breast carcinoma MDA-MB-435 cells. Anticancer Res. 1999 May-Jun;19(3A):1657-62.

298. Bopanna K, Kannan L, Gadgil, et al. Antidiabetic and antihyperlipaemic effects of neem seed kernal powder on alloxan diabetic rabbits. Indian Journal of Pharmacology. 1997;29:162-167.

299. Hayakawa-Fujii Y, Iida H, Dohi S. Propofol anesthesia enhances pressor response to ephedrine in patients given clonidine. Anesth Analg 1999 Jul;89(1):37-41.

300. Debersac P, Vernevaut MF, Amiot MJ, et al. Effects of a water-soluble extract of rosemary and its purified component rosmarinic acid on xenobiotic-metabolizing enzymes in rat liver. Food Chem Toxicol. 2001 Feb;39(2):109-17.

301. Benwahhoud M, Jouad H, Eddouks M, et al. Hypoglycemic effect of in streptozotocin-induced diabetic rats. J Ethnopharmacol. 2001 Jun;76(1):35-8.

302. Kim M, Shin HK. The water-soluble extract of chicory reduces glucose uptake from the perfused jejunum in rats. J Nutr. 1996 Sep;126(9):2236-42.

303. Nishimura N, Naora K, Hirano H, et al. Effects of Sho-saiko-to on the pharmacokinetics and pharmacodynamics of tolbutamide in rats. J Pharm Pharmacol. 1998 Feb;50(2):231-6.

304. Vikrant V, Grover JK, Tandon N, et al. Treatment with extracts of *Momordica charantia* and *Eugenia jambolana* prevents hyperglycemia and hyperinsulinemia in fructose fed rats. J Ethnopharmacol. 2001 Jul;76(2):139-43.

305. Callaway JC, Grob CS. Ayahuasca preparations and serotonin reuptake inhibitors: a potential combination for severe adverse interactions. J Psychoactive Drugs. 1998 Oct-Dec;30(4):367-9.

306. Scambia G, De Vincenzo R, Ranelletti FO, et al. Antiproliferative effect of silybin on gynaecological malignancies: synergism with cisplatin and doxorubicin. Eur J Cancer. 1996 May;32A(5):877-82.

307. Ang-Lee MK, Moss J, Yuan CS. Herbal medicines and perioperative care. JAMA. 2001 Jul 11;286(2):208-16.

308. Caltagirone S, Ranelletti FO, Rinelli A, et al. Interaction with type II estrogen binding sites and antiproliferative activity of tamoxifen and quercetin in human non-small-cell lung cancer. Am J Respir Cell Mol Biol. 1997 Jul;17(1):51-9.

309. Grover JK, Vats V, Rathi SS. Anti-hyperglycemic effect of *Eugenia jambolana* and *Tinospora cordifolia* in experimental diabetes and their effects on key metabolic enzymes involved in carbohydrate metabolism. J Ethnopharmacol. 2000 Dec;73(3):461-70.

310. Dhuley J. Protective effect of Rhinax, a herbal formulation against physical and chemical gastric induced duodenal ulcers in rats. Indian Journal of Pharmacoology. 1999;31:128-32.

311. Saraswathy V, Suji V, Gurumurthy P, et al. Effect of LIV.100 against antitubercular drugs (isoniazid, rifampicin and pyrazinamide) induced hepatotoxicity in rats. Indian Journal of Pharmacoology. 1998;30:233-238.

312. Karan R, Bhargava V, Garg S. Effect of trikatu (piperine) on the pharmacokinetic profile of isoniazid in rabbits. Indian Journal of Pharmacology. 1998;30:254-256.

313. Mallkajal S, Wanwimolruk S. Effect of herbal teas on hepatic drug metabolizing enzymes in rats. J Pharm Pharmacol 2001 Oct;53(10):1323-9

314. Devi Priya S, Shyamala Devi C. Protective effect of quercetin in cisplatin - induced cell injury in the rat kidney. Indian Journal of Pharmacology. 1999;31:422-426.

315. Scaglione F, Cattaneo G, Alessandria M, et al. Efficacy and safety of the standardised Ginseng extract G115 for potentiating vaccination against the influenza syndrome and protection against the common cold. Drugs Exp Clin Res. 1996;22(2):65-72.

316. Lin RC, Li TK. Effects of isoflavones on alcohol pharmacokinetics and alcohol-drinking behavior in rats. Am J Clin Nutr. 1998 Dec;68(6 Suppl):1512S-1515S.

317. Avallone R, Zanoli P, Puia G, et al. Pharmacological profile of apigenin, a flavonoid isolated from Matricaria chamomilla. Biochem Pharmacol 2000 Jun 1;59(11):1387-94.

318. Sun GY, Xia J, Xu J, et al. Dietary supplementation of grape polyphenols to rats ameliorates chronic ethanol-induced changes in hepatic morphology without altering changes in hepatic lipids. J Nutr. 1999 Oct;129(10):1814-9.

319. Keung WM, Lazo O, Kunze L, et al. Potentiation of the bioavailability of daidzin by an extract of Radix puerariae. Proc Natl Acad Sci U S A. 1996 Apr 30;93(9):4284-8.

320. Gyamfi MA, Hokama N, Oppong-Boachie K, et al. Inhibitory effects of the medicinal herb, Thonningia sanguinea, on liver drug metabolizing enzymes of rats. Hum Exp Toxicol. 2000 Nov;19(11):623-31.

321. Yamada T, Hoshino M, Hayakawa T, et al. Dietary diosgenin attenuates subacute intestinal inflammation associated with indomethacin in rats. Am J Physiol. 1997 Aug;273(2 Pt 1):G355-64.

325

322. Duke J. Plants containing diosgenin. Dr. Dukes Phytochemical and Ethnobotanical Databases.

323. Torrado S, Torrado S, Agis A, Jimenez ME, Cadorniga R. Effect of dissolution profile and (-)-alpha-bisabolol on the gastrotoxicity of acetylsalicylic acid. Pharmazie 1995 Feb;50(2):141-3

324. Jayasooriya AP, Sakono M, Yukizaki C, et al. Effects of *Momordica charantia* powder on serum glucose levels and various lipid parameters in rats fed with cholesterol-free and cholesterol-enriched diets. J Ethnopharmacol. 2000 Sep;72(1-2):331-6.

325. Smith TJ, Yang CS. Effect of organosulfur compounds from garlic and cruciferous vegetables on drug metabolism enzymes. Drug Metabol Drug Interact. 2000;17(1-4):23-49.

326. Viola H, Wasowski C, Levi de Stein M, et al. Apigenin, a component of *Matricaria recutita* flowers, is a central benzodiazepine receptors-ligand with anxiolytic effects. Planta Med 1995 Jun;61(3):213-6.

327. Suleyman H, Emin Buyukokuroglu M, Koruk M, et al. The effects of *Hippophae rhamnoides L.* Indian Journal of Pharmacology. 2001;33:77-81.

328. Briggs WH, Xiao H, Parkin KL, et al. Differential inhibition of human platelet aggregation by selected Allium thiosulfinates. J Agric Food Chem. 2000 Nov;48(11):5731-5.

329. Skim F, Lazrek HB, Kaaya A, et al. Pharmacological studies of two antidiabetic plants: *Globularia alypum* and *Zygophyllum gaetulum*. Therapie. 1999 Nov-Dec;54(6):711-5.

330. Chen HW, Yang JJ, Tsai CW, et al. Dietary fat and garlic oil independently regulate hepatic cytochrome p(450) 2B1 and the placental form of glutathione S-transferase expression in rats. J Nutr. 2001 May;131(5):1438-43.

331. Wang J, Xu R, Jin R, et al. Immunosuppressive activity of the Chinese medicinal plant *Tripterygium wilfordii*. II. Prolongation of hamster-to-rat cardiac xenograft survival by combination therapy with the PG27 extract and cyclosporine. Transplantation. 2000 Aug 15;70(3):456-64.

332. Duffy SJ, Vita JA, Holbrook M, et al. Effect of acute and chronic tea consumption on platelet aggregation in patients with coronary artery disease. Arterioscler Thromb Vasc Biol. 2001 Jun;21(6):1084-9.

333. Meckes-Lozoya M, Roman-Ramos R. *Opuntia streptacantha*: a coadjutor in the treatment of diabetes mellitus. Am J Chin Med. 1986;14(3-4):116-8.

334. Bargossi AM, Grossi G, Fiorella PL, et al. Exogenous CoQ10 supplementation prevents plasma ubiquinone reduction induced by HMG-CoA reductase inhibitors. Mol Aspects Med 1994;15 Suppl:s187-93.

335. Fernando MR, Wickramasinghe N, Thabrew MI, et al. A preliminary investigation of the possible hypoglycaemic activity of *Asteracanthus longifolia*. J Ethnopharmacol. 1989 Nov;27(1-2):7-14.

336. Freedman JE, Parker C 3rd, Li L, et al. Select flavonoids and whole juice from purple grapes inhibit platelet function and enhance nitric oxide release. Circulation. 2001 Jun 12;103(23):2792-8.

337. Menendez JA, del Mar Barbacid M, Montero S, et al. Effects of gamma-linolenic acid and oleic acid on paclitaxel cytotoxicity in human breast cancer cells. Eur J Cancer. 2001 Feb;37(3):402-13.

338. Liu F, Ng TB. Antioxidative and free radical scavenging activities of selected medicinal herbs. Life Sci. 2000 Jan 14;66(8):725-35.

339. Kavvadias D, Abou-Mandour AA, Czygan FC, et al. Identification of benzodiazepines in *Artemisia dracunculus* and *Solanum tuberosum* rationalizing their endogenous formation in plant tissue. Biochem Biophys Res Commun. 2000 Mar 5;269(1):290-5.

340. Cheng JH. [Clinical study on prevention and treatment to chemotherapy caused nephrotoxicity with jian-pi yi-qi li-shui Decoction]. [Article in Chinese] Zhongguo Zhong Xi Yi Jie He Za Zhi.. 1994 Jun;14(6):331-3, 323. Abstract.

341. Cheng JH. [Effect of preventive and therapeutical function of jian-pi yi-qi li-shui decoction on cisplatin nephrotoxicity in rats]. [Article in Chinese] Zhongguo Zhong Xi Yi Jie He Za Zhi.. 1992 Oct;12(10):614-6, 581-2. Abstract.

342. Yang D, Lee J, Lee K, et al. Effect of Leuca-F-a herbal concentrated granules on the white blood cells and platelets during chemotherapy. 2000 AAPS Annual meeting. October 29 – November 2, 2000. Abstract.

343. Luccia B, Kunkel M. Assessment of calcium bioavailability from psyllium. FASEB Experimental Biology Meeting. March 31 – April 4, 2001. Abstract B258.

344. Kudolo G. Ingestion of *Ginkgo biloba* extract significantly inhibits collagen – induced platelet aggregation and thromboxane A_2 synthesis. An International Conference on Complementary, Alternative, and Integrative Medicine Research. Alternative Therapies. 2001;7(3):105. Abstract.

345. Gundling K, Brodsky Z, Robbins J, et al. *Panax ginseng* enhances IGM and IGA antibody titers after influenza vaccination. An International Conference on Complementary, Alternative, and Integrative Medicine Research. Alternative Therapies. 2001;7(3):104. Abstract.

346. Duke J. Plants containing quercetin. Dr. Dukes Phytochemical and Ethnobotanical Databases.

347 . Hauns B, Haring B, Kohler S, et al. Phase II study of combined 5-fluorouracil/ Ginkgo biloba extract (GBE 761 ONC) therapy in 5-fluorouracil pretreated patients with advanced colorectal cancer. Phytother Res. 2001 Feb;15(1):34-8.

348. Joshi SS, Kuszynski CA, Benner EJ, et al. Amelioration of the cytotoxic effects of chemotherapeutic agents by grape seed proanthocyanidin extract. Antioxid Redox. Signal 1999 Winter;1(4):563-70.

349. Naidu MU, Shifow AA, Kumar KV, et al. Ginkgo biloba extract ameliorates gentamicin-induced nephrotoxicity in rats. Phytomedicine. 2000 Jun;7(3):191-7.

350. Duke J. Plants containing caffeine. Dr. Dukes Phytochemical and Ethnobotanical Databases.

351. Jeong TC, Gu HK, Chun YJ, et al. Effects of beta-ionone on the expression of cytochrome P450s and NADPH-cytochrome P450 reductase in Sprague Dawley rats. Chem Biol Interact 1998 Jul 3;114(1-2):97-107.

352. Hakas JF Jr. Topical capsaicin induces cough in patient receiving ACE inhibitor. Ann Allergy 1990 Oct;65(4):322-3.

353. Tsuchiya H. Biphasic membrane effects of capsaicin, an active component in *Capsicum* species. J Ethnopharmacol 2001 May;75(2-3):295-9.

354. Jancso-Gabor A. Anaesthesia-like condition and/or potentiation of hexobarbital sleep produced by pungent agents in normal and capsaicin-desensitized rats. Acta Physiol Acad Sci Hung 1980;55(1):57-62.

355. Yeoh KG, Kang JY, Yap I, et al. Chili protects against aspirin-induced gastroduodenal mucosal injury in humans. Dig Dis Sci 1995 Mar;40(3):580-3.

356. Cruz L, Castaneda-Hernandez G, Navarrete A. Ingestion of chilli pepper (*Capsicum annuum*) reduces salicylate bioavailability after oral asprin administration in the rat. Can J Physiol Pharmacol 1999 Jun;77(6):441-6.

357. Kim KM, Kawada T, Ishihara K, et al. Increase in swimming endurance capacity of mice by capsaicin-induced adrenal catecholamine secretion. Biosci Biotechnol Biochem 1997 Oct;61(10):1718-23.

358. Miller MS, Brendel K, Burks TF, Sipes IG. Interaction of capsaicinoids with drug-metabolizing systems. Relationship to toxicity. Biochem Pharmacol 1983 Feb 1;32(3):547-51.

359. Miller CH, Zhang Z, Hamilton SM, Teel RW. Effects of capsaicin on liver microsomal metabolism of the tobacco-specific nitrosamine NNK. Cancer Lett 1993 Nov 30;75(1):45-52.

360. Zhang Z, Hamilton SM, Stewart C, Strother A, Teel RW. Inhibition of liver microsomal cytochrome P450 activity and metabolism of the tobacco-specific nitrosamine NNK by capsaicin and ellagic acid. Anticancer Res 1993 Nov-Dec;13(6A):2341-6.

361. Norred CL, Brinker F. Potential coagulation effects of preoperative complementary and alternative medicines. Altern Ther Health Med 2001 Nov-Dec;7(6):58-67.

362. Stickel F, Egerer G, Seitz HK. Hepatotoxicity of botanicals. Public Health Nutr 2000 Jun;3(2):113-24.

328

363. Sliutz G, Speiser P, Schultz AM, Spona J, Zeillinger R. *Agnus castus* extracts inhibit prolactin secretion of rat pituitary cells. Horm Metab Res 1993 May;25(5):253-5.

329

364. Jarry H, Leonhardt S, Gorkow C, Wuttke W. In vitro prolactin but not LH and FSH release is inhibited by compounds in extracts of *Agnus castus*: direct evidence for a dopaminergic principle by the dopamine receptor assay. Exp Clin Endocrinol 1994;102(6):448-54.

365. Liu J, Burdette JE, Xu H, et al. Evaluation of estrogenic activity of plant extracts for the potential treatment of menopausal symptoms. J Agric Food Chem 2001 May;49(5):2472-9.

366. Tanaka S, Yoon YH, Fukui H, et al. Antiulcerogenic compounds isolated from Chinese cinnamon. Planta Med 1989 Jun;55(3):245-8.

367. Choi J, Lee KT, Ka H, et al. Constituents of the essential oil of the *Cinnamomum cassia* stem bark and the biological properties. Arch Pharm Res 2001 Oct;24(5):418-23.

368. Gallaher CM, Munion J, Hesslink R Jr, Wise J, Gallaher DD. Cholesterol reduction by glucomannan and chitosan is mediated by changes in cholesterol absorption and bile acid and fat excretion in rats. J Nutr 2000 Nov;130(11):2753-9.

369. Mazieres B, Combe B, Phan Van A, Tondut J, Grynfeltt M. Chondroitin sulfate in osteoarthritis of the knee: a prospective, double blind, placebo controlled multicenter clinical study. J Rheumatol 2001 Jan;28(1):173-81.

370. Leeb BF, Schweitzer H, Montag K, Smolen JS. A metaanalysis of chondroitin sulfate in the treatment of osteoarthritis. J Rheumatol 2000 Jan;27(1):205-11.

371. Embriano PJ. Postoperative pressures after phacoemulsification: sodium hyaluronate vs. sodium chondroitin sulfate-sodium hyaluronate. Ann Ophthalmol 1989 Mar;21(3):85-8, 90.

372. Bangchang KN, Karbwang J, Back DJ. Mefloquine metabolism by human liver microsomes. Effect of other antimalarial drugs. Biochem Pharmacol 1992 May 8;43(9):1957-61.

373. Shah BH, Nawaz Z, Virani SS, et al. The inhibitory effect of cinchonine on human platelet aggregation due to blockade of calcium influx. Biochem Pharmacol 1998 Oct 15;56(8):955-60.

374. Kambam JR, Franks JJ, Naukam R, Sastry BV. Effect of quinidine on plasma cholinesterase activity and succinylcholine neuromuscular blockade. Anesthesiology 1987 Nov;67(5):858-60.

375. Pedersen KE, Lysgaard Madsen J, et al. Effect of quinine on plasma digoxin concentration and renal digoxin clearance. Acta Med Scand 1985;218(2):229-32.

376. Srivastava KC. Antiplatelet principles from a food spice clove (*Syzygium aromaticum* L). Prostaglandins Leukot

Essent Fatty Acids 1993 May;48(5):363-72.

377. Kumar GP, Sudheesh S, Vijayalakshmi NR. Hypoglycaemic effect of *Coccinia indica*: mechanism of action. Planta Med 1993 Aug;59(4):330-2.

378. Rein D, Paglieroni TG, Wun T, et al. Cocoa inhibits platelet activation and function. Am J Clin Nutr 2000 Jul;72(1):30-5.

379. Spigset O. Reduced effect of warfarin caused by ubidecarenone. Lancet 1994 Nov 12;344(8933):1372-3.

380. Barbieri B, Lund B, Lundstrom B, Scaglione F. Coenzyme Q10 administration increases antibody titer in hepatitis B vaccinated volunteers—a single blind placebo-controlled and randomized clinical study. Biofactors 1999;9(2-4):351-7.

381. Ohhara H, Kanaide H, Nakamura M. A protective effect of coenzyme Q10 on the adriamycin-induced cardiotoxicity in the isolated perfused rat heart. J Mol Cell Cardiol 1981 Aug;13(8):741-52.

382. Singh RB, Niaz MA, Rastogi SS, Shukla PK, Thakur AS. Effect of hydrosoluble coenzyme Q10 on blood pressures and insulin resistance in hypertensive patients with coronary artery disease. J Hum Hypertens 1999 Mar;13(3):203-8.

383. Langsjoen H, Langsjoen P, Langsjoen P, Willis R, Folkers K. Usefulness of coenzyme Q10 in clinical cardiology: a long-term study. Mol Aspects Med 1994;15 Suppl:s165-75.

384. Bleske BE, Willis RA, Anthony M, et al. The effect of pravastatin and atorvastatin on coenzyme Q10. Am Heart J 2001 Aug;142(2):E2.

385. Ghirlanda G, Oradei A, Manto A, et al. Evidence of plasma CoQ10-lowering effect by HMG-CoA reductase inhibitors: a double-blind, placebo-controlled study. J Clin Pharmacol 1993 Mar;33(3):226-9.

386. Mortensen SA, Leth A, Agner E, Rohde M. Dose-related decrease of serum coenzyme Q10 during treatment with HMG-CoA reductase inhibitors. Mol Aspects Med 1997;18 Suppl:S137-44.

387. Landbo C, Almdal TP. [Interaction between warfarin and coenzyme Q10.] Ugeskr Laeger 1998 May 25;160(22):3226-7. Abstract.

388. Zhou S, T, Watanabe T, Folkers K. Bioenergetics in clinical medicine XV. Inhibition of coenzyme Q10-enzymes by clinically used adrenergic blockers of beta-receptors. Res Commun Chem Pathol Pharmacol 1977 May;17(1):157-64.

389. Kishi T, Walanabe T, Folkers K. Bioenergetics in clinical medicine XV. Imhibition of coenzyme Q10-enzymes by clinially used adrenergic blockers of beta-receptors. Res Commun Chem Pathol Pharmacol. 1977 May;17(1):157-64.

390. Valls V, Castelluccio C, Fato R, et al. Protective effect of exogenous coenzyme Q against damage by adriamycin in perfused rat liver. Biochem Mol Biol Int 1994 Jul;33(4):633-42.

391. Adachi K, Fujiwara Y, Mayumi F, et al. A deletion of mitochondrial DNA in murine doxorubicin-induced cardiotoxi-city. Biochem Biophys Res Commun 1993 Sep 15;195(2):945-51.

392. Iarussi D, Auricchio U, Agretto A, et al. Protective effect of coenzyme Q10 on anthracyclines cardiotoxicity: control study in children with acute lymphoblastic leukemia and non-Hodgkin lymphoma. Mol Aspects Med 1994;15 Suppl:S207-12.

393. Iqbal N, Ahmad B, Janbaz KH, Gilani AU, Niazi SK. The effect of caffeine on the pharmacokinetics of acetaminophen in man. Biopharm Drug Dispos 1995 Aug;16(6):481-7.

394. Strubelt O, Diederich KW. Experimental treatment of the acute cardiovascular toxicity of caffeine. J Toxicol Clin Toxicol 1999;37(1):29-33.

395. Agarwal KC, Zielinski BA, Maitra RS. Significance of plasma adenosine in the antiplatelet activity of forskolin: potentiation by dipyridamole and dilazepam. Thromb Haemost 1989 Feb 28;61(1):106-10.

396. Ahmad F, Khan MM, Rastogi AK, Kidwai JR. Insulin and glucagon releasing activity of coleonol (forskolin) and its effect on blood glucose level in normal and alloxan diabetic rats. Acta Diabetol Lat 1991 Jan-Mar;28(1):71-7.

397. Hirono I, Mori H, Culvenor CC. Carcinogenic activity of coltsfoot, *Tussilago farfara* l. Gann 1976 Feb;67(1):125-9.

398. Li YP, Wang YM. Evaluation of tussilagone: a cardiovascular-respiratory stimulant isolated from Chinese herbal medicine. Gen Pharmacol 1988;19(2):261-3.

399. Culvenor CC, Clarke M, Edgar JA, et al. Structure and toxicity of the alkaloids of Russian comfrey (*Symphytum x uplandicum Nyman*), a medicinal herb and item of human diet. Experientia 1980 Apr 15;36(4):377-9.

400. Hikino H, Yoshizawa M, Suzuki Y, Oshima Y, Konno C. Isolation and hypoglycemic activity of trichosans A, B, C, D, and E: glycans of *Trichosanthes kirilowii* roots. Planta Med 1989 Aug;55(4):349-50.

401. Swanston-Flatt SK, Day C, Bailey CJ, Flatt PR. Traditional plant treatments for diabetes. Studies in normal and streptozotocin diabetic mice. Diabetologia 1990 Aug;33(8):462-4.

402. Saltzman JR, Kemp JA, Golner BB, et al. Effect of hypochlorhydria due to omeprazole treatment or atrophic gastritis on protein-bound vitamin B12 absorption. J Am Coll Nutr 1994 Dec;13(6):584-91.

403. Vandenberghe K, Gillis N, Van Leemputte M, et al. Caffeine counteracts the ergogenic action of muscle creatine loading. J Appl Physiol 1996 Feb;80(2):452-7.

404. Dutt MK, Moody P, Northfield TC. Effect of cimetidine on renal function in man. Br J Clin Pharmacol 1981 Jul;12(1):47-50.

405. Lampe JW, King IB, Li S, et al. *Brassica* vegetables increase and apiaceous vegetables decrease cytochrome P450 1A2 activity in humans: changes in caffeine metabolite ratios in response to controlled vegetable diets. Carcinogenesis 2000 Jun;21(6):1157-62.

406. Couris RR, Tataronis GR, Booth SL, et al. Development of a self-assessment instrument to determine daily intake and variability of dietary vitamin K. J Am Coll Nutr 2000 Nov-Dec;19(6):801-7.

407. Srivastava KC. Extracts from two frequently consumed spices—cumin (*Cuminum cyminum*) and turmeric (*Curcuma longa*)—inhibit platelet aggregation and alter eicosanoid biosynthesis in human blood platelets. Prostaglandins Leukot Essent Fatty Acids 1989 Jul;37(1):57-64.

408. Chan TY. Interaction between warfarin and danshen (*Salvia miltiorrhiza*). Ann Pharmacother 2001 Apr;35(4):501-4.

409. Wahed A, Dasgupta A. Positive and negative in vitro interference of Chinese medicine dan shen in serum digoxin measurement. Elimination of interference by monitoring free digoxin concentration. Am J Clin Pathol 2001 Sep;116(3):403-8.

410. Neef H, Cilli F, Declerck P, Laekeman G. Platelet anti-aggregating activity of *Taraxacum officinale* Weber. Phytotherapy Research. 1996;10(suppl 1): S138-S140.

411. Racz-Kotilla E, Racz G, Solomon A. The action of *Taraxacum officinale* extracts on the body weight and diuresis of laboratory animals. Planta Med 1974 Nov;26(3):212-7.

412. Liapina LA, Koval'chuk GA. [A comparative study of the action on the hemostatic system of extracts from the flowers and seeds of the meadowsweet (*Filipendula ulmaria* (L.) Maxim.)]. Izv Akad Nauk Ser Biol 1993 Jul-Aug;(4):625-8. Abstract.

413. Circosta C, Occhiuto F, Ragusa S, et al. A drug used in traditional medicine: *Harpagophytum procumbens* DC. II. Cardiovascular activity. J Ethnopharmacol 1984 Aug;11(3):259-74.

414. Costa De Pasquale R, Busa G, Circosta C, et al. A drug used in traditional medicine: *Harpagophytum procumbens* DC. III. Effects on hyperkinetic ventricular arrhythmias by reperfusion. J Ethnopharmacol 1985 May;13(2):193-9.

415. Rosenberg Zand RS, Jenkins DJ, Diamandis EP. Effects of natural products and nutraceuticals on steroid hormone-regulated gene expression. Clin Chim Acta 2001 Oct;312(1-2):213-9.

416. Page RL 2nd, Lawrence JD. Potentiation of warfarin by dong quai. Pharmacotherapy 1999 Jul;19(7):870-6.

417. Ellis G, Stephens M. Minerva. BMJ 1999;319:650.

418. Wang H, Peng RX. [Sodium ferulate alleviated paracetamol-induced liver toxicity in mice.] Zhongguo Yao Li

Xue Bao 1994 Jan;15(1):81-3. Abstract.

419. Lersch C, Zeuner M, Bauer A, et al. Stimulation of the immune response in outpatients with hepatocellular carcinomas by low doses of cyclophosphamide (LDCY), *Echinacea purpurea* extracts (Echinacin) and thymostimulin. Arch Geschwulstforsch 1990;60(5):379-83.

420. Lersch C, Zeuner M, Bauer A, et al. Nonspecific immunostimulation with low doses of cyclophosphamide (LDCY), thymostimulin, and *Echinacea purpurea* extracts (echinacin) in patients with far advanced colorectal cancers: preliminary results. Cancer Invest 1992;10(5):343-8.

421. Gray AM, Abdel-Wahab YH, Flatt PR. The traditional plant treatment, *Sambucus nigra* (elder), exhibits insulin-like and insulin-releasing actions in vitro. J Nutr 2000 Jan;130(1):15-20.

422. Knoll Pharmaceutical Company. Meridia Healthcare Professional. Meridia can help your patients. http://www.4meridia.com/hcprof/fin.htm

423. Kuntzman RG, Tsai I, Brand L, Mark LC. The influence of urinary pH on the plasma half-life of pseudoephedrine in man and dog and a sensitive assay for its determination in human plasma. Clin Pharmacol Ther 1971 Jan-Feb;12(1):62-7.

424. Young R, Glennon RA. Discriminative stimulus properties of (-)-ephedrine. Pharmacol Biochem Behav 1998 Jul;60(3):771-5.

425. Boada S, Solsona B, Papaceit J, Saludes J, Rull M. [Hypotension refractory to ephedrine after sympathetic blockade in a patient on long-term therapy with tricyclic antidepressants]. Rev Esp Anestesiol Reanim 1999 Oct;46(8):364-6.

426. Jubiz W, Meikle AW. Alterations of glucocorticoid actions by other drugs and disease states. Drugs 1979 Aug;18(2):113-21.

427. Reeves RR, Pinkofsky HB. Postpartum psychosis induced by bromocriptine and pseudoephedrine. J Fam Pract 1997 Aug;45(2):164-6.

428. Dingemanse J, Guentert T, Gieschke R, Stabl M. Modification of the cardiovascular effects of ephedrine by the reversible monoamine oxidase A-inhibitor moclobemide. J Cardiovasc Pharmacol 1996 Dec;28(6):856-61.

429. Renfrew C, Dickson R, Schwab C. Severe hypertension following ephedrine administration in a patient receiving entacapone. Anesthesiology 2000 Dec;93(6):1562.

430. Hendershot PE, Antal EJ, Welshman IR, Batts DH, Hopkins NK. Linezolid: pharmacokinetic and pharmacodynamic evaluation of coadministration with pseudoephedrine HCl, phenylpropanolamine HCl, and dextromethorphan HBr. J Clin Pharmacol 2001 May;41(5):563-72.

431. Pederson KJ, Kuntz DH, Garbe GJ. Acute myocardial ischemia associated with ingestion of bupropion and pseudoephedrine in a 21-year-old man. Can J Cardiol 2001 May;17(5):599-601.

432. Brooks SM, Sholiton LJ, Werk EE Jr, Altenau P. The effects of ephedrine and theophylline on dexamethasone metabolism in bronchial asthma. J Clin Pharmacol 1977 May-Jun;17(5-6):308-18.

433. Tekol Y, Tercan E, Esmaoglu A. Ephedrine enhances analgesic effect of morphine. Acta Anaesthesiol Scand 1994 May;38(4):396-7.

434. Kockler D, McCarthy W, Lawson C. Seizure activity and unresponsiveness after hydroxycut ingestion. 2001;21(5):647-51

435. Wilson BE, Hobbs WN. Case report: pseudoephedrine-associated thyroid storm: thyroid hormone-catecholamine interactions. Am J Med Sci 1993 Nov;306(5):317-9.

436. De-Oliveira AC, Fidalgo-Neto AA, Paumgartten FJ. In vitro inhibition of liver monooxygenases by beta-ionone, 1,8-cineole, (-)-menthol and terpineol. Toxicology 1999 Jul 1;135(1):33-41.

437. Abdul-Ghani AS, Amin R. The vascular action of aqueous extracts of *Foeniculum vulgare* leaves. J Ethnopharmacol 1988 Dec;24(2-3):213-8.

438. Zhu M, Wong PY, Li RC. Effect of oral administration of fennel (*Foeniculum vulgare*) on ciprofloxacin absorption and disposition in the rat. J Pharm Pharmacol 1999 Dec;51(12):1391-6.

439. El Bardai S, Lyoussi B, Wibo M, Morel N. Eadie Pharmacological evidence of hypotensive activity of *Marrubium vulgare* and *Foeniculum vulgare* in spontaneously hypertensive rat. Clin Exp Hypertens 2001 May;23(4):329-43.

440. Sowmya P, Rajyalakshmi P. Hypocholesterolemic effect of germinated fenugreek seeds in human subjects. Plant Foods Hum Nutr 1999;53(4):359-65.

441. Abdel-Barry JA, Abdel-Hassan IA, Jawad AM, al-Hakiem MH. Hypoglycaemic effect of aqueous extract of the leaves of *Trigonella foenum-graecum* in healthy volunteers. East Mediterr Health J 2000 Jan;6(1):83-8.

442. Groenewegen WA, Heptinstall S. A comparison of the effects of an extract of feverfew and parthenolide, a component of feverfew, on human platelet activity in-vitro. J Pharm Pharmacol 1990 Aug;42(8):553-7.

443. Hutchins AM, Martini MC, Olson BA, Thomas W, Slavin JL. Flaxseed consumption influences endogenous hormone concentrations in postmenopausal women. Nutr Cancer 2001;39(1):58-65.

444. Cunnane SC, Ganguli S, Menard C, et al. High alpha-linolenic acid flaxseed (*Linum usitatissimum*): some nutritional properties in humans. Br J Nutr 1993 Mar;69(2):443-53.

445 Nordstrom DC, Honkanen VE, Nasu Y, et al. Alpha-linolenic acid in the treatment of rheumatoid arthritis. A double-blind, placebo-controlled and randomized study: flaxseed vs. safflower seed. Rheumatol Int 1995;14(6):231-4.

446 Allman MA, Pena MM, Pang D. Supplementation with flaxseed oil versus sunflower seed oil in healthy young men consuming a low fat diet: effects on platelet composition and function. Eur J Clin Nutr 1995 Mar;49(3):169-78.

447 Dec GW, Jenike MA, Stern TA. Trazodone-digoxin interaction in an animal model. J Clin Psychopharmacol 1984 Jun;4(3):153-5.

448 Dockens RC, Greene DS, Barbhaiya RH. Assessment of pharmacokinetic and pharmacodynamic drug interactions between nefazodone and digoxin in healthy male volunteers. J Clin Pharmacol 1996 Feb;36(2):160-7.

449 Andersson TL, Zygmunt P, Vinge E. Some substances with proposed digitalis-like effects evaluated on platelet functions sensitive for cardiac glycosides. Gen Pharmacol 1991;22(4):749-53.

450 Durig J, Bruhn J, Zurborn KH, et al. Anticoagulant fucoidan fractions from *Fucus vesiculosus* induce platelet activation in vitro. Thromb Res 1997 Mar 15;85(6):479-91.

451 Leutgeb U. Ambient iodine and lithium-associated with clinical hypothyroidism. Br J Psychiatry 2000 May;176:495-6.

452 Kenny FS, Pinder SE, Ellis IO, et al. Gamma linolenic acid with tamoxifen as primary therapy in breast cancer. Int J Cancer 2000 Mar 1;85(5):643-8.

453 Guivernau M, Meza N, Barja P, Roman O. Clinical and experimental study on the long-term effect of dietary gamma-linolenic acid on plasma lipids, platelet aggregation, thromboxane formation, and prostacyclin production. Prostaglandins Leukot Essent Fatty Acids 1994 Nov;51(5):311-6.

454 Piscitelli SC, Burstein AH, Welden N, Gallicano KD, Falloon J. The effect of garlic supplements on the pharmacokinetics of saquinavir. Clin Infect Dis 2002 Jan 15;34(2):234-238.

455 Hoshino T, Kashimoto N, Kasuga S. Effects of garlic preparations on the gastrointestinal mucosa. J Nutr 2001 Mar;131(3s):1109S-13S.

456 Shweita SA, Abd El-Gabar M, Bastawy M. Carbon tetrachloride changes the activity of cytochrome P450 system in the liver of male rats: role of antioxidants. Toxicology 2001 Dec 14;169(2):83-92.

457 Martin N, Bardisa L, Pantoja C, et al. Anti-arrhythmic profile of a garlic dialysate assayed in dogs and isolated atrial preparations. J Ethnopharmacol 1994 Jun;43(1):1-8.

458 Sheela CG, Augusti KT. Antidiabetic effects of S-allyl cysteine sulphoxide isolated from garlic *Allium sativum* Linn. Indian J Exp Biol 1992 Jun;30(6):523-6.

459. Mostafa MG, Mima T, Ohnishi ST, Mori K. S-allylcysteine ameliorates doxorubicin toxicity in the heart and liver in mice. Planta Med 2000 Mar;66(2):148-51.

460. Li G, Shi Z, Jia H, et al. A clinical investigation on garlicin injectio for treatment of unstable angina pectoris and its actions on plasma endothelin and blood sugar levels. J Tradit Chin Med 2000 Dec;20(4):243-6.

461. Zhang XH, Lowe D, Giles P, et al. Gender may affect the action of garlic oil on plasma cholesterol and glucose levels of normal subjects. J Nutr 2001 May;131(5):1471-8.

462. Fujita K, Kamataki T, et al. Screening of organosulfur compounds as inhibitors of human CYP2A6. Drug Metab Dispos 2001 Jul;29(7):983-9.

463. Foster BC, Foster MS, Vandenhoek S, et al. An in vitro evaluation of human cytochrome p450 3a4 and p-glycoprotein inhibition by garlic. J Pharm Pharm Sci 2001 May-Aug;4(2):176-84.

464. Steiner M, Li W. Aged garlic extract, a modulator of cardiovascular risk factors: a dose-finding study on the effects of AGE on platelet functions. J Nutr 2001 Mar;131(3s):980S-4S.

465. Rahman K, Billington D. Dietary supplementation with aged garlic extract inhibits ADP-induced platelet aggregation in humans. J Nutr 2000 Nov;130(11):2662-5.

466. Elkayam A, Mirelman D, Peleg E, et al. The effects of allicin and enalapril in fructose-induced hyperinsulinemic hyperlipidemic hypertensive rats. Am J Hypertens 2001 Apr;14(4 Pt 1):377-81.

467. Ali M, Bordia T, Mustafa T. Effect of raw versus boiled aqueous extract of garlic and onion on platelet aggregation. Prostaglandins Leukot Essent Fatty Acids 1999 Jan;60(1):43-7.

468. Auer W, Eiber A, Hertkorn E, et al. Hypertension and hyperlipidaemia: garlic helps in mild cases. Br J Clin Pract Suppl 1990 Aug;69:3-6.

469. al-Yahya MA, Rafatullah S, Mossa JS, et al. Gastroprotective activity of ginger *Zingiber officinale* rosc., in albino rats. Am J Chin Med 1989;17(1-2):51-6.

470. Yamahara J, Rong HQ, Naitoh Y, Kitani T, Fujimura H. Inhibition of cytotoxic drug-induced vomiting in suncus by a ginger constituent. J Ethnopharmacol 1989 Dec;27(3):353-5.

471. Suekawa M, Ishige A, Yuasa K, et al. Pharmacological studies on ginger. I. Pharmacological actions of pungent constitutents, (6)-gingerol and (6)-shogaol. J Pharmacobiodyn 1984 Nov;7(11):836-48.

472. Ahmed RS, Sharma SB. Biochemical studies on combined effects of garlic (*Allium sativum* Linn) and ginger (*Zingiber officinale* Rosc) in albino rats. Indian J Exp Biol 1997 Aug;35(8):841-3.

473. Verma SK, Singh J, Khamesra R, Bordia A. Effect of ginger on platelet aggregation in man. Indian J Med Res 1993 Oct;98:240-2.

474. Lumb AB. Effect of dried ginger on human platelet function. Thromb Haemost 1994 Jan;71(1):110-1.

475. Sharma SS, Gupta YK. Reversal of cisplatin-induced delay in gastric emptying in rats by ginger (*Zingiber officinale*). J Ethnopharmacol 1998 Aug;62(1):49-55.

476. Meyer K, Schwartz J, Crater D, Keyes B. *Zingiber officinale* (ginger) used to prevent 8-Mop associated nausea. Dermatol Nurs 1995 Aug;7(4):242-4.

477. Bordia A, Verma SK, Srivastava KC. Effect of ginger (*Zingiber officinale* Rosc.) and fenugreek (*Trigonella foenum-graecum* L.) on blood lipids, blood sugar and platelet aggregation in patients with coronary artery disease. Prostaglandins Leukot Essent Fatty Acids 1997 May;56(5):379-84.

478. al-Zuhair H, Abd el-Fattah A, el-Sayed MI. The effect of meclofenoxate with *Ginkgo biloba* extract or zinc on lipid peroxide, some free radical scavengers and the cardiovascular system of aged rats. Pharmacol Res 1998 Jul;38(1):65-72.

479. Gurley B. Clinical assessment of potential cytochrome P450-mediated herb-drug interactions. 2000 AAPS Annual meeting. October 29 – November 2, 2000. Abstract.

480. Granger AS. *Ginkgo biloba* precipitating epileptic seizures. Age Ageing 2001 Nov;30(6):523-525.

481. Sloley BD, Urichuk LJ, Morley P, et al. Identification of kaempferol as a monoamine oxidase inhibitor and potential neuroprotectant in extracts of *Ginkgo biloba* leaves. J Pharm Pharmacol 2000 Apr;52(4):451-9.

482. Kudolo GB. The effect of 3-month ingestion of *Ginkgo biloba* extract on pancreatic beta-cell function in response to glucose loading in normal glucose tolerant individuals. J Clin Pharmacol 2000 Jun;40(6):647-54.

483. Agha AM, El-Fattah AA, Al-Zuhair HH, Al-Rikabi AC. Chemopreventive effect of *Ginkgo biloba* extract against benzo(a)pyrene-induced forestomach carcinogenesis in mice: amelioration of doxorubicin cardiotoxicity. J Exp Clin Cancer Res 2001 Mar;20(1):39-50.

484. Barth SA, Inselmann G, Engemann R, Heidemann HT. Influences of *Ginkgo biloba* on cyclosporin A induced lipid peroxidation in human liver microsomes in comparison to vitamin E, glutathione and N-acetylcysteine. Biochem Pharmacol 1991 May 15;41(10):1521-6.

485. Mahmoud F, Abul H, Onadeko B, et al. In vitro effects of Ginkgolide B on lymphocyte activation in atopic asthma: comparison with cyclosporin A. Jpn J Pharmacol 2000 Jul;83(3):241-5.

486. Kim YS, Pyo MK, Park KM, et al. Antiplatelet and antithrombotic effects of a combination of ticlopidine and *Ginkgo* *biloba* ext (EGb 761). Thromb Res 1998 Jul 1;91(1):33-8.

487. Ellison JM, DeLuca P. Fluoxetine-induced genital anesthesia relieved by *Ginkgo biloba* extract. J Clin Psychiatry 1998 Apr;59(4):199-200.

488. Cohen AJ, Bartlik B. *Ginkgo biloba* for antidepressant-induced sexual dysfunction. J Sex Marital Ther 1998 Apr-Jun;24(2):139-43.

489. Hemmeter U, Annen B, Bischof R, et al. Polysomnographic effects of adjuvant *Ginkgo biloba* therapy in patients with major depression medicated with trimipramine. Pharmacopsychiatry 2001 Mar;34(2):50-9.

490. Ashton AK, Ahrens K, Gupta S, Masand PS. Antidepressant-induced sexual dysfunction and *Ginkgo Biloba*. Am J Psychiatry 2000 May;157(5):836-7.

491. Wada K, Sasaki K, Miura K, et al. Isolation of bilobalide and ginkgolide A from *Ginkgo biloba* L. shorten the sleeping time induced in mice by anesthetics. Biol Pharm Bull 1993 Feb;16(2):210-2.

492. Hauns B, Haring B, Kohler S, et al. et al. Phase II study with 5-fluorouracil and ginkgo biloba extract (GBE 761 ONC) in patients with pancreatic cancer. Arzneimittelforschung 1999 Dec;49(12):1030-4.

493. Li Z, Xu NJ, Wu CF, et al. Pseudoginsenoside-F11 attenuates morphine-induced signalling in Chinese hamster ovary-mu cells. Neuroreport 2001 May 25;12(7):1453-6.

494. Bhattacharya SK, Mitra SK. Anxiolytic activity of *Panax ginseng* roots: an experimental study. J Ethnopharmacol 1991 Aug;34(1):87-92.

495. Han KH, Choe SC, Kim HS, et al. Effect of red ginseng on blood pressure in patients with essential hypertension and white coat hypertension. Am J Chin Med 1998;26(2):199-209.

496. Janetzky K, Morreale AP. Probable interaction between warfarin and ginseng. Am J Health Syst Pharm 1997 Mar 15;54(6):692-3.

497. Kim JY, Germolec DR, Luster MI. *Panax ginseng* as a potential immunomodulator: studies in mice. Immunopharmacol Immunotoxicol 1990;12(2):257-76.

498. Cho YK, Sung H, Lee HJ, Joo CH, Cho GJ. Long-term intake of Korean red ginseng in HIV-1-infected patients: development of resistance mutation to zidovudine is delayed. Int Immunopharmacol 2001 Jul;1(7):1295-1305.

499. Kim YR, Lee SY, Shin BA, Kim KM. Panax ginseng blocks morphine-induced thymic apoptosis by lowering plasma corticosterone level. Gen Pharmacol 1999 Jun;32(6):647-52.

500. Konno C, Murakami M, Oshima Y, Hikino H. Isolation and hypoglycemic activity of panaxans Q, R, S, T and glycans of *Panax ginseng* roots. J Ethnopharmacol 1985 Sep;14(1):69-74.

501. Park HJ, Lee JH, Song YB, Park KH. Effects of dietary supplementation of lipophilic fraction from *Panax ginseng* on cGMP and cAMP in rat platelets and on blood coagulation. Biol Pharm Bull 1996 Nov;19(11):1434-9.

502. Gokhale SD, Gulati OD, Udwadia BP. Antagonism of the adrenergic neurone blocking action of guanethidine by certain antidepressant and antihistamine drugs. Arch Int Pharmacodyn Ther 1966 Apr;160(2):321-9.

503. Ding DZ, Shen TK, Cui YZ. [Effects of red ginseng on the congestive heart failure and its mechanism.] Zhongguo Zhong Xi Yi Jie He Za Zhi 1995 Jun;15(6):325-7. Abstract.

504. Vereshchagin IA, Geskina OD, Bukhteeva ER. [Increased effectiveness of antibiotic therapy with adaptogens in dysentery and Proteus infection in children]. Antibiotiki 1982 Jan;27(1):65-9. Abstract.

505. Person correspondence with B. Gurley.

506. Setnikar I, Rovati LC. Absorption, distribution, metabolism and excretion of glucosamine sulfate. A review. Arzneimittelforschung 2001 Sep;51(9):699-725.

507. Pouwels MJ, Jacobs JR, Span PN, et al. Short-term glucosamine infusion does not affect insulin sensitivity in humans. J Clin Endocrinol Metab 2001 May;86(5):2099-103.

508. Atanasov AT, Spasov V. Inhibiting and disaggregating effect of gel-filtered *Galega officinalis* L. herbal extract on platelet aggregation. J Ethnopharmacol 2000 Mar;69(3):235-40.

509. Chodera A, Dabrowska K, Sloderbach A, Skrzypczak L, Budzianowski J. [Effect of flavonoid fractions of *Solidago virgaurea* L on diuresis and levels of electrolytes]. Acta Pol Pharm 1991;48(5-6):35-7. Abstract.

510. Pyevich D, Bogenschutz MP. Herbal diuretics and lithium toxicity. Am J Psychiatry 2001 Aug;158(8):1329.

511. Rabbani GH, Butler T, Knight J, Sanyal SC, Alam K. Randomized controlled trial of berberine sulfate therapy for diarrhea due to enterotoxigenic *Escherichia coli* and *Vibrio cholerae*. J Infect Dis 1987 May;155(5):979-84.

512. Lin HL, Liu TY, Wu CW, Chi CW. Berberine modulates expression of mdr1 gene product and the responses of digestive track cancer cells to Paclitaxel. Br J Cancer 1999 Oct;81(3):416-22.

513. Ford JM, Hait WN, Matlin SA, Benz CC. Modulation of resistance to alkylating agents in cancer cell by gossypol enantiomers. Cancer Lett 1991 Jan;56(1):85-94.

514. Messiha FS. Behavioral and metabolic interaction between gossypol and ethanol. Toxicol Lett 1991 Jul;57(2):175-81.

515. Sairam K, Rao CV, Goel RK. Effect of *Centella asiatica* Linn on physical and chemical factors induced gastric ulceration and secretion in rats. Indian J Exp Biol 2001 Feb;39(2):137-42.

516. Johansen RL, Misra HP. Effects of gossypol on the hepatic drug metabolizing system in rats. Contraception 1990 Dec;42(6):683-90.

517. Rikihisa Y, Lin YC. Effect of gossypol on the thyroid in young rats. J Comp Pathol 1989 May;100(4):411-7.

518. Ye YX, Akera T, Ng YC. Modification of the positive inotropic effects of catecholamines, cardiac glycosides and Ca2+ by the orally active male contraceptive, gossypol, in isolated guinea-pig heart. Life Sci 1989;45(20):1853-61.

519. Kumar M, Sharma S, Lohiya NK. Gossypol-induced hypokalemia and role of exogenous potassium salt supplementation when used as an antispermatogenic agent in male langur monkey. Contraception 1997 Oct;56(4):251-6.

520. Seo K, Jung S, Park M, Song Y, Choung S. Effects of leucocyanidines on activities of metabolizing enzymes and antioxidant enzymes. Biol Pharm Bull 2001 May;24(5):592-3.

521. Roder E. Medicinal plants in Europe containing pyrrolizidine alkaloids. Pharmazie. 1995;50:83-98.

522. Luksa-Lichtenthaeler GL, Ladutko EI, Nowicky JW. Radiomodification effects of Ukrain, a cytostatic and immunomodulating drug, on intracellular glucocorticoid reception during short-term gamma-irradiation. Drugs Exp Clin Res 2000;26(5-6):311-5.

523. Homann HH, Kemen M, Fuessenich C, Senkal M, Zumtobel V. Reduction in diarrhea incidence by soluble fiber in patients receiving total or supplemental enteral nutrition. JPEN J Parenter Enteral Nutr 1994 Nov-Dec;18(6):486-90.

524. Soci MM, Parrott EL. Influence of viscosity on absorption from nitrofurantoin suspensions. J Pharm Sci 1980 Apr;69(4):403-6.

525. Jenkins DJ, Wolever TM, Nineham R, et al. Improved glucose tolerance four hours after taking guar with glucose. Diabetologia 1980 Jul;19(1):21-4.

526. Reppas C, Eleftheriou G, Macheras P, Symillides M, Dressman JB. Effect of elevated viscosity in the upper gastrointestinal tract on drug absorption in dogs. Eur J Pharm Sci 1998 Apr;6(2):131-9.

527. Holt S, Heading RC, Carter DC, Prescott LF, Tothill P. Effect of gel fibre on gastric emptying and absorption of glucose and paracetamol. Lancet 1979 Mar 24;1(8117):636-9.

528. Garcia JJ, Fernandez N, Diez MJ, et al. Influence of two dietary fibers in the oral bioavailability and other pharmacokinetic parameters of ethinyloestradiol. Contraception 2000 Nov;62(5):253-7.

529. Sierra M, Garcia JJ, Fernandez N, et al. Effects of ispaghula husk and guar gum on postprandial glucose and insulin concentrations in healthy subjects. Eur J Clin Nutr 2001 Apr;55(4):235-43.

530. Bydlowski SP, D'Amico EA, Chamone DA. An aqueous extract of guarana (*Paullinia cupana*) decreases platelet thromboxane synthesis. Braz J Med Biol Res 1991;24(4):421-4.

531. Notarianni LJ, Oliver SE, Dobrocky P, Bennett PN, Silverman BW. Caffeine as a metabolic probe: a comparison of the metabolic ratios used to assess CYP1A2 activity. Br J Clin Pharmacol 1995 Jan;39(1):65-9.

532. Chatopadhyay RR. Possible mechanism of antihyperglycemic effect of *Gymnema sylvestre* leaf extract, part I. Gen Pharmacol 1998 Sep;31(3):495-6.

533. Wang LF, Luo H, Miyoshi M, et al. Inhibitory effect of gymnemic acid on intestinal absorption of oleic acid in rats. Can J Physiol Pharmacol 1998 Oct-Nov;76(10-11):1017-23.

534. al Makdessi S, Sweidan H, Dietz K, Jacob R. Protective effect of *Crataegus oxyacantha* against reperfusion arrhythmias after global no-flow ischemia in the rat heart. Basic Res Cardiol 1999 Apr;94(2):71-7.

535. Rothfuss MA, Pascht U, Kissling G. Effect of long-term application of *Crataegus oxyacantha* on ischemia and reperfusion induced arrhythmias in rats. Arzneimittelforschung 2001 Jan;51(1):24-8.

536. Della Loggia R, Tubaro A, Redaelli C. [Evaluation of the activity on the mouse CNS of several plant extracts and a combination of them]. Riv Neurol 1981 Sep-Oct;51(5):297-310. Abstract.

537. Kim SH, Kang KW, Kim KM, ND. Procyanidins in crataegus extract evoke endothelium-dependent vasorelaxation in rat aorta. Life Sci 2000;67(2):121-31.

538. Vibes J, Lasserre B, Gleye J, Declume C. Inhibition of thromboxane A2 biosynthesis in vitro by the main components of *Crataegus oxyacantha* (Hawthorn) flower heads. Prostaglandins Leukot Essent Fatty Acids 1994 Apr;50(4):173-5.

539. Jaffe AM, Gephardt D, Courtemanche L. Poisoning due to ingestion of *Veratrum viride* (false hellebore). J Emerg Med 1990 Mar-Apr;8(2):161-7.

540. Penttila J, Vesalainen R, Helminen A, et al. Spontaneous baroreflex sensitivity as a dynamic measure of cardiac anticholinergic drug effect. J Auton Pharmacol 2001 Apr;21(2):71-8.

541. Liu J, Burdette JE, Xu H, et al. Evaluation of estrogenic activity of plant extracts for the potential treatment of menopausal symptoms. J Agric Food Chem 2001 May;49(5):2472-9.

542. Hansel R, Wohlfart R, Coper H. [Sedative-hypnotic compounds in the exhalation of hops, II]. Z Naturforsch [C] 1980 Nov-Dec;35(11-12):1096-7.

543. Milligan SR, Kalita JC, Heyerick A, et al. Identification of a potent phytoestrogen in hops (*Humulus lupulus* L.) and beer. J Clin Endocrinol Metab 1999 Jun;84(6):2249-52.

544. El Bardai S, Lyoussi B, Wibo M, Morel N. Pharmacological evidence of hypotensive activity of *Marrubium vulgare* and *Foeniculum vulgare* in spontaneously hypertensive rat. Clin Exp Hypertens 2001 May;23(4):329-43.

545. Novaes AP, Rossi C, Poffo C, et al. Preliminary evaluation of the hypoglycemic effect of some Brazilian medicinal plants. Therapie 2001 Jul-Aug;56(4):427-30.

546. Matsuda H, Murakami T, Li Y, Yamahara J, Yoshikawa M. Mode of action of escins Ia and IIa and E,Z-senegin II on glucose absorption in gastrointestinal tract. Bioorg Med Chem 1998 Jul;6(7):1019-23.

547. Yoshikawa M, Murakami T, Matsuda H, et al. Bioactive saponins and glycosides. III. Horse chestnut. (1): The structures, inhibitory effects on ethanol absorption, and hypoglycemic activity of escins Ia, Ib, IIa, IIb, and IIIa from the seeds of *Aesculus hippocastanum* L. Chem Pharm Bull (Tokyo) 1996 Aug;44(8):1454-64.

548. Yoshikawa M, Harada E, Murakami T, et al. Escins-Ia, Ib, IIa, IIb, and IIIa, bioactive triterpene oligoglycosides from the seeds of *Aesculus hippocastanum* L.: their inhibitory effects on ethanol absorption and hypoglycemic activity on glucose tolerance test. Chem Pharm Bull (Tokyo) 1994 Jun;42(6):1357-9.

549. Sekiya K, Okuda H, Arichi S. Selective inhibition of platelet lipoxygenase by esculetin. Biochim Biophys Acta 1982 Oct 14;713(1):68-72.

550. Marhuenda E, Alarcon de la Lastra C, Martin MJ. Antisecretory and gastroprotective effects of aescine in rats. Gen Pharmacol 1994 Oct;25(6):1213-9.

551. Martin MJ, Alarcon C, Motilva V. [Effects of aescine and aesculine on kidney excretion of water and electrolytes in rats.] Ann Pharm Fr 1990;48(6):306-11. Abstract.

552. Divi RL, Doerge DR. Inhibition of thyroid peroxidase by dietary flavonoids. Chem Res Toxicol 1996 Jan-Feb;9(1):16-23.

553. Lin JH, Hu GY, Tang XC. Comparison between huperzine A, tacrine, and E2020 on cholinergic transmission at mouse neuromuscular junction in vitro. Zhongguo Yao Li Xue Bao 1997 Jan;18(1):6-10.

554. Mash DC, Kovera CA, Pablo J, et al. Ibogaine: complex pharmacokinetics, concerns for safety, and preliminary efficacy measures. Ann N Y Acad Sci 2000;914:394-401.

555. Glick SD, Maisonneuve IM. Development of novel medications for drug addiction. The legacy of an African shrub. Ann N Y Acad Sci 2000;909:88-103.

556. Neuman J, de Engel AM, Neuman MP. Pilot study of the effect of raubasine on platelet biological activity. Arzneimittelforschung 1986 Sep;36(9):1394-8.

557. Smith WM. Treatment of mild hypertension: results of a ten-year intervention trial. Circ Res 1977 May;40(5 Suppl 1):I98-105.

558. Chaveron M, Assie MB, Stenger A, Briley M. Benzodiazepine agonist-type activity of raubasine, a *Rauwolfia serpentina* alkaloid. Eur J Pharmacol 1984 Nov 13;106(2):313-7.

559. Wang EJ, Lew K, Barecki M, et al. Quantitative distinctions of active site molecular recognition by P-glycoprotein and cytochrome P450 3A4. Chem Res Toxicol 2001 Dec 17;14(12):1596-1603.

560. Kumar GP, Sudheesh S, Vijayalakshmi NR. Hypoglycaemic effect of *Coccinia indica*: mechanism of action. Planta Med 1993 Aug;59(4):330-2.

561. Azad Khan AK, Akhtar S, Mahtab H. *Coccinia indica* in the treatment of patients with diabetes mellitus. Bangladesh Med Res Counc Bull 1979 Dec;5(2):60-6.

562. Kamble SM, Kamlakar PL, Vaidya S, Bambole VD. Influence of *Coccinia indica* on certain enzymes in glycolytic and lipolytic pathway in human diabetes. Indian J Med Sci 1998 Apr;52(4):143-6.

563. de Medeiros JM, Macedo M, Contancia JP, et al. Antithrombin activity of medicinal plants of the Azores. J Ethnopharmacol 2000 Sep;72(1-2):157-65.

564. Della Loggia R, Tubaro A, Redaelli C. [Evaluation of the activity on the mouse CNS of several plant extracts and a combination of them] Riv Neurol 1981 Sep-Oct;51(5):297-310. Abstract.

565. Chang WC, Hsu FL. Inhibition of platelet activation and endothelial cell injury by polyphenolic compounds isolated from *Lonicera japonica* Thunb. Prostaglandins Leukot Essent Fatty Acids 1992 Apr;45(4):307-12.

566. Kitagawa I, Mahmud T, Simanjuntak P, et al. Chemical structures of three new triterpenoids, brucealavanin A, and dihydrobrucealavanin A, and brucealavanin B, and a new alkaloidal glycoside, brucealanthinoside, from the stems of *Brucea javanica* (Simaroubaceae). Chem Pharm Bull (Tokyo) 1994 Jul;42(7):1416-21.

567. Beaux D, Fleurentin J, Mortier F. Effect of extracts of *Orthosiphon stamineus* Benth, *Hieracium pilosella* L., *Sambucus nigra* L. and *Arctostaphylos uva-ursi* (L.) Spreng. in rats. Phytother Res 1999 May;13(3):222-5.

568. Guharoy SR, Barajas M. Atropine intoxication from the ingestion and smoking of jimson weed (*Datura stramonium*). Vet Hum Toxicol 1991 Dec;33(6):588-9.

569. Sanchez de Medina F, Gamez MJ, Jimenez I, Osuna JI, Zarzuelo A. Hypoglycemic activity of juniper "berries". Planta Med 1994 Jun;60(3):197-200.

570. Jussofie A, Schmiz A, Hiemke C. Kavapyrone enriched extract from *Piper methysticum* as modulator of the GABA binding site in different regions of rat brain. Psychopharmacology (Berl) 1994 Dec;116(4):469-74.

571. De Leo V, la Marca A, Morgante G, et al. Evaluation of combining kava extract with hormone replacement therapy in the treatment of postmenopausal anxiety. Maturitas 2001 Aug 25;39(2):185-8.

572. Gleitz J, Beile A, Wilkens P, Ameri A, Peters T. Antithrombotic action of the kava pyrone (+)-kavain prepared from *Piper methysticum* on human platelets. Planta Med 1997 Feb;63(1):27-30.

573. Herberg KW. [Effect of Kava-Special Extract WS 1490 combined with ethyl alcohol on safety-relevant performance parameters.] Blutalkohol 1993 Mar;30(2):96-105

574. Mauray S, De Raucourt E, Chaubet F, Maiga-Revel O, Sternberg C, Fischer AM. Comparative anticoagulant activity and influence on thrombin generation of dextran derivatives and of a fucoidan fraction. J Biomater Sci Polym Ed 1998;9(4):373-87.

575. Jamieson DD, Duffield PH. Positive interaction of ethanol and kava resin in mice. Clin Exp Pharmacol Physiol 1990 Jul;17(7):509-14.

576. Jamieson DD, Duffield PH, Cheng D, Duffield AM. Comparison of the central nervous system activity of the aqueous and lipid extract of kava (*Piper methysticum*). Arch Int Pharmacodyn Ther 1989 Sep-Oct;301:66-80.

577. Schelosky L, Raffauf C, Jendroska K, Poewe W. Kava and dopamine antagonism. J Neurol Neurosurg Psychiatry 1995 May;58(5):639-40.

578. Leutgeb U. Ambient iodine and lithium-associated with clinical hypothyroidism. Br J Psychiatry 2000 May;176:495-6.

579. Kalix P. Cathinone, an alkaloid from khat leaves with an amphetamine-like releasing effect. Psychopharmacology (Berl) 1981;74(3):269-70.

580. Wagner GC, Preston K, Ricaurte GA, Schuster CR, Seiden LS. Neurochemical similarities between d,l-cathinone and d-amphetamine. Drug Alcohol Depend 1982 Aug;9(4):279-84.

581. Nasher AA, Qirbi AA, Ghafoor MA, et al. Khat chewing and bladder neck dysfunction. A randomized controlled trial of alpha 1-adrenergic blockade. Br J Urol 1995 May;75(5):597-8.

582. Islam MW, Tariq M, el-Feraly FS, al-Meshal IA. Effect of khatamines and their enantiomers on plasma triiodothyronine and thyroxine levels in normal Wistar rats. Am J Chin Med 1990;18(1-2):71-6.

583. Attef OA, Ali AA, Ali HM. Effect of khat chewing on the bioavailability of ampicillin and amoxycillin. J Antimicrob Chemother 1997 Apr;39(4):523-5.

584. Duarte J, Vallejo I, Perez-Vizcaino F, et al. Effects of visnadine on rat isolated vascular smooth muscles. Planta Med 1997 Jun;63(3):233-6.

585. Schimmer O, Rauch P. Inhibition of metabolic activation of the promutagens, benzo[a]pyrene, 2-aminofluorene and 2-aminoanthracene by furanochromones in *Salmonella typhimurium*. Mutagenesis 1998 Jul;13(4):385-9.

586. Duarte J, Torres AI, Zarzuelo A. Cardiovascular effects of visnagin on rats. Planta Med 2000 Feb;66(1):35-9.

587. Pan JX, Han ZH, Miao JL, et al. Furanochromone radical cations: generation, characterization and interaction with DNA. Biophys Chem 2001 Jul 2;91(2):105-13.

588. Harvengt C, Desager JP. HDL-cholesterol increase in normolipaemic subjects on khellin: a pilot study. Int J Clin Pharmacol Res 1983;3(5):363-6.

589. Rauwald HW, Brehm O, Odenthal KP. The involvement of a Ca2+ channel blocking mode of action in the pharmacology of *Ammi visnaga* fruits. Planta Med 1994 Apr;60(2):101-5.

590. Duarte J, Vallejo I, Perez-Vizcaino F, Jimenez R, Zarzuelo A, Tamargo J. Effects of visnadine on rat isolated vascular smooth muscles. Planta Med 1997 Jun;63(3):233-6.

591. Hennessy M, Kelleher D, Spiers JP, et al. St John's Wort increases expression of P-glycoprotein: implications for drug interactions. Br J Clin Pharmacol 2002 Jan;53(1):75-82.

592. Shaheen SM, Fleming SE. High-fiber foods at breakfast: influence on plasma glucose and insulin responses to lunch. Am J Clin Nutr 1987 Nov;46(5):804-11.

593. Vuksan V, Sievenpiper JL, Owen R, et al. Beneficial effects of viscous dietary fiber from Konjac-mannan in subjects with the insulin resistance syndrome: results of a controlled metabolic trial. Diabetes Care 2000 Jan;23(1):9-14.

594. Liu F, Kim J, Li Y, et al. An extract of *Lagerstroemia speciosa* L. has insulin-like glucose uptake-stimulatory and adipocyte differentiation-inhibitory activities in 3T3-L1 cells. J Nutr 2001 Sep;131(9):2242-7.

595. Guillemain J, Rousseau A, Delaveau P. [Neurodepressive effects of the essential oil of *Lavandula angustifolia* Mill.] Ann Pharm Fr 1989;47(6):337-43. Abstract.

596. Delaveau P, Guillemain J, Narcisse G, Rousseau A. [Neuro-depressive properties of essential oil of lavender.] C R Seances Soc Biol Fil 1989;183(4):342-8. Abstract.

597. Soulimani R, Fleurentin J, Mortier F, et al. Neurotropic action of the hydroalcoholic extract of *Melissa officinalis* in the mouse. Planta Med 1991 Apr;57(2):105-9.

598. Aufmkolk M, Kohrle J, Gumbinger H, Winterhoff H, Hesch RD. Antihormonal effects of plant extracts: iodothyronine deiodinase of rat liver is inhibited by extracts and secondary metabolites of plants. Horm Metab Res 1984 Apr;16(4):188-92.

599. Zhang H, Teng Y. Effect of li ren (semen litchi) anti-diabetes pills in 45 cases of diabetes mellitus. J Tradit Chin Med 1986 Dec;6(4):277-8.

600. Hatano T, Fukuda T, Miyase T, Noro T, Okuda T. Phenolic constituents of licorice. III. Structures of glicoricone and licofuranone, and inhibitory effects of licorice constituents on monoamine oxidase. Chem Pharm Bull (Tokyo) 1991 May;39(5):1238-43.

601. Takii H, Kometani T, Nishimura T, et al. Antidiabetic effect of glycyrrhizin in genetically diabetic KK-Ay mice. Biol Pharm Bull 2001 May;24(5):484-7.

602. Fujiwara Y, Kikkawa R, Nakata K, et al. Hypokalemia and sodium retention in patients with diabetes and chronic hepatitis receiving insulin and glycyrrhizin. Endocrinol Jpn 1983 Apr;30(2):243-9.

603. Bernardi M, D'Intino PE, Trevisani F, et al. Effects of prolonged ingestion of graded doses of licorice by healthy volunteers. Life Sci 1994;55(11):863-72.

604. Wang JY, Guo JS, Li H, Liu SL, Zern MA. Inhibitory effect of glycyrrhizin on NF-kappaB binding activity in CCl4- plus ethanol-induced liver cirrhosis in rats. Liver 1998 Jun;18(3):180-5.

605. Razina TG, Zueva EP, Amosova EN, Krylova SG. [Medicinal plant preparations used as adjuvant therapeutics in experimental oncology]. Eksp Klin Farmakol 2000 Sep-Oct;3(5):59-61.

606. Moon A, Kim SH. Effect of *Glycyrrhiza glabra* roots and glycyrrhizin on the glucuronidation in rats. Planta Med 1997 Apr;63(2):115-9.

607. Liu J, Liu Y, Mao Q, Klaassen CD. The effects of 10 triterpenoid compounds on experimental liver injury in mice. Fundam Appl Toxicol 1994 Jan;22(1):34-40.

608. Ojima M, Satoh K, Gomibuchi T, et al. [The inhibitory effects of glycyrrhizin and glycyrrhetinic acid on the metabolism of cortisol and prednisolone—in vivo and in vitro studies]. Nippon Naibunpi Gakkai Zasshi 1990 May 20;66(5):584-96. Abstract.

609. Eisenburg J. [Treatment of chronic hepatitis B. Part 2: Effect of glycyrrhizic acid on the course of illness]. Fortschr Med 1992 Jul 30;110(21):395-8.

610. Abe Y, Ueda T, Kato T, Kohli Y. [Effectiveness of interferon, glycyrrhizin combination therapy in patients with chronic hepatitis C]. Nippon Rinsho 1994 Jul;52(7):1817-22. Abstract.

611. Paolini M, Barillari J, Broccoli M, et al. Effect of liquorice and glycyrrhizin on rat liver carcinogen metabolizing enzymes. Cancer Lett 1999 Oct 18;145(1-2):35-42.

612. Serra A, Uehlinger DE, Ferrari P, et al. Glycyrrhetinic acid decreases plasma potassium concentrations in patients with anuria. J Am Soc Nephrol 2002 Jan;13(1):191-6.

613. Eriksson JW, Carlberg B, Hillorn V. Life-threatening ventricular tachycardia due to liquorice-induced hypokalaemia. J Intern Med 1999 Mar;245(3):307-10.

614. Datla R, Rao SR, Murthy KJ. Excretion studies of nitrofurantoin and nitrofurantoin with deglycyrrhizinated liquorice. Indian J Physiol Pharmacol 1981 Jan-Mar;25(1):59-63.

615. Sigurjonsdottir HA, Franzson L, Manhem K, Ragnarsson J, Sigurdsson G, Wallerstedt S. Liquorice-induced rise in blood pressure: a linear dose-response relationship. J Hum Hypertens 2001 Aug;15(8):549-52.

616. Bennett A, Clark-Wibberley T, Stamford IF, Wright JE. Aspirin-induced gastric mucosal damage in rats: cimetidine and deglycyrrhizinated liquorice together give greater protection than low doses of either drug alone. J Pharm Pharmacol 1980 Feb;32(2):151.

617. Doll R, Langman MJ, Shawdon HH. Treatment of gastric ulcer with carbenoxolone: antagonistic effect of spironolactone. Gut 1968 Feb;9(1):42-5.

618. Itoh K, Hayasaka M, Niizeki M, et al. Direct determination of serum glycyrrhetic acid by a monoclonal antibody-based inhibition ELISA using ibuprofen for releasing serum albumin-bound glycyrrhetic acid. J Immunoassay 1996 Nov;17(4):343-52.

619. Tanaka M, Takahashi M, Kuwahara E, et al. Effect of glycyrrhizinate on dissolution behavior and rectal absorption of amphotericin B in rabbits. Chem Pharm Bull (Tokyo) 1992 Jun;40(6):1559-62.

620. Reed PI, Lewis SI, Vincent-Brown A, et al. The influence of amiloride on the therapeutic and metabolic effects of carbenoxolone in patients with gastric ulcer. A double-blind controlled trial. Scand J Gastroenterol Suppl 1980;65:51-7.

621. Greaves MW. Potentiation of hydrocortisone activity in skin by glycerrhetinic acid. Lancet 1990 Oct 6;336(8719):876.

622. Chen MF, Shimada F, Kato H, Yano S, Kanaoka M. Effect of oral administration of glycyrrhizin on the pharmacokinetics of prednisolone. Endocrinol Jpn 1991 Apr;38(2):167-74.

623. Hatano T, Fukuda T, Miyase T, Noro T, Okuda T. Phenolic constituents of licorice. III. Structures of glicoricone and licofuranone, and inhibitory effects of licorice constituents on monoamine oxidase. Chem Pharm Bull (Tokyo) 1991 May;39(5):1238-43.

624. Shintani S, Murase H, Tsukagoshi H, Shiigai T. Glycyrrhizin (licorice)-induced hypokalemic myopathy. Report of 2 cases and review of the literature. Eur Neurol 1992;32(1):44-51.

625. Folkersen L, Knudsen NA, Teglbjaerg PS. [Licorice. A basis for precautions one more time!] Ugeskr Laeger 1996 Dec 16;158(51):7420-1. Abstract.

626. Rees WD, Rhodes J, Wright JE, Stamford LF, Bennett A. Effect of deglycyrrhizinated liquorice on gastric mucosal damage by aspirin. Scand J Gastroenterol 1979;14(5):605-7.

627. Tawata M, Yoda Y, Aida K, et al. Anti-platelet action of GU-7, a 3-arylcoumarin derivative, purified from glycyrrhizae radix. Planta Med 1990 Jun;56(3):259-63.

628. Francischetti IM, Monteiro RQ, Guimaraes JA, et al. Identification of glycyrrhizin as a thrombin inhibitor. Biochem Biophys Res Commun 1997 Jun 9;235(1):259-63.

629. Agrawal AK, Rao CV, Sairam K, Joshi VK, Goel RK. Effect of *Piper longum* Linn, *Zingiber officinalis* Linn and *Ferula* species on gastric ulceration and secretion in rats. Indian J Exp Biol 2000 Oct;38(10):994-8.

630. Lamela M, Cadavid I, Calleja JM. Effects of *Lythrum salicaria* extracts on hyperglycemic rats and mice. J Ethnopharmacol 1986 Feb;15(2):153-60.

631. Torres IC, Suarez JC. A preliminary study of hypoglycemic activity of *Lythrum salicaria*. J Nat Prod 1980 Sep-Oct;43(5):559-63.

632. Chen IS, Chang CT, Sheen WS, et al. Coumarins and antiplatelet aggregation constituents from Formosan Peucedanum japonicum. Phytochemistry 1996 Feb;41(2):525-30.

633. Lam AY, Elmer GW, Mohutsky MA. Possible interaction between warfarin and *Lycium barbarum* L. Ann Pharmacother 2001 Oct;35(10):1199-201.

634. Singh SN, Vats P, Suri S, et al. Effect of an antidiabetic extract of Catharanthus roseus on enzymic activities in streptozotocin induced diabetic rats. J Ethnopharmacol 2001 Aug;76(3):269-77.

635. Horio H, Ohtsuru M. Maitake (*Grifola frondosa*) improve glucose tolerance of experimental diabetic rats. J Nutr Sci Vitaminol (Tokyo) 2001 Feb;47(1):57-63.

636. Migliardi JR, Armellino JJ, Friedman M, Gillings DB, Beaver WT. Caffeine as an analgesic adjuvant in tension headache. Clin Pharmacol Ther 1994 Nov;56(5):576-86.

637. Rush CR C, Higgins ST S, Bickel WK W, Hughes JR J. Acute behavioral effects of lorazepam and caffeine, alone and in combination, in humans. Behav Pharmacol 1994 Jun;5(3):245-254.

348

349

638. Fiebich BL, Lieb K, Hull M, et al. Effects of caffeine and paracetamol alone or in combination with acetylsali-cylic acid on prostaglandin E(2) synthesis in rat microglial cells. Neuropharmacology 2000 Aug 23;39(11):2205-13.

639. Sugiyama T, Sadzuka Y. Enhancing effects of green tea components on the antitumor activity of adriamycin against M5076 ovarian sarcoma. Cancer Lett 1998 Nov 13;133(1):19-26.

640. Sadzuka Y, Sugiyama T, Sonobe T. Efficacies of tea components on doxorubicin induced antitumor activity and reversal of multidrug resistance. Toxicol Lett 2000 Apr 3;114(1-3):155-62.

641. Hodgson JM, Puddey IB, Mori TA, et al. Effects of regular ingestion of black tea on haemostasis and cell adhesion molecules in humans. Eur J Clin Nutr 2001 Oct;55(10):881-6.

642. Kudriashov BA, Liapina LA, Azieva LD. [The content of a heparin-like anticoagulant in the flowers of the meadowsweet (Filipendula ulmaria).] Farmakol Toksikol 1990 Jul-Aug;53(4):39-41. Abstract.

643. Cheeseman HJ, Neal MJ. Interaction of chlorpromazine with tea and coffee. Br J Clin Pharmacol 1981 Aug;12(2):165-9.

644. Kang WS, Lim IH, Yuk DY, Chung KH, Park JB, Yoo HS, Yun YP. Antithrombotic activities of green tea catechins and (-)-epigallocatechin gallate. Thromb Res 1999 Nov 1;96(3):229-37.

645. Csaba G, Nagy ZU. Effect of TSH and melatonin on thyroid activity in the rat. Acta Physiol Acad Sci Hung 1976;48(2-3):101-3.

646. Taylor JR, Wilt VM. Probable antagonism of warfarin by green tea. Ann Pharmacother 1999 Apr;33(4):426-8.

647. Sohn OS, Surace A, Fiala ES, et al. Effects of green and black tea on hepatic xenobiotic metabolizing systems in the male F344 rat. Xenobiotica 1994 Feb;24(2):119-27.

648. Maliakal PP, Coville PF, Wanwimolruk S. Tea consumption modulates hepatic drug metabolizing enzymes in Wistar rats. J Pharm Pharmacol 2001 Apr;53(4):569-77.

649. Chang MC, Bailey JW, Collins JL. Dietary tannins from cowpeas and tea transiently alter apparent calcium absorption but not absorption and utilization of protein in rats. J Nutr 1994 Feb;124(2):283-8.

650. Sparano N. Is the combination of ibuprofen and caffeine effective for the treatment of a tension-type headache? J Fam Pract 2001 Jan;50(1):10.

651. Graham TE, Sathasivam P, Rowland M, et al. Caffeine ingestion elevates plasma insulin response in humans during an oral glucose tolerance test. Can J Physiol Pharmacol 2001 Jul;79(7):559-65.

652. Uchida K, Aoki T, Satoh H, Tajiri O. [Effects of melatonin on muscle contractility and neuromuscular blockade produced by muscle relaxants]. Masui 1997 Feb;46(2):205-12. Abstract

653. Eadie MJ. Clinically significant drug interactions with agents specific for migraine attacks. CNS Drugs 2001;15(2):105-18.

654. Beach CA, Mays DC, Guiler RC, Jacober CH, Gerber N. Inhibition of elimination of caffeine by disulfiram in normal subjects and recovering alcoholics. Clin Pharmacol Ther 1986 Mar;39(3):265-70.

655. Gibb JW, Bush L, Hanson GR. Exacerbation of methamphetamine-induced neurochemical deficits by melatonin. J Pharmacol Exp Ther 1997 Nov;283(2):630-5.

656. Labbe L, Turgeon J. Clinical pharmacokinetics of mexiletine. Clin Pharmacokinet 1999 Nov;37(5):361-84.

657 Food and Drug Administration Public Health Advisory Subject: Safety of Phenylpropanolamine 11/6/00.

658. Carrillo JA, Benitez J. Clinically significant pharmacokinetic interactions between dietary caffeine and medications. Clin Pharmacokinet 2000 Aug;39(2):127-53.

659. Drago F, Frisina M, Grech M, et al. Dual effects of melatonin on barbiturate-induced narcosis in rats. Neurosci Lett 2001 Mar 16;300(3):176-8.

660. Pang CS, Tsang SF, Yang JC. Effects of melatonin, morphine and diazepam on formalin-induced nociception in mice. Life Sci 2001 Jan 12;68(8):943-51.

661. Manzana EJ, Chen WJ, Champney TH. Acute melatonin and para-chloroamphetamine interactions on pineal, brain and serum serotonin levels as well as stress hormone levels. Brain Res 2001 Aug 3;909(1-2):127-37.

662. Currier NL, Sicotte M, Miller SC. Deleterious effects of *Echinacea purpurea* and melatonin on myeloid cells in mouse spleen and bone marrow. J Leukoc Biol 2001 Aug;70(2):274-6.

663. Raghavendra V, Naidu PS, Kulkarni SK. Reversal of reserpine-induced vacuous chewing movements in rats by melatonin: involvement of peripheral benzodiazepine receptors. Brain Res 2001 Jun 15;904(1):149-52.

664. Futagami M, Sato S, Sakamoto T, Yokoyama Y, Saito Y. Effects of melatonin on the proliferation and cis-diamminedichloroplatinum (CDDP) sensitivity of cultured human ovarian cancer cells. Gynecol Oncol 2001 Sep;82(3):544-9.

665. Gurdol F, Genc S, Oner-Iyidogan Y, Suzme R. Coadministration of melatonin and estradiol in rats: effects on oxidant status. Horm Metab Res 2001 Oct;33(10):608-11.

666. Agapito MT, Antolin Y, del Brio MT, et al. Protective effect of melatonin against adriamycin toxicity in the rat. J Pineal Res 2001 Aug;31(1):23-30.

667. Othman AI, El-Missiry MA, Amer MA. The protective action of melatonin on indomethacin-induced gastric and testicular oxidative stress in rats. Redox Rep 2001;6(3):173-7.

668. Xu MF, Ho S, Qian ZM, Tang PL. Melatonin protects against cardiac toxicity of doxorubicin in rat. J Pineal Res 2001 Nov;31(4):301-7.

669. Hartter S, Ursing C, Morita S, et al. Orally given melatonin may serve as a probe drug for cytochrome P450 1A2 activity in vivo: a pilot study. Clin Pharmacol Ther 2001 Jul;70(1):10-6.

670. Shear NH, Malkiewicz IM, Klein D, et al. Acetaminophen-induced toxicity to human epidermoid cell line A431 and hepatoblastoma cell line Hep G2, in vitro, is diminished by silymarin. Skin Pharmacol 1995;8(6):279-91.

671. Lusardi P, Piazza E, Fogari R. Cardiovascular effects of melatonin in hypertensive patients well controlled by nifedipine: a 24-hour study. Br J Clin Pharmacol 2000 May;49(5):423-7.

672. Allain H, Schuck S, Lebreton S, et al. Aminotransferase levels and silymarin in de novo tacrine-treated patients with Alzheimer's disease. Dement Geriatr Cogn Disord 1999 May-Jun;10(3):181-5.

673. Kim DH, Jin YH, Park JB, Kobashi K. Silymarin and its components are inhibitors of beta-glucuronidase. Biol Pharm Bull 1994 Mar;17(3):443-5.

674. Venkataramanan R, Komoroski BJ, et al. Milk thistle, a herbal supplement, decreases the activity of CYP3A4 and uridine diphosphoglucuronosyl transferase in human hepatocyte cultures. Drug Metab Dispos 2000 Nov;28(11):1270-3.

675. Sonnenbichler J, Scalera F, Sonnenbichler I, Weyhenmeyer R. Stimulatory effects of silibinin and silicristin from the milk thistle *Silybum marianum* on kidney cells. J Pharmacol Exp Ther 1999 Sep;290(3):1375-83.

676. Siegers CP, Fruhling A, Younes M. Influence of dithiocarb (+)-catechin and silybine on halothane hepatotoxicity in the hypoxic rat model. Acta Pharmacol Toxicol (Copenh) 1983 Aug;53(2):125-9.

677. Mourelle M, Favari L. Silymarin improves metabolism and disposition of aspirin in cirrhotic rats. Life Sci 1988;43(3):201-7.

678. Soto CP, Perez BL, Favari LP, Reyes JL. Prevention of alloxan-induced diabetes mellitus in the rat by silymarin. Comp Biochem Physiol C Pharmacol Toxicol Endocrinol 1998 Feb;119(2):125-9.

679. Maitrejean M, Comte G, Barron D, et al. The flavonolignan silybin and its hemisynthetic derivatives, a novel series of potential modulators of P-glycoprotein. Bioorg Med Chem Lett 2000 Jan 17;10(2):157-60.

680. Venkataramanan R, Komoroski BJ, et al. Milk thistle, a herbal supplement, decreases the activity of CYP3A4 and uridine diphosphoglucuronosyl transferase in human hepatocyte cultures. Drug Metab Dispos 2000 Nov;28(11):1270-3.

681. Velussi M, Cernigoi AM, De Monte A, et al. Long-term (12 months) treatment with an anti-oxidant drug (silymarin) is effective on hyperinsulinemia, exogenous insulin need and malondialdehyde levels in cirrhotic diabetic patients. J Hepatol 1997 Apr;26(4):871-9.

682. von Schonfeld J, Weisbrod B, Muller MK. Silibinin, a plant extract with antioxidant and membrane stabilizing properties, protects exocrine pancreas from cyclosporin A toxicity. Cell Mol Life Sci 1997 Dec;53(11-12):917-20.

683. Gaedeke J, Fels LM, Bokemeyer C, et al. Cisplatin nephrotoxicity and protection by silibinin. Nephrol Dial Transplant 1996 Jan;11(1):55-62.

684. Zima T, Kamenikova L, Janebova M, et al. The effect of silibinin on experimental cyclosporine nephrotoxicity. Ren Fail 1998 May;20(3):471-9.

685. Bantel H, Engels IH, Voelter W, et al. Mistletoe lectin activates caspase-8/FLICE independently of death receptor signaling and enhances anticancer drug-induced apoptosis. Cancer Res 1999 May 1;59(9):2083-90.

686. Timoshenko AV, Lan Y, Gabius HJ, Lala PK. Immunotherapy of C3H/HeJ mammary adenocarcinoma with interleukin-2, mistletoe lectin or their combination. effects on tumour growth, capillary leakage and nitric oxide (NO) production. Eur J Cancer 2001 Oct;37(15):1910-20.

687. Zou QZ, Bi RG, Li JM, et al. Effect of motherwort on blood hyperviscosity. Am J Chin Med 1989;17(1-2):65-70.

688. Chen F, Nakashima N, Kimura I, Kimura M. [Hypoglycemic activity and mechanisms of extracts from mulberry leaves (folium mori) and cortex *mori radicis* in streptozotocin-induced diabetic mice]. Yakugaku Zasshi 1995 Jun;115(6):476-82. Abstract.

689. al-Harbi MM, Qureshi S, Raza M, et al. Gastric antiulcer and cytoprotective effect of *Commiphora molmol* in rats. J Ethnopharmacol 1997 Jan;55(2):141-50.

690. al-Harbi MM, Qureshi S, Ahmed MM, et al. Effect of *Commiphora molmol* (oleo-gum-resin) on the cytological and biochemical changes induced by cyclophosphamide in mice. Am J Chin Med 1994;22(1):77-82.

691. Elfellah MS, Akhter MH, Khan MT. Anti-hyperglycaemic effect of an extract of *Myrtus communis* in streptozotocin-induced diabetes in mice. J Ethnopharmacol 1984 Aug;11(3):275-81.

692. Tepel M, van der Giet M, Schwarzfeld C, et al. Prevention of radiographic-contrast-agent-induced reductions in renal function by acetylcysteine. N Engl J Med 2000 Jul 20;343(3):180-4.

353

693. Ruiz FJ, Salom MG, Ingles AC, et al. N-acetyl-L-cysteine potentiates depressor response to captopril and enalaprilat in SHRs. Am J Physiol 1994 Sep;267(3 Pt 2):R767-72.

694. D'Agostini F, Bagnasco M, Giunciuglio D, Albini A, De Flora S. Inhibition by oral N-acetylcysteine of doxorubicin-induced clastogenicity and alopecia, and prevention of primary tumors and lung micrometastases in mice. Int J Oncol 1998 Aug;13(2):217-24.

695. Tariq M, Morais C, Sobki S, Al Sulaiman M, Al Khader A. N-acetylcysteine attenuates cyclosporin-induced nephrotoxicity in rats. Nephrol Dial Transplant 1999 Apr;14(4):923-9.

696. Attri S, Rana SV, Vaiphei K, et al. Isoniazid- and rifampicin-induced oxidative hepatic injury—protection by N-acetylcysteine. Hum Exp Toxicol 2000 Sep;19(9):517-22.

697. Neri S, Ierna D, Antoci S, et al. Association of alpha-interferon and acetyl cysteine in patients with chronic C hepatitis. Panminerva Med 2000 Sep;42(3):187-92.

698. Bach SP, Williamson SE, Marshman E, et al. The antioxidant n-acetylcysteine increases 5-fluorouracil activity against colorectal cancer xenografts in nude mice. J Gastrointest Surg 2001 Jan-Feb;5(1):91-7.

699. Neuwelt EA, Pagel MA, Hasler BP, Deloughery TG, Muldoon LL. Therapeutic efficacy of aortic administration of N-acetylcysteine as a chemoprotectant against bone marrow toxicity after intracarotid administration of alkylators, with or without glutathione depletion in a rat model. Cancer Res 2001 Nov 1;61(21):7868-74.

700. Clark J. Acetaminophen poisoning and the use of intravenous N-acetylcysteine. Air Med J 2001 Jul-Aug;20(4):16-7.

701. Kaneto H, Kajimoto Y, Miyagawa J, et al. Beneficial effects of antioxidants in diabetes: possible protection of pancreatic beta-cells against glucose toxicity. Diabetes 1999 Dec;48(12):2398-406.

702. Chirkov YY, Horowitz JD. N-Acetylcysteine potentiates nitroglycerin-induced reversal of platelet aggregation. J Cardiovasc Pharmacol 1996 Sep;28(3):375-80.

703. Khosla P, Bhanwra S, Singh J, Seth S, Srivastava RK. A study of hypoglycaemic effects of Azadirachta indica (Neem) in normal and alloxan diabetic rabbits. Indian J Physiol Pharmacol 2000 Jan;44(1):69-74.

704. Chattopadhyay RR. Possible mechanism of antihyperglycemic effect of Azadirachta indica leaf extract: part V. J Ethnopharmacol 1999 Nov 30;67(3):373-6.

705. Saprionova N, Grinkevich I, Orlova L, Kucherova T. The content of vitamin K-1 and some trace elements in Urtica dioica L. Rastit Resur. 1989;25(2):243-7.

705. Tahri A, Yamani S, Legssyer A, et al. Acute diuretic, natriuretic and hypotensive effects of a continuous perfusion of

aqueous extract of *Urtica dioica* in the rat. J Ethnopharmacol 2000 Nov;73(1-2):95-100.

707. Stein U, Greyer H, Hentschel H. Nutmeg (myristicin) poisoning—report on a fatal case and a series of cases recorded by a poison information centre. Forensic Sci Int 2001 Apr 15;118(1):87-90.

708. Jeong HG, Yun CH. Induction of rat hepatic cytochrome P450 enzymes by myristicin. Biochem Biophys Res Commun 1995 Dec 26;217(3):966-71.

709. Connor J, Connor T, Marshall PB, Reid A, Turnbull MJ. The pharmacology of *Avena sativa*. J Pharm Pharmacol 1975 Feb;27(2):92-8.

710. Richter WO, Jacob BG, Schwandt P. Interaction between fibre and lovastatin. Lancet 1991 Sep 14;338(8768):706.

711. Smith JA, Madden T, Vijjeswarapu M, Newman RA. Inhibition of export of fibroblast growth factor-2 (FGF-2) from the prostate cancer cell lines PC3 and DU145 by Anvirzel and its cardiac glycoside component, oleandrin. Biochem Pharmacol 2001 Aug 15;62(4):469-72.

712. Teyssier C, Amiot MJ, Mondy N, et al. Effect of onion consumption by rats on hepatic drug-metabolizing enzymes. Food Chem Toxicol 2001 Oct;39(10):981-7.

713. Morimoto S, Suemori K, Moriwaki J, et al. Morphine metabolism in the opium poppy and its possible physiological function. Biochemical characterization of the morphine metabolite, bismorphine. J Biol Chem 2001 Oct 12;276(41):38179-84.

714. Sripanidkulchai B, Wongpanich V, Laupattarakasem P, Suwansaksri J, Jirakulsomchok D. Diuretic effects of selected Thai indigenous medicinal plants in rats. J Ethnopharmacol 2001 May;75(2-3):185-90.

715. Sulkowska M, Sulkowski S. Apoptosis-like changes in the lungs induced by cyclophosphamide and papain. I. An ultrastructural study. J Submicrosc Cytol Pathol 1998 Jan;30(1):105-16.

716. United States Department of Agriculture. Agricultural Research Service. Provisional table on the vitamin k content of foods, Revised 1994. HNIS/PT-104. http://www.nal.usda.gov/fnic/foodcomp/Data/Other/pt104.pdf.

717. Griffiths IB, Douglas RG. Phytophotodermatitis in pigs exposed to parsley (*Petroselinum crispum*). Vet Rec 2000 Jan 15;146(3):73-4.

718. Soulimani R, Younos C, Jarmouni S, et al. Behavioural effects of *Passiflora incarnata* L. and its indole alkaloid and flavonoid derivatives and maltol in the mouse. J Ethnopharmacol 1997 Jun;57(1):11-20.

719. Argento A, Tiraferri E, Marzaloni M. [Oral anticoagulants and medicinal plants. An emerging interaction]. Ann Ital Med Int 2000 Apr-Jun;15(2):139-43. Abstract.

720. Akhondzadeh S, Kashani L, Mobaseri M, et al. Passionflower in the treatment of opiates withdrawal: a double-blind randomized controlled trial. J Clin Pharm Ther 2001 Oct;26(5):369-73.

721. Dhawan K, Kumar S, Sharma A. Anxiolytic activity of aerial and underground parts of *Passiflora incarnata*. Fitoterapia 2001 Dec;72(8):922-6.

722. Preusch PC, Suttie JW. Lapachol inhibition of vitamin K epoxide reductase and vitamin K quinone reductase. Arch Biochem Biophys 1984 Nov 1;234(2):405-12.

723. Richter WO, Jacob BG, Schwandt P. Interaction between fibre and lovastatin. Lancet 1991 Sep 14;338(8768):706.

724. Holt S, Heading RC, Carter DC, et al. Effect of gel fibre on gastric emptying and absorption of glucose and paracetamol. Lancet 1979 Mar 24;1(8117):636-9.

725. Thomassen D, Slattery JT, Nelson SD. Menthofuran-dependent and independent aspects of pulegone hepatotoxicity: roles of glutathione. J Pharmacol Exp Ther 1990 May;253(2):567-72.

726. Noble RL. The discovery of the vinca alkaloids—chemotherapeutic agents against cancer. Biochem Cell Biol 1990 Dec;68(12):1344-51.

727. Bjornsson TD, Huang AT, Roth P, Jacob DS, Christenson R. Effects of high-dose cancer chemotherapy on the absorption of digoxin in two different formulations. Clin Pharmacol Ther 1986 Jan;39(1):25-8.

728. The European Agency for the Evaluation of Medicinal Products. Veterinary Medicines Evaluation Unit. Committee for Veterinary Medicinal Products. *Adonis vernalis* summary report. December 1998. http://www.emea.eu.int/pdfs/vet/mrls/054398en.pdf.

729. Rovenska E, Svik K, Stancikova M, Rovensky J. Inhibitory effect of enzyme therapy and combination therapy with cyclosporin A on collagen-induced arthritis. Clin Exp Rheumatol 2001 May-Jun;19(3):303-9.

730. Srividya N, Periwal S. Diuretic, hypotensive and hypoglycaemic effect of *Phyllanthus amarus*. Indian J Exp Biol 1995 Nov;33(11):861-4.

731. Plantain. The Reiew of Natural Products. Jan 1998:4.

732. Trejo-Gonzalez A, Gabriel-Ortiz G, Puebla-Perez AM, Huizar-Contreras MD, et al. A purified extract from prickly pear cactus (*Opuntia fuliginosa*) controls experimentally induced diabetes in rats. J Ethnopharmacol 1996 Dec;55(1):27-33.

733. Garcia JJ, Fernandez N, Diez MJ, et al. Influence of two dietary fibers in the oral bioavailability and other pharmacokinetic parameters of ethinyloestradiol. Contraception 2000 Nov;62(5):253-7.

734. Nordstrom M, Melander A, Robertsson E, Steen B. Influence of wheat bran and of a bulk-forming ispaghula cathartic on the bioavailability of digoxin in geriatric in-patients. Drug Nutr Interact 1987;5(2):67-9.

735. Maciejko JJ, Brazg R, Shah A, Patil S, Rubenfire M. Psyllium for the reduction of cholestyramine-associated gastrointestinal symptoms in the treatment of primary hypercholesterolemia. Arch Fam Med 1994 Nov;3(11):955-60.

736. Spence JD, Huff MW, Heidenheim P, et al. Combination therapy with colestipol and psyllium mucilloid in patients with hyperlipidemia. Ann Intern Med 1995 Oct 1;123(7):493-9.

737. Turley SD, Daggy BP, Dietschy JM. Effect of feeding psyllium and cholestyramine in combination on low density lipoprotein metabolism and fecal bile acid excretion in hamsters with dietary-induced hypercholesterolemia. J Cardiovasc Pharmacol 1996 Jan;27(1):71-9.

738. Sierra M, Garcia JJ, Fernandez N, et al. Effects of ispaghula husk and guar gum on postprandial glucose and insulin concentrations in healthy subjects. Eur J Clin Nutr 2001 Apr;55(4):235-43.

739. Cavaliere H, Floriano I, Medeiros-Neto G. Gastrointestinal side effects of orlistat may be prevented by concomitant prescription of natural fibers (psyllium mucilloid). Int J Obes Relat Metab Disord 2001 Jul;25(7):1095-9.

740. Frati Munari AC, Benitez Pinto W, Raul Ariza Andraca C, Casarrubias M. Lowering glycemic index of food by acarbose and *Plantago psyllium* mucilage. Arch Med Res 1998 Summer;29(2):137-41

741. Perlman BB. Interaction between lithium salts and ispaghula husk. Lancet 1990 Feb 17;335(8686):416.

742. Rodriguez-Moran M, Guerrero-Romero F, Lazcano-Burciaga G. Lipid- and glucose-lowering efficacy of *Plantago psyllium* in type II diabetes. J Diabetes Complications 1998 Sep-Oct;12(5):273-8.

743. Anderson JW, Allgood LD, Turner J, Oeltgen PR, Daggy BP. Effects of psyllium on glucose and serum lipid responses in men with type 2 diabetes and hypercholesterolemia. Am J Clin Nutr 1999 Oct;70(4):466-73.

744. Li Y, Wang E, Patten CJ, Chen L, Yang CS. Effects of flavonoids on cytochrome P450-dependent acetaminophen metabolism in rats and human liver microsomes. Drug Metab Dispos 1994 Jul-Aug;22(4):566-71.

745. Widyarini S, Spinks N, Husband AJ, Reeve VE. Isoflavonoid compounds from red clover (Trifolium pratense) protect from inflammation and immune suppression induced by UV radiation. Photochem Photobiol 2001 Sep;74(3):465-70.

746. Kanathur N, Mathai MG, Byrd RP Jr, Fields CL, Roy TM. Simvastatin-diltiazem drug interaction resulting in rhabdomyolysis and hepatitis. Tenn Med 2001 Sep;94(9):339-41.

747. Wakatsuki A, Okatani Y, Ikenoue N. Effects of combination therapy with estrogen plus simvastatin on lipoprotein metabolism in postmenopausal women with type IIa hypercholesterolemia. Atherosclerosis 2000 May;150(1):103-11.

748. Lin JC, Ito MK, Stolley SN, Morreale AP, Marcus DB. The effect of converting from pravastatin to simvastatin on the pharmacodynamics of warfarin. J Clin Pharmacol 1999 Jan;39(1):86-90.

749. Tavintharan S, Kashyap ML. The benefits of niacin in atherosclerosis. Curr Atheroscler Rep 2001 Jan;3(1):74-82.

750. SoRelle R. Niacin-simvastatin combination benefits patients with coronary artery disease. Circulation 2001 Dec 11;104(24):E9050-60.

751. Heber D, Yip I, Ashley JM, et al. Cholesterol-lowering effects of a proprietary Chinese red-yeast-rice dietary supplement. Am J Clin Nutr 1999 Feb;69(2):231-6.

752. Federman DG, Hussain F, Walters AB. Fatal rhabdomyolysis caused by lipid-lowering therapy. South Med J 2001 Oct;94(10):1023-6.

753. Pataik GK, Kohler E. Pharmacological investigation on asclepin—a new cardenolide from Asclepias currassavica. Part II. Comparative studies on the inotropic and toxic effects of asclepin, g-strophanthin, digoxin and digitoxin). Arzneimittelforschung 1978;28(8):1368-72.

754. Gau JP, Lin CK, Lee SS, Wang SR. The lack of antiplatelet effect of crude extracts from ganoderma lucidum on HIV-positive hemophiliacs. Am J Chin Med 1990;18(3-4):175-9.

755. Komoda Y, Shimizu M, Sonoda Y, Sato Y. Ganoderic acid and its derivatives as cholesterol synthesis inhibitors. Chem Pharm Bull (Tokyo) 1989 Feb;37(2):531-3.

756. Yoon SY, Eo SK, Kim YS, Lee CK, Han SS. Antimicrobial activity of Ganoderma lucidum extract alone and in combination with some antibiotics. Arch Pharm Res 1994 Dec;17(6):438-42.

757. Kim YS, Eo SK, Oh KW, Lee C, Han SS. Antiherpetic activities of acidic protein bound polysacchride isolated from Ganoderma lucidum alone and in combinations with interferons. J Ethnopharmacol 2000 Oct;72(3):451-8.

758. Bao X, Duan J, Fang X, Fang J. Chemical modifications of the (1—>3)-alpha-D-glucan from spores of Ganoderma lucidum and investigation of their physicochemical properties and immunological activity. Carbohydr Res 2001 Nov 8;336(2):127-40.

759. Hikino H, Ishiyama M, Suzuki Y, Konno C. Mechanisms of hypoglycemic activity of ganoderan B: a glycan of Ganoderma lucidum fruit bodies. Planta Med 1989 Oct;55(5):423-8.

760. Oh KW, Lee CK, Kim YS, Eo SK, Han SS. Antiherpetic activities of acidic protein bound polysacchride isolated from Ganoderma lucidum alone and in combinations with acyclovir and vidarabine. J Ethnopharmacol 2000 Sep;72(1-2):221-7.

761. Su C, Shiao M, Wang C. Potentiation of ganodermic acid S on prostaglandin E(1)-induced cyclic AMP elevation in human platelets. Thromb Res 2000 Jul 15;99(2):135-45.

762. Rossi T, Melegari M, Bianchi A, Albasini A, Vampa G. Sedative, anti-inflammatory and anti-diuretic effects induced in rats by essential oils of varieties of *Anthemis nobilis*: a comparative study. Pharmacol Res Commun 1988 Dec;20 Suppl 5:71-4.

763. Debersac P, Heydel JM, Amiot MJ, et al. Induction of cytochrome P450 and/or detoxication enzymes by various extracts of rosemary: description of specific patterns. Food Chem Toxicol 2001 Sep;39(9):907-18.

764. Fahim FA, Esmat AY, Fadel HM, Hassan KF. Allied studies on the effect of *Rosmarinus officinalis* L. on experimental hepatotoxicity and mutagenesis. Int J Food Sci Nutr 1999 Nov;50(6):413-27.

765. Haloui M, Louedec L, Michel JB, Lyoussi B. Experimental diuretic effects of *Rosmarinus officinalis* and *Centaurium erythraea*. J Ethnopharmacol 2000 Aug;71(3):465-72.

766. Plouzek CA, Ciolino HP, Clarke R, Yeh GC. Inhibition of P-glycoprotein activity and reversal of multidrug resistance in vitro by rosemary extract. Eur J Cancer 1999 Oct;35(10):1541-5.

767. Kamel MS, Assaf MH, Abe Y, et al. Cardiac glycosides from *Cryptostegia grandiflora*. Phytochemistry 2001 Oct;58(4):537-42.

768. Ojala T, Vuorela P, Kiviranta J, Vuorela H, Hiltunen R. A bioassay using *Artemia salina* for detecting phototoxicity of plant coumarins. Planta Med 1999 Dec;65(8):715-8.

769. Rhiouani H, Lyoussi B, Settaf A, Cherrah Y, Hassar M. [Antihypertensive effect of *Herniaria glabra* saponins in the spontaneously hypertensive rat] Ann Pharm Fr 2001 May;59(3):211-4. Abstract.

770. Sakina MR, Dandiya PC, Hamdard ME, Hameed A. Preliminary psychopharmacological evaluation of *Ocimum sanctum* leaf extract. J Ethnopharmacol 1990 Feb;28(2):143-50.

771. Balanehru S, Nagarajan B. Intervention of adriamycin induced free radical damage. Biochem Int 1992 Dec;28(4):735-44.

772. Vats V, Grover JK, Rathi SS. Evaluation of anti-hyperglycemic and hypoglycemic effect of *Trigonella foenum-graecum* Linn, *Ocimum sanctum* Linn and *Pterocarpus marsupium* Linn in normal and alloxanized diabetic rats. J Ethnopharmacol 2002 Feb;79(1):95-100.

773. Singh S, Rehan HM, Majumdar DK. Effect of *Ocimum sanctum* fixed oil on blood pressure, blood clotting time and pentobarbitone-induced sleeping time. J Ethnopharmacol 2001 Dec;78(2-3):139-43.

774. Sharma M, Kishore K, Gupta SK, Joshi S, Arya DS. Cardioprotective potential of *Ocimum sanctum* in

358

775. Agrawal P, Rai V, Singh RB. Randomized placebo-controlled, single blind trial of holy basil leaves in patients with noninsulin-dependent diabetes mellitus. Int J Clin Pharmacol Ther 1996 Sep;34(9):406-9.

776. Panda S, Kar A. Ocimum sanctum leaf extract in the regulation of thyroid function in the male mouse. Pharmacol Res 1998 Aug;38(2):107-10.

777. Ohno I, Shibasaki T, Nakano H, et al. Effect of sairei-to on gentamicin nephrotoxicity in rats. Arch Toxicol 1993;67(2):145-7.

778. Mertz W, Roginski EE, Gordon WA, et al. In vitro potentiation of insulin by ash from saltbush (Atriplex halimus). Arch Int Pharmacodyn Ther 1973 Nov;206(1):121-8.

779. Di Rocco A, Rogers JD, Brown R, Werner P, Bottiglieri T. S-Adenosyl-Methionine improves depression in patients with Parkinson's disease in an open-label clinical trial. Mov Disord 2000 Nov;15(6):1225-9.

780. Benson R, Crowell B, Hill B, Doonquah K, Charlton C. The effects of L-dopa on the activity of methionine adenosyl-transferase: relevance to L-dopa therapy and tolerance. Neurochem Res 1993 Mar;18(3):325-30.

781. Fernández E, Galan AI, Moran D, et al. Reversal of cyclosporine-A-induced alterations in biliary secretion by S-adenosyl-L-methionine in rats. J Pharmacol Exp Ther 1995 Oct;275(1):442-9.

782. Muriel P, Castro V. Effects of S-adenosyl-L-methionine and interferon-alpha2b on liver damage induced by bile duct ligation in rats. J Appl Toxicol 1998 Mar-Apr;18(2):143-7.

783. Di Padova C, Tritapepe R, Di Padova F, Frezza M, Stramentinoli G. S-adenosyl-L-methionine antagonizes oral contraceptive-induced bile cholesterol supersaturation in healthy women: preliminary report of a controlled randomized trial. Am J Gastroenterol 1984 Dec;79(12):941-4.

784. Carrasco J, Perez-Mateo M, Gutierrez T, et al. Effect of different doses of S-adenosyl-L-methionine on paracetamol hepatotoxicity in a mouse model. Methods Find Exp Clin Pharmacol 2000 Dec;22(10):737-40.

785. Berlanga C, Ortega-Soto HA, Ontiveros M, Senties H. Efficacy of S-adenosyl-l-methionine in speeding the onset of action of imipramine. Psychiatry Res 1992 Dec;44(3):257-62.

786. Kumaravelu P, Dakshinamoorthy DP, Subramaniam S, Devaraj H, Devaraj NS. Effect of eugenol on drug-metabolizing enzymes of carbon tetrachloride-intoxicated rat liver. Biochem Pharmacol 1995 May 26;49(11):1703-7.

787. Rompelberg CJ, Verhagen H, van Bladeren PJ. Effects of the naturally occurring alkenylbenzenes eugenol and trans-anethole on drug-metabolizing enzymes in the rat liver. Food Chem Toxicol 1993 Sep;31(9):637-45.

isoproterenol induced myocardial infarction in rats. Mol Cell Biochem 2001 Sep;225(1-):75-83.

788. Ioannides C, Delaforge M, Parke DV. Interactions of safrole and isosafrole and their metabolites with cytochromes P-450. Chem Biol Interact 1985 May;53(3):303-11.

789. Cheema P, El-Mefty O, Jazieh AR. Intraoperative haemorrhage associated with the use of extract of Saw Palmetto herb: a case report and review of literature. J Intern Med 2001 Aug;250(2):167-9.

790. Di Silverio F, Monti S, Sciarra A, et al. Effects of long-term treatment with *Serenoa repens* (Permixon) on the concentrations and regional distribution of androgens and epidermal growth factor in benign prostatic hyperplasia. Prostate 1998 Oct 1;37(2):77-83.

791. el-Sheikh MM, Dakkak MR, Saddique A. The effect of Permixon on androgen receptors. Acta Obstet Gynecol Scand 1988;67(5):397-9.

792. Northover BJ. Effect of pre-treating rat atria with potassium channel blocking drugs on the electrical and mechanical responses to phenylephrine. Biochem Pharmacol 1994 Jun 15;47(12):2163-9.

793. Flockhart, D. Cytochrome P450 drug interaction table. http://medicine.iupui.edu/flockhart/.

794. Kako M, Miura T, Nishiyama Y, et al. Hypoglycemic effect of the rhizomes of *Polygala senega* in normal and diabetic mice and its main component, the triterpenoid glycoside senegin-II. Planta Med 1996 Oct;62(5):440-3.

795. Gordon M, Guralnik M, Kaneko Y, et al. A phase II controlled study of a combination of the immune modulator, lentinan, with didanosine (ddI) in HIV patients with CD4 cells of 200-500/mm3. J Med 1995;26(5-6):193-207.

796. Hokama Y, Hokama JL. In vitro inhibition of platelet aggregation with low dalton compounds from aqueous dialysates of edible fungi. Res Commun Chem Pathol Pharmacol 1981 Jan;31(1):177-80.

797. Qing ZJ, Ming QX, Zhong TF. Clinical evaluation of anti-tumor effects of lentinan combined with chemotherapy in the treatment of various malignancies. Gan To Kagaku Ryoho 1997 May;24 Suppl 1:1-8.

798. Nakagawa A, Yamaguchi T, Takao T, Amano H. [Five cases of drug-induced pneumonitis due to Sho-saiko-to or interferon-alpha or both.] Nihon Kyobu Shikkan Gakkai Zasshi 1995;Dec;33(12):1361-1366.

799. Piras G, Makino M, Baba M. Sho-saiko-to, a traditional Kampo medicine, enhances the anti-HIV-1 activity of lamivudine (3TC) in vitro. Microbiol Immunol 1997;41(10):835-9.

800. Ueng YF, Shyu CC, Lin YL, et al. Effects of baicalein and wogonin on drug-metabolizing enzymes in C57BL/6J mice. Life Sci 2000 Sep 22;67(18):2189-200.

801. Goto M, Hayashi M, Todoroki T, Seyama Y, Yamashita S. [Effects of traditional Chinese medicines (dai-saiko-to,

361 sho-saiko-to and hachimi-zio-gan) on spontaneously diabetic rat (WBN/Kob) with experimentally induced lipid and mineral disorders]. Nippon Yakurigaku Zasshi 1992 Oct;100(4):353-8. Abstract.

802. Vereshchagin IA, Geskina EN, Bukhteeva ER. [Increased effectiveness of antibiotic therapy with adaptogens in dysentery and *Proteus* infection in children]. Antibiotiki 1982 Jan;27(1):65-9. Abstract.

803. Hikino H, Takahashi M, Otake K, Konno C. Isolation and hypoglycemic activity of eleutherans A, B, C, D, E, F, and G: glycans of *Eleutherococcus senticosus* roots. J Nat Prod 1986 Mar-Apr;49(2):293-7.

804. Medon PJ, Ferguson PW, Watson CF. Effects of *Eleutherococcus senticosus* extracts on hexobarbital metabolism in vivo and in vitro. J Ethnopharmacol 1984 Apr;10(2):235-41.

805. Hacker B, Medon PJ. Cytotoxic effects of *Eleutherococcus senticosus* aqueous extracts in combination with N6-(delta 2-isopentenyl)-adenosine and 1-beta-D-arabinofuranosylcytosine against L1210 leukemia cells. J Pharm Sci 1984 Feb;73(2):270-2.

806. Martini MC, Dancisak BB, Haggans CJ, Thomas W, Slavin JL. Effects of soy intake on sex hormone metabolism in premenopausal women. Nutr Cancer 1999;34(2):133-9.

807. Khoshyomn S, Manske GC, Lew SM, Wald SL, Penar PL. Synergistic action of genistein and cisplatin on growth inhibition and cytotoxicity of human medulloblastoma cells. Pediatr Neurosurg 2000 Sep;33(3):123-31.

808. Jabbar MA, Larrea J, Shaw RA. Abnormal thyroid function tests in infants with congenital hypothyroidism: the influence of soy-based formula. J Am Coll Nutr 1997 Jun;16(3):280-2.

809. Persky VW, Turyk ME, Wang L, et al. Effect of soy protein on endogenous hormones in postmenopausal women. Am J Clin Nutr 2002 Jan;75(1):145-53.

810. Shulman KI, Walker SE. Refining the MAOI diet: tyramine content of pizzas and soy products. J Clin Psychiatry 1999 Mar;60(3):191-3.

811. Knight D, Eden J. A review of the clinical effects of phytoestrogens. *Obstet Gynecol.* 1996;87:897-904.

812. Bell DS, Ovalle F. Use of soy protein supplement and resultant need for increased dose of levothyroxine. Endocr Pract 2001 May-Jun;7(3):193-4.

813. Hiroyuki F, Tomohide Y, Kazunori O. Efficacy and safety of Touchi extract, an alpha-glucosidase inhibitor derived from fermented soybeans, in non-insulin-dependent diabetic mellitus. J Nutr Biochem 2001 Jun;12(6):351-356.

814. Ahmed SM, Banner NR, Dubrey SW. Low cyclosporin-A level due to Saint-John's-wort in heart transplant patients. J Heart Lung Transplant 2001 Jul;20(7):795.

815. Barone GW, Gurley BJ, Ketel BL, et al. Drug interaction between St. John's wort and cyclosporine. Ann Pharmacother. 2000 Sep;34(9):1013-6.

816. Beckman SE, Sommi RW, Switzer J. Consumer use of St. John's wort: a survey on effectiveness, safety, and tolerability. Pharmacotherapy. 2000 May;20(5):568-74.

817. Beer AM, Ostermann T. [St. John's wort: interaction with cyclosporine increases risk of rejection for the kidney transplant and raises daily cost of medication.] Med Klin 2001 Aug 15;96(8):480-3. Abstract.

818. Breidenbach T, Hoffmann MW, Becker T, et al. Drug interaction of St John's wort with cyclosporin. Lancet. 2000 May 27;355(9218):1912.

819. Breidenbach T, Kliem V, Burg M, et al. Letter to the editor. Correspondence. Profound drop of cyclosporin A whole blood trough levels caused by St. John's wort (*Hypericum perforatum*) Transplantation. 2000 May 27;69(10):2229-30.

820. Brockmoller J, Reum T, Bauer S, et al. Hypericin and pseudohypericin: pharmacokinetics and effects on photosensitivity in humans. Pharmacopsychiatry. 1997 Sep;30 Suppl 2:94-101.

821. Burstein A, Horton R, Dunn T, et al. Lack of effect of St. John's wort on carbamazepine pharmacokinetics in healthy volunteers. Clin Pharmacol Ther. 2000;68(6):605-12.

822. Carson SW, Hill-Zabala CE, Blalock SB, et al. Constituents of St. John's wort inhibit cytochrome P450 3A4 and P450 reductase activity in human liver microsomes. 2001 Annual Meeting of the American Society for Clinical Pharmacology and Therapeutics. Orlando, Florida, USA. March 6-10, 2001. Clin Pharmacol Ther. 2001 Feb;69(2):Abstract PI-28.

823. Carson SW, Hill-Zabala CE, Roberts SH, et al. Inhibitory effect of methanolic solution of St. John's wort (*hypericum perforatum*) on cytochrome P450 3A4 activity in human liver microsomes. 2000 Annual Meeting of the American Society for Clinical Pharmacology and Therapeutics. Los Angeles, California, USA. March 14-18, 2000. Clin Pharmacol Ther. 2000 Feb;67(2):Abstract PI-39.

824. de Maat MM, Hoetelmans RM, Math t RA, et al. Drug interaction between St John's wort and nevirapine. AIDS 2001 Feb 16;15(3):420-1.

825. Demott K. St. John's wort tied to serotonin syndrome. Clin Psychiatry News 1998;26:28.

826. Dürr D, Stieger B, Kullak-Ublick G, et al. St. John's wort induces intestinal P-glycoprotein/MDR1 and intestinal and hepatic CYP 3A4. Clin Pharmacol Ther. 2000;68(6):598-604.

827. Ereshefsky B, Gerwertz N, Lam Y, et al. Determination of SJW differential metabolism at CYP2D6 and

CYP3A4, using dextromethorphan probe methodology. 1999:poster 130.

828. Gewertz N, Ereshefsky B, Lam Y, et al. Determination of the differential effects of St. John's wort on the CYP1A2 and NAT2 metabolic pathways using caffeine probe methodology. 39th New Clinical Drug Evaluation Unit Program Annual Meeting. 1999:poster 131.

829. Hussain MD, Teixeira MG. Saint John's wort and analgesia: Effect of Saint John's wort on morphine induced analgesia. 2000 AAPS Annual meeting, November 20, 2000. Abstract.

830. Irefin S, Sprung J. A possible cause of cardiovascular collapse during anesthesia: long-term use of St. John's wort. J Clin Anesth. 2000 Sep;12(6):498-9.

831. Jacobson JM, Feinman L, Liebes L, et al. Pharmacokinetics, safety, and antiviral effects of hypericin, a derivative of St. John's wort plant, in patients with chronic hepatitis C virus infection. Antimicrob Agents Chemother 2001 Feb;45(2):517-24.

832. Johne A, Schmider J, Brockmoller J, et al. Decreased plasma levels of amitriptyline and its metabolites on comedication with an extract from St. John's wort (Hypericum perforatum). J Clin Psychopharmacol 2002 Feb;22(1):46-54.

833. Karliova M, Treichel U, Malago M, et al. Interaction of Hypericum perforatum (St. John's wort) with cyclosporin A metabolism in a patient after liver transplantation. J Hepatol. 2000;33:853-5.

834. Lam Y. St. John's wort may decrease efficacy of digoxin. Psychopharmacology Update. 1999;10:2-3.

835. Lane-Brown M. Photosensitivity associated with herbal preparations of St. John's wort (Hypericum perforatum). Med J Aust. 2000;172(6):302.

836. Mai I, Kruger H, Budde K, et al. Hazardous pharmacokinetic interaction of St. John's wort (Hypericum perforatum) with the immunosuppressant cyclosporin. Int J Clin Pharmacol Ther. 2000;38(10):500-2.

837. Maurer A, Johne A, Bauer S, et al. Interaction of St. John's wort with extract with phenprocoumon. Eur J Clin Pharmacol. 1999;55:A22.

838. Moore L, Goodwin B, Jones S, Wisely G, Serabjit-Singh C, Kliewer S. St. John's wort induces hepatic drug metabolism through activation of the pregnane X receptor. Proc Natl Acad Sci U S A. 2000;97:7500-2.

839. Moschella C, Jaber BL. Interaction between cyclosporine and Hypericum perforatum (St. John's wort) after organ transplantation. Am J Kidney Dis 2001 Nov;38(5):1105-7.

840. Nathan P. The experimental and clinical pharmacology of St John's Wort (*Hypericum perforatum* L.). Mol Psychiatry. 1999 Jul;4(4):333-8. Review.

841. Nebel A, Schneider B, Baker R, Kroll D. Potential metabolic interaction between St. John's wort and theophylline. Ann Pharmacother. 1999;33(4):502.

842. Obach R. Inhibition of human cytochrome P450 enzymes by constituents of St. John's wort, an herbal preparation used in the treatment of depression. Pharmacol Exp Ther. 2000;294:88-95.

843. Okpanyi SN, Weischer ML. [Animal experiments on the psychotropic action of a *Hypericum* extract]. Arzneimittelforschung. 1987 Jan;37(1):10-3. (abstract).

844. Peebles KA, Baker RK, Kurz EU, Schneider BJ, Kroll DJ. Catalytic inhibition of human DNA topoisomerase IIalpha by hypericin, a naphthodianthrone from St. John's wort (*Hypericum perforatum*). Biochem Pharmacol 2001 Oct 15;62(8):1059-70.

845. Rey JM, Walter G. *Hypericum perforatum* (St John's wort) in depression: pest or blessing? Med J Aust. 1998 Dec 7-21;169(11-12):583-6. Review.

846. Roby C, Anderson G, Kantor E, Dryer D, Burstein A. St. John's Wort: effect on CYP3A4 activity. Clin Pharmacol Ther. 2000:67;451-7.

847. Schempp CM, Muller K, Winghofer B, Schulte-Monting J, Simon JC. Single-dose and steady-state administration of *Hypericum perforatum* extract (St John's Wort) does not influence skin sensitivity to UV radiation, visible light, and solar-simulated radiation. Arch Dermatol 2001 Apr;137(4):512-3.

848. Sugimoto Ki K, Ohmori M, Tsuruoka S, et al. Different effects of St John's Wort on the pharmacokinetics of simvastatin and pravastatin. Clin Pharmacol Ther 2001 Dec;70(6):518-24.

849. Walter G, Rey JM, Harding A. Psychiatrists' experience and views regarding St John's Wort and 'alternative' treatments. Aust N Z J Psychiatry. 2000 Dec;34(6):992-6.

850. Wang Z, Gorski JC, Hamman MA, et al. The effects of St John's wort (*Hypericum perforatum*) on human cytochrome P450 activity. Clin Pharmacol Ther 2001 Oct;70(4):317-26.

851. Wentworth JM, Agostini M, Love J, et al. St John's wort, a herbal antidepressant, activates the steroid X receptor. J Endocrinol. 2000 Sep;166(3):R11-6.

852. Dresser G, Schwarz U, Wilkinson G, et al. St. John's wort induces intestinal and hepatic CYP3A4 and

364

P-glycoprotein in healthy volunteers. 2001 Annual Meeting of the American Society for Clinical Pharmacology and Therapeutics. Orlando, Florida. USA. March 6–10, 2001. Clin Pharmacol Ther. Abstract.

853. Gordon J. SSRIs and St. John's wort: possible toxicity? (letter) Am Fam Physician. 1998;57:950,953.

854. Yue Q, Bergquist C, Gerden B. Commentary. Lancet. 2000;355(9203):576-7.

855. Kim HS, Zhang YH, Fang LH, Yun YP, Lee HK. Effects of tetrandrine and fangchinoline on human platelet aggregation and thromboxane B2 formation. J Ethnopharmacol 1999 Aug;66(2):241-6.

856. Weinsberg F, Bickmeyer U, Wiegand H. Effects of tetrandrine on calcium channel currents of bovine chromaffin cells. Neuropharmacology 1994 Jul;33(7):885-90.

857. Houghton PJ, Skari KP. The effect on blood clotting of some west African plants used against snakebite. J Ethnopharmacol 1994 Oct;44(2):99-108.

858. Davies MK, Hollman A. Digitalis and strophanthus—cardiac glycosides. Heart 1998 Jul;80(1):4.

859. Kusamran WR, Ratanavila A, Tepsuwan A. Effects of neem flowers, Thai and Chinese bitter gourd fruits and sweet basil leaves on hepatic monooxygenases and glutathione S-transferase activities, and in vitro metabolic activation of chemical carcinogens in rats. Food Chem Toxicol 1998 Jun;36(6):475-84.

860. Ahmed M, Shikha HA, Sadhu SK, Rahman MT, Datta BK. Analgesic, diuretic, and anti-inflammatory principles from *Scoparia dulcis*. Pharmazie 2001 Aug;56(8):657-60.

861. Nur-E-Alam M, Rokeya B, Chowdhury N. Effects of three Nepalese plants on serum glucose levels of normal and diabetic model rats. Diabetologia. 1997;40(Suppl. 1):A369.

862. Stirling Y. Warfarin-induced changes in procoagulant and anticoagulant proteins. Blood Coagul Fibrinolysis 1995 Jul;6(5):361-73.

863. Yaniv Z, Dafni A, Friedman J, Palevitch D. Plants used for the treatment of diabetes in Israel. J Ethnopharmacol 1987 Mar-Apr;19(2):145-51.

864. Wanwimoluruk S, Wong SM, Zhang H, Coville PF, Walker RJ. Metabolism of quinine in man: identification of a major metabolite, and effects of smoking and rifampicin pretreatment. J Pharm Pharmacol 1995 Nov;47(11):957-63.

865. Chetty M, Miller R, Moodley SV. Smoking and body weight influence the clearance of chlorpromazine. Eur J Clin Pharmacol 1994;46(6):523-6.

866. Miller LG. Cigarettes and drug therapy: pharmacokinetic and pharmacodynamic considerations. Clin Pharm 1990 Feb;9(2):125-35.

867. Gomita Y, Eto K, Furuno K, Araki Y. Effects of exposure to standard- and nicotine-reduced-cigarette smoke on pharmacokinetics of theophylline and cimetidine in rats. J Pharm Sci 1992 Nov;81(11):1132-5.

868. Zevin S, Benowitz NL. Drug interactions with tobacco smoking. An update. Clin Pharmacokinet 1999 Jun;36(6):425-38.

869. Callaghan JT, Bergstrom RF, Ptak LR, Beasley CM. Olanzapine. Pharmacokinetic and pharmacodynamic profile. Clin Pharmacokinet 1999 Sep;37(3):177-93.

870. Bondy SC, Ali SF, Kleinman MT. Exposure of mice to tobacco smoke attenuates the toxic effect of methamphetamine on dopamine systems. Toxicol Lett 2000 Dec 20;118(1-2):43-6.

871. Jokinen MJ, Olkkola KT, Ahonen J, Neuvonen PJ. Effect of rifampin and tobacco smoking on the pharmacokinetics of ropivacaine. Clin Pharmacol Ther 2001 Oct;70(4):344-50.

872. Decreased clinical efficacy of propoxyphene in cigarette smokers. Clin Pharmacol Ther 1973 Mar-Apr;14(2):259-63.

873. Hokama Y, Hokama JL. In vitro inhibition of platelet aggregation with low dalton compounds from aqueous dialysates of edible fungi. Res Commun Chem Pathol Pharmacol 1981 Jan;31(1):177-80.

874. Karan RS, Bhargava VK, Garg SK. Effect of trikatu, an Ayurvedic prescription, on the pharmacokinetic profile of rifampicin in rabbits. J Ethnopharmacol 1999 Mar;64(3):259-64.

875. Ranjan D, Johnston TD, Wu G, Elliott L, et al. Curcumin blocks cyclosporine A-resistant CD28 costimulatory pathway of human T-cell proliferation. J Surg Res 1998 Jul 1;77(2):174-8.

876. Verma SP, Salamone E, Goldin B. Curcumin and genistein, plant natural products, show synergistic inhibitory effects on the growth of human breast cancer MCF-7 cells induced by estrogenic pesticides. Biochem Biophys Res Commun 1997 Apr 28;233(3):692-6.

877. Rafatullah S, Tariq M, Al-Yahya MA, Mossa JS, Ageel AM. Evaluation of turmeric (*Curcuma longa*) for gastric and duodenal antiulcer activity in rats. J Ethnopharmacol 1990 Apr;29(1):25-34.

878. Shoba G, Joy D, Joseph T, et al. Influence of piperine on the pharmacokinetics of curcumin in animals and human volunteers. Planta Med 1998 May;64(4):353-6.

879. Thapliyal R, Maru GB. Inhibition of cytochrome P450 isozymes by curcumins in vitro and in vivo. Food Chem Toxicol 2001 Jun;39(6):541-7.

880. Thapliyal R, Deshpande SS, Maru GB. Effects of turmeric on the activities of benzo(a)pyrene-induced cytochrome P-450 isozymes. J Environ Pathol Toxicol Oncol 2001;20(1):59-63.

881. Srivastava KC, Bordia A, Verma SK. Curcumin, a major component of food spice turmeric (*Curcuma longa*) inhibits aggregation and alters eicosanoid metabolism in human blood platelets. Prostaglandins Leukot Essent Fatty Acids 1995 Apr;52(4):223-7.

882. Srivastava KC. Extracts from two frequently consumed spices—cumin (*Cuminum cyminum*) and turmeric (*Curcuma longa*)—inhibit platelet aggregation and alter eicosanoid biosynthesis in human blood platelets. Prostaglandins Leukot Essent Fatty Acids 1989 Jul;37(1):57-64.

883. Shimizu M, Shiota S, Mizushima T, et al. Marked potentiation of activity of beta-lactams against methicillin-resistant *Staphylococcus aureus* by Corilagin. Antimicrob Agents Chemother 2001 Nov;45(11):3198-201.

884. Matsuda H, Nakata H, Tanaka T, Kubo M. [Pharmacological study on *Arctostaphylos uva-ursi* (L.) Spreng. II. Combined effects of arbutin and prednisolone or dexamethasone on immuno-inflammation.] Yakugaku Zasshi 1990 Jan;110(1):68-76. Abstract.

885. Matsuda H, Tanaka T, Kubo M. [Pharmacological studies on leaf of *Arctostaphylos uva-ursi* (L.) Spreng. III. Combined effect of arbutin and indomethacin on immuno-inflammation.] Yakugaku Zasshi 1991 Apr-May;111(4-5):253-8. Abstract.

886. Matsuda H, Nakamura S, Tanaka T, Kubo M. [Pharmacological studies on leaf of *Arctostaphylos uva-ursi* (L.) Spreng. V. Effect of water extract from *Arctostaphylos uva-ursi* (L.) Spreng. (bearberry leaf) on the antiallergic and antiinflammatory activities of dexamethasone ointment.] Yakugaku Zasshi 1992 Sep;112(9):673-7. Abstract.

887. Ortiz JG, Nieves-Natal J, Chavez P. Effects of *Valeriana officinalis* extracts on [3H]flunitrazepam binding, synaptosomal [3H]GABA uptake, and hippocampal [3H]GABA release. Neurochem Res 1999 Nov;24(11):1373-8.

888. Houghton PJ. The scientific basis for the reputed activity of Valerian. J Pharm Pharmacol 1999 May;51(5):505-12.

889. Andreatini R, Leite JR. Effect of valepotriates on the behavior of rats in the elevated plus-maze during diazepam withdrawal. Eur J Pharmacol 1994 Aug 1;260(2-3):233-5.

890. Leuschner J, Muller J, Rudmann M. Characterisation of the central nervous depressant activity of a commercially available valerian root extract. Arzneimittelforschung 1993 Jun;43(6):638-41.

891. Chen L, Mohr SN, Yang CS. Decrease of plasma and urinary oxidative metabolites of acetaminophen after consumption of watercress by human volunteers. Clin Pharmacol Ther 1996 Dec;60(6):651-60.

892. Leclercq I, Desager JP, Horsmans Y. Inhibition of chlorzoxazone metabolism, a clinical probe for CYP2E1, by a single ingestion of watercress. Clin Pharmacol Ther 1998 Aug;64(2):144-9.

893. Hamilton SM, Teel RW. Effects of isothiocyanates on cytochrome P-450 1A1 and 1A2 activity and on the mutagenicity of heterocyclic amines. Anticancer Res 1996 Nov-Dec;16(6B):3597-602.

894. Gilani AH, Shaheen E, Saeed SA, et al. Hypotensive action of coumarin glycosides from *Daucus carota*. Phytomedicine 2000 Oct;7(5):423-6.

895. Cayen MN, Dvornik D. Combined effects of clofibrate and diosgenin on cholesterol metabolism in rats. Atherosclerosis 1978 Mar;29(3):317-27.

896. Yamada T, Hoshino M, Hayakawa T, et al. Dietary diosgenin attenuates subacute intestinal inflammation associated with indomethacin in rats. Am J Physiol 1997 Aug;273(2 Pt 1):G355-4.

897. Schmid B, Kotter I, Heide L. Pharmacokinetics of salicin after oral administration of a standardised willow bark extract. Eur J Clin Pharmacol 2001 Aug;57(5):387-91.

898. Chan TY. Drug interactions as a cause of overanticoagulation and bleedings in Chinese patients receiving warfarin. Int J Clin Pharmacol Ther 1998 Jul;36(7):403-5.

899. Gilani AH, Janbaz KH. Preventive and curative effects of *Artemisia absinthium* on acetaminophen and CCl4-induced hepatotoxicity. Gen Pharmacol 1995 Mar;26(2):309-15.

900. Charney DS, Heninger GR, Sternberg DE. Assessment of alpha 2 adrenergic autoreceptor function in humans: effects of oral yohimbine. Life Sci 1982 Jun 7;30(23):2033-41.

901. Jacobsen FM. Fluoxetine-induced sexual dysfunction and an open trial of yohimbine. J Clin Psychiatry 1992 Apr;53(4):119-22.

902. Henry B, Fox SH, Peggs D, Crossman AR, Brotchie JM. The alpha2-adrenergic receptor antagonist idazoxan reduces dyskinesia and enhances anti-parkinsonian actions of L-dopa in the MPTP-lesioned primate model of Parkinson's disease. Mov Disord 1999 Sep;14(5):744-53.

903. Schreiber S, Backer MM, Pick CG. The antinociceptive effect of venlafaxine in mice is mediated through opioid and adrenergic mechanisms. Neurosci Lett 1999 Oct 1;273(2):85-8.

904. Morales L, Perez-Garcia C, Alguacil LF. Effects of yohimbine on the antinociceptive and place conditioning effects of opioid agonists in rodents. Br J Pharmacol 2001 May;133(1):172-8

905. Ndeereh DR, Mbithi PM, Kihurani DO. The reversal of xylazine hydrochloride by yohimbine and 4-aminopyridine in goats. J S Afr Vet Assoc 2001 Jun;72(2):64-7.

906. Charney DS, Heninger GR, Redmond DE Jr. Yohimbine induced anxiety and increased noradrenergic function in humans: effects of diazepam and clonidine. Life Sci 1983 Jul 4;33(1):19-29.

907. Abdel-Zaher AO, Ahmed IT, El-Koussi Ael-D. The potential antidiabetic activity of some alpha-2 adrenoceptor antagonists. Pharmacol Res 2001 Nov;44(5):397-409.

908. Jaouhari JT, Lazrek HB, Seddik A, Jana M. Hypoglycaemic response to *Zygophyllum gaetulum* extracts in patients with non-insulin-dependent diabetes mellitus. J Ethnopharmacol 1999 Mar;64(3):211-7.

909. Martin WR, Sloan JW, Sapira JD, Jasinski DR. Physiologic, subjective, and behavioral effects of amphetamine, methamphetamine, ephedrine, phenmetrazine, and methylphenidate in man. Clin Pharmacol Ther 1971 Mar-Apr;12(2):245-58.

910. Edner M, Jogestrand T, Dahlqvist R. Effect of salbutamol on digoxin pharmacokinetics. Eur J Clin Pharmacol 1992;42(2):197-201.

911. Katzung B. *Basic & Clinical Pharmacology*. 8th edition. New York:Lange MedicalBooks/McGraw-Hill. 2001.

912. The Medical Letter. *Handbook of Adverse Drug Interactions*. New York:The Medical Letter, Inc. 2001.

913. Alvarez-Cedron L, Lopez FG, Lanao JM. Influence of verapamil and digoxin on the in vitro binding of doxorubicin to the rat heart. Biol Pharm Bull 1998 Aug;21(8):839-43.

914. Kuhlmann J. Inhibition of digoxin absorption but not of digitoxin during cytostatic drug therapy. Arzneimittelforschung 1982;32(6):698-704.

915. Rodin SM, Johnson BF. Pharmacokinetic interactions with digoxin. Clin Pharmacokinet 1988 Oct;15(4):227-44.

916. Dr. Duke's Phytochemical and Ethnobotanical Databases. http://www.ars-grin.gov/duke/.

917. Longwood Herbal Taskforce. In-depth Monograph (rhubarb). http://www.mcp.edu/herbal/rhubarb/rhubarb.pdf.

918. Fosamax package insert. Available at http://www.druginfonet.com/pi_mfr/pi/merck/fosamax/fosamax.htm.

919. *Merck Manual* 17th ed. NJ:Merck Research Laboratories. 1999.

920. American Botanical Council. Press release announcing new safety information on kava. Dec. 20, 2001.

921. Smolinske SC. Dietary supplement-drug interactions. J Am Med Womens Assoc 1999 Fall;54(4):191-2,195.

922. Norton S. Raw animal tissues and dietary supplements. N Engl J Med 2000 Jul 27;343(4):304-5.

923. Gundling K, Ernst E. Herbal medicines: influences on blood coagulation. Perfusion 2001;14:336-342.

924. Izzo A, Ernst E. Interactions between herbal medicines and prescribed drugs. Drugs 2001;61(15):2163-75.

925. Fugh-Berman A, Ernst E. Herb-drug interactions: review and assessment of report reliability. Br J Clin Pharmacol

2001;52:587-95.

926. Ernst E. Possible interactions between synthetic and herbal medicinal products part 1: a systematic review of the indirect evidence. Perfusion. 2000;13:4-15.

927. Ernst E. Possible interactions between synthetic and herbal medicinal products part 2: a systematic review of the indirect evidence. Perfusion. 2000;13:60-70.

928. Krishnaswamy K, Raghuramulu N. Bioactive phytochemicals with emphasis on dietary practices. Indian J Med Res 1998 Nov;108:167-81.

929. Gorski J, Hamman M, Wang Z, etal. The effect of St. John's wort on the efficacy of oral contraception. American Society for Clinical Pharmacology and Therapeutics. Clin Pharmacol Ther. 2002; 71(2):MPI-106. Abstract

930. Argento A, Tiraferri E, Marzaloni M. [Oral anticoagulants and medicinal plants. An emerging interaction]. Ann Ital Med Int 2000 Apr-Jun;15(2):139-43. Abstract.

931. Stoschitzky K, Sakotnik A, Lercher P, et al. Influence of beta-blockers on melatonin release. Eur J Clin Pharmacol 1999 Apr;55(2):111-5.

932. Nathan PJ, Maguire KP, Burrows GD, Norman TR. The effect of atenolol, a beta1-adrenergic antagonist, on nocturnal plasma melatonin secretion: evidence for a dose-response relationship in humans. J Pineal Res 1997 Oct;23(3):131-5.

933. Van Den Heuvel CJ, Reid KJ, Dawson D. Effect of atenolol on nocturnal sleep and temperature in young men: reversal by pharmacological doses of melatonin. Physiol Behav 1997 Jun;61(6):795-802.

934. Wiid I, Hoal-van Helden E, Hon D, Lombard C, van Helden P. Potentiation of isoniazid activity against Mycobacterium tuberculosis by melatonin. Antimicrob Agents Chemother 1999 Apr;43(4):975-7.

935. Hartter S, Grozinger M, Weigmann H, Roschke J, Hiemke C. Increased bioavailability of oral melatonin after fluvoxamine coadministration. Clin Pharmacol Ther 2000 Jan;67(1):1-6.

936. von Bahr C, Ursing C, Yasui N, et al. Fluvoxamine but not citalopram increases serum melatonin in healthy subjects-- an indication that cytochrome P450 CYP1A2 and CYP2C19 hydroxylate melatonin. Eur J Clin Pharmacol 2000 May;56(2):123-7.

937. Dolberg OT, Hirschmann S, Grunhaus L. Melatonin for the treatment of sleep disturbances in major depressive disorder. Am J Psychiatry 1998 Aug;155(8):1119-21.

938. Childs PA, Rodin I, Martin NJ, et al. Effect of fluoxetine on melatonin in patients with seasonal affective disorder and matched controls. Br J Psychiatry 1995 Feb;166(2):196-8.

INDEX

372

374

378

German

Terazosin (Hytrin) 234, 290

Terbinafine (Lamisil) 2, 77, 83, 86, 140, 181, 261, 295

Terbutaline (Brethine, Bricanyl) 299

Terfenadine 301, 302

Terminalia chebula 223

Testolactone (Teslac) 293

Testosterone 301

Tetracycline (Achromycin) 1, 37, 54, 71, 110, 130, 201, 202, 211, 288, 298

Teucrium chamaedrys 116

Theobroma cacao 74

Theophylline (Elixophyllin, Slo-bid, Theo-Dur, Uniphyl, Uni-Dur) 5, 47, 64, 77, 83, 86, 101, 140, 174, 181, 196, 253, 261, 264, 266, 299, 300, 301

Thevetia peruviana 278

Thiazide diuretics 122, 171

Thioacetamine 37, 65

Thioctic acid see Alpha-lipoic acid

Thioguanine 293

Thiopental (Pentothal) 291

Thioridazine (Mellaril) 297, 300

Thiotepa (Thioplex) 293

Thonningia sanguinea 269

Thorn Apple see Jimsonweed

Thorny Burnet 262

Thoroughwort see Boneset

Thyroid replacement therapy 29, 41, 56, 65, 90, 101, 113, 132, 141, 148, 161, 162, 166, 184, 192, 229, 244

Thyroidal radioactive isotopes 56

Thyroxine (Levothyroid, Levoxyl, Synthroid) see Thryoid replacement therapy

Tiagabine (Gabitril) 290

Ticarcillin (Ticar) 287

Tickweed see Pennyroyal

Ticlopidine (Ticlid) 2, 288

Tilia cordata 172

Timolol (Blocadren) 290, 300

Tinospora cordifolia 142

Tipton Weed see St. John's wort

Tirofiban (Aggrastat) 288

TJ-114 231

TJ-9 240

Tobacco 2, 262

Tobramycin (Nebcin) 287, 297

Tocainide (Tonocard) 286

Tolazamide (Tolinase) 296

Tolazoline (Priscoline) 291

Tolbutamide (Orinase) 31, 240, 253, 296, 298, 300

Tolmetin (Tolectin) 288

Tolterodine (Detrol) 286